"Radically open dialectical behavior therapy (RO DBT) is a truly innovative treatment, developed through translation of neuroscience into clinical practice, integrating various influences from dialectical behavior therapy (DBT), mindfulness-based approaches, emotion, personality and developmental theory, evolutionary theory, and Malamati Sufism. RO DBT is applicable to a spectrum of disorders characterized by excessive inhibitory control or *overcontrol* (OC). This is the first treatment that directly targets social signaling and nonverbal aspects of communication not only in clients but also in therapists.…This book on the theory and practice of RO DBT, together with the skills training manual that describes the content of skills classes, are excellent guides for clinicians who want to embark in delivering transdiagnostic treatments based on science and clinical practice."

> —**Mima Simic, MD, MRCPsych**, joint head of the child and adolescent eating disorder service, and consultant child and adolescent psychiatrist at the Maudsley Hospital in London, UK

"A new and comprehensive statement from one of the more creative minds in evidence-based clinical intervention today, RO DBT brings together a contemporary focus on a limited set of key transdiagnostic processes, with new assessment and intervention techniques for moving them in a positive direction. Emphasizing flexibility, openness, connection, and attention to social signaling, RO DBT specifies the details that can matter, from how you arrange your consulting room furniture to how nonverbal cues signal social information. RO DBT seems destined to make an impact on evidence-based care in many corners of clinical work. Highly recommended."

> —**Steven C. Hayes, PhD**, codeveloper of acceptance and commitment therapy (ACT); Foundation Professor of psychology at the University of Nevada, Reno; and author of *Get Out of Your Mind and Into Your Life*

"RO DBT offers an intriguing reconceptualization of traditional views of internalizing and externalizing disorders, and provides the clinician with valuable new tools to address a number of problems that have been particularly resistant to standard CBT approaches. I will definitely include RO DBT theory and techniques in my graduate-level intervention class. I know beginning clinicians in particular will be grateful to have a systematic way to approach these slow-to-warm-up clients who are difficult to establish rapport with. Their early termination from therapy and failure to respond to traditional approaches often leaves clinicians befuddled and critical of their own skills. RO DBT provides a compassionate way for clinicians to view this type of resistant client, as well as to work on some areas that are likely to benefit them. A very welcome addition to any clinician's toolbox."

> —**Linda W. Craighead, PhD**, professor of psychology and director of clinical training at Emory University, and author of *The Appetite Awareness Workbook*

RADICALLY OPEN

DIALECTICAL BEHAVIOR THERAPY

THEORY *and* PRACTICE *for* TREATING DISORDERS *of* OVERCONTROL

THOMAS R. LYNCH, PhD

CONTEXT PRESS

An Imprint of New Harbinger Publications, Inc.

Publisher's Note

NEW HARBINGER PUBLICATIONS is a registered trademark of New Harbinger Publications, Inc.

Distributed in Canada by Raincoast Books

Copyright © 2018 by Thomas R. Lynch
        Context Press
        An imprint of New Harbinger Publications, Inc.
        5674 Shattuck Avenue
        Oakland, CA 94609
        www.newharbinger.com

Figure 6.3, "Prototypical Emotional Expressions," from Keltner, D., Young, R. C., & Buswell, B. N. (1997). "Appeasement in human emotion, social practice, and personality." *Aggressive Behavior, 23*(5), 359–374. Copyright © 1988 by Wiley. Used with permission.

Images in figure 6.5, "Polite Smile vs. Genuine Smile," © Vladimir Gjorgiev and Monkey Business Images/Shutterstock.

Figure 6.12, "Subtle, Low-Intensity Social Signals Are Powerful," from EMOTIONS REVEALED: RECOGNIZING FACES AND FEELINGS TO IMPROVE COMMUNICATION AND EMOTIONAL LIFE by Paul Ekman, copyright © 2003 by Paul Ekman. Used by permission of Paul Ekman.

Lines from "A Man and a Woman Arguing" from THE ESSENTIAL RUMI by Jalal al-Din Rumi, translated by Coleman Barks. Copyright © 1997 by Coleman Barks. Used by permission.

Illustrations on pages 163, 164, and 168 by Henrietta Hellard

Cover design by Amy Shoup; Acquired by Catharine Meyers;
Edited by Xavier Callahan; Indexed by James Minkin

Library of Congress Cataloging-in-Publication Data

Names: Lynch, Thomas R. (Professor of clinical psychology), author.
Title: Radically open dialectical behavior therapy : theory and practice for treating disorders of overcontrol /
    Thomas R. Lynch.
Description: Oakland, CA : New Harbinger Publications, Inc., [2018] | Includes bibliographical references and index.
Identifiers: LCCN 2017040500 (print) | LCCN 2017042252 (ebook) | ISBN 9781626259294 (pdf e-book) | ISBN
    9781626259300 (ePub) | ISBN 9781626259287 (hardcover : alk. paper)
Subjects: | MESH: Behavior Therapy--methods | Compulsive Personality Disorder--therapy | Self-Control--psychology
Classification: LCC RC489.B4 (ebook) | LCC RC489.B4 23 (print) | NLM WM 425 | DDC 616.89/142--dc23
LC record available at https://lccn.loc.gov/2017040500

Printed in the United States of America

23   22   21

10   9   8   7   6   5   4

Contents

Acknowledgments

This work could not have been accomplished without a tribe. I would like to begin by thanking our patients for their willingness to share their personal struggles and insights—they have been my teachers and the *raison d'être* behind it all.

However, without doubt, I am most grateful for the tremendous amount of support, energy, and intellectual contributions made by my wife, best friend, and colleague Erica Smith-Lynch. Without her insight into human nature and willingness to question existing paradigms (most often those I held dearly), much of what is written would not exist. Erica helped develop and refine the core philosophical premises underlying the treatment and was seminal in the development of novel therapist training methods, as well as new RO skills. Erica is *the rock* of RO DBT.

I am also indebted to Roelie Hempel, who has been our research lab's senior scientist and associate director for the past 10 years. Her basic science background in psychophysiology, her analytic brain, and her keen curiosity have been essential in our mechanisms of change research. She was the clinical trial manager for our MRC funded multi-center randomized controlled trial and primary driver behind most of our bio-behavioral and experimental research (and that's just before breakfast). Roelie is the *roll* to Erica's *rock*.

Importantly, this work would also not be same without the time invested and gentle challenges made by Lee Anna Clark in helping refine and strengthen the neuroregulatory model that underlies the treatment—e.g. insights regarding optimal self-regulation, the importance of accounting for bio-temperament, and the utility of undercontrol and overcontrol as multi-dimensional constructs. Finally, when it comes to core contributors, I am grateful for the wide range of intellectual and instrumental contributions made by Jennifer S. Cheavens during the early years of treatment development at Duke University—e.g., help with the development of new skills linked to openness, flexibility, and forgiveness.

In addition, I have been very fortunate to have been mentored by a number of exceptional clinical academic researchers—five of whom I consider most influential in the development of RO DBT. First, I learned most of what I know about radical behaviorism from Alan Fruzzetti—my PhD advisor at Kent State University. Alan introduced me to Marsha Linehan, who trained me in standard DBT, and I was grateful when she also began collaborating with me in research—resulting in the first multi-site RCT of standard DBT funded by NIDA (PIs: Linehan, UW; Lynch, Duke). While this was going on, I was simultaneously running several other funded studies, including an NIMH K23 career development award that afforded me the opportunity of meeting and learning from two prominent psychiatric researchers—Ranga Krishnan and Chip Reynolds. Ranga was the Chair of the Department of Psychiatry Department at Duke University Medical Center and a world-leading depression researcher. It would be impossible for me to outline all the ways Ranga encouraged, advised, and supported me during my tenure at Duke. He invited me to be part of a number of large-scale initiatives including the NIMH funded Conte Neuroscience Center as a co-investigator, which is where I met Kevin LaBar and Greg McCarthy and started to work on models of depression that integrated brain and behavioral science. It was also during this time that I met my other primary mentor for my NIMH K23 award—Charles (Chip) F. Reynolds—a world-leading clinical trial and depression researcher who was located at the University of Pittsburgh's Western Psychiatric Institute. Chip somehow seemed to recognize something useful in me, because he spent an enormous amount of his valuable time helping me refine my grant submissions and articles, including a visit to my clinic and lab at Duke accompanied by my NIMH program officer. One of the things I admire most about Ranga and Chip was how they managed their research teams and collaborations—always with humility and openness to differing points of view.

I am also grateful to a number of key influencers who have contributed in smaller yet powerful ways to RO DBT over the years. For starters, Sophie Rushbrook was pivotal in helping me formulate the final version of the skills manual and improving our methods of training and supervision. Our dissemination work has become vastly more sophisticated under the leadership of R. Trent Codd III and Jason Luoma. Plus, I am also enormously grateful to Jackie Persons for her perspicacious read of earlier versions of this book and encouragement to "find my voice" when describing RO DBT rather than comparing it to others. Plus, the clinical observations and insights made by Christine Dunkley during the initial phases of our multi-site RCT were seminal in helping me refine a number of key concepts and treatment targets. During the early treatment development years, one of the most important influencers was Clive Robins. Clive was my primary clinical supervisor and research mentor during my clinical internship and postdoctoral training at Duke University. He was the yang to my yin—encouraging yet critical and challenging of my novel ideas. Similarly, the supportive yet oftentimes challenging feedback from Martin Bohus helped me better articulate how RO DBT differed from standard DBT. Our work with eating disorders and subsequent empirical support has largely been due to the efforts and continued enthusiastic support from Eunice Chen, Mimi Simic, Martina Wolf, and Marian Titley. A special thanks to Laura Hamilton and her team who have been instrumental in applying RO DBT in forensic settings. Plus, a note of gratitude goes out to Richard Booth and his research team who have been the driving force behind novel research testing the efficacy of RO skills alone approaches. I also wish to thank Frank Keefe, who was instrumental in the development and research of the RO loving kindness meditation protocol—whereby Frank obtained grant funding that allowed us to run a randomized controlled trial testing our LKM protocol and providing the empirical basis for adopting it in RO DBT.

Of course, those mentioned above represent only a subset of all of the people involved in this work over the years. The remaining list is too long for me to describe each person's unique contribution—but suffice it to say the contributions were substantial, and I am grateful for each. These individuals include (and hopefully I have not left anyone out): Zach Rosenthal, Linda Craighead, Ian Russell, Ben Whalley, Alex Chapman, Heather O'Mahen, Vanessa Ford, Linda George, Sue Clarke, David Kingdon, Michaela Swales, John Beyers, Jim Carson, Leslie Bronner, David Steffens, Carl Lejuez, Dan Blazer, Steve Hollon, Mark Williams, Sarah Burford, Kate Tchanturia, and Bob Remington. In addition, I am also enormously grateful for the enthusiasm, energy, and feedback I have received from our ever-expanding tribe of senior clinician trainers, trainers-in-training, and supervisors from around the world; including Pip Thomas, Maggie Stanton, Nicole Little, Alex Fowke, Kristi Colwell, Lexi Giblin, Ann Gresham, Chris Kvidera, Michel Masler, Nate Tomcik, Jimmy Portner, Karyn Hall, Kristen Fritsinger, Kirsten McAteer, Katrina Hunt, and Amy Gaglia.

I would also like to acknowledge the wide range of instrumental and intellectual input, support, and new ideas generated from my prior students, postdocs, residents, and interns who I have mentored over the years, many of whom are now in senior positions, including; Kirsten Gilbert, Sara Beth Austin, Emily Vanderbleek, Guy Mizon, Davina Wong, Kelly Cukrowicz, Moria Smoski, Sammy Banawan, Lorie Ritschel, Steven Thorp, Megan Barnsley, Dionysis Seretis, Prue Cuper, Kristin Schneider, Ann Aspnes, Caroline Cozza, Daniel Dillon, Christine Vitt-Ferri, Beth Krause, Tamar Mendelson, and Jen Morse.

It is unlikely that our evidence base for RO DBT would be where it stands at the launch of the manual without noting the support I have been fortunate to have received over the years from a wide-range of external grant funding agencies, including NIMH, NARSAD, AFSP, MRC-EME (UK), Conte Neuroscience Centre (Duke), Centre for Aging (Duke), and the Hartford Foundation. In particular, my NIMH program officer, Enid Light, was exceptionally helpful in guiding me through the funding maze during the earlier developmental years of RO DBT. Lastly, I am grateful for the editorial expertise, practical suggestions, and wit that helped make the final product much improved—that being my senior editor, Xavier Callahan, as well as the overall support from New Harbinger—in particular that of Catherine Meyers, Erin Heath, and Matt McKay. Their flexibility, experience, and belief in this work helped me finally get it off the typewriter and out the door. I hope you enjoy reading the text and that you find the material beneficial.

Key Terms

approach coping: a strategy for reducing distress by engaging directly with its source or actively attempting to solve the problem that has triggered the distress

biotemperament: genetic and biological predispositions that affect one's perception and regulation of emotions (compare *trait*)

detail-focused processing: a style of integrating sensory stimuli that is characterized by paying much more attention to the parts than to the whole ("missing the forest for the trees")

dorsal vagal complex: the branch of the vagus nerve that is evolutionarily older and associated with physiological and emotional shutdown, immobilization, and numbing of pain (compare *ventral vagal complex*)

edge: in RO DBT, a term that refers to actions, thoughts, feelings, images, or sensations that we want to avoid, feel embarrassed about, or prefer not to admit to others (see also *outing oneself; personal unknown*)

emotional leakage: the expression of emotion at higher intensity than one would generally feel comfortable exhibiting

flat face: a facial expression devoid of perceptible emotion

outing oneself: revealing vulnerability, fallibility, or one's personal edge to someone else in order to locate the point where one's personal growth can occur (see also *edge; personal unknown*)

personal unknown: the far edge of psychological growth, where learning can take place

smuggle: the RO DBT therapist's practice of introducing new information to a client by planting a seed or a small part of a new idea, without telling the entire story, so that the client has an opportunity to reflect on the information without feeling compelled to immediately accept or reject it

social safety system: neural substrate associated with feelings of contentment, relaxation, and desire to affiliate (see also *ventral vagal complex*)

social signal: any action or overt behavior, regardless of its form, its intent, or the performer's awareness, that is carried out in the presence of another person

trait: a stable pattern of behavior moderated by biology as well as by the environment (compare *biotemperament*)

turn the heat on/take the heat off: increasing or decreasing the amount of therapist attention—such as eye contact—directed toward a client in order to enhance client engagement, provide opportunities for learning, or reinforce therapeutic progress

urge-surfing: the practice of noticing but not acting on a compulsive desire or action urge, and, instead, mindfully observing the compulsion or desire as it rises, crests, and falls away—like a wave—without trying to change it

valued goal: a personal objective that has emotional significance, is aligned with one's core principles, and guides one's actions

ventral vagal complex: the branch of the vagus nerve that is evolutionarily newer and associated with feelings of safety and affiliation as well as with urges toward exploration (compare *dorsal vagal complex*)

Introduction

This book presents a new transdiagnostic treatment, *radically open dialectical behavior therapy* (RO DBT), which targets a spectrum of disorders characterized by excessive inhibitory control, or *overcontrol* (OC). It is intended for clinicians treating clients with such chronic problems as refractory depression, anorexia nervosa, and obsessive-compulsive personality disorder. Although the book can be read alone, it is best used in tandem with *The Skills Training Manual for Radically Open Dialectical Behavior Therapy: A Clinician's Guide for Treating Disorders of Overcontrol* (T. R. Lynch, 2018), referred to throughout this volume as "the skills training manual." In thirty lessons, the skills training manual presents twenty skills of radical openness (RO) along with class exercises, user-friendly handouts and worksheets, and detailed notes for instructors.

Radical openness, the concept at the foundation of RO DBT, is a way of behaving. But it is also a state of mind informed by the central premise that emotional well-being involves the confluence of three features: *openness*, *flexibility*, and *social connectedness*. As a state of mind, radically open living involves actively seeking our personal unknown in order to learn from an ever-changing environment. Radical openness also enhances relationships because it models humility and the willingness to learn from what the world has to offer. As such, radical openness often requires us to sacrifice our firmly held convictions and self-constructs—and this is why the practice of radical openness can be painful.

Overview of Core RO DBT Tenets

RO DBT is supported by twenty years of clinical experience and translational research that parallels established guidelines for treatment development (Rounsaville, Carroll, & Onken, 2001). As a new treatment, it is both similar and dissimilar to its predecessors.

The decision to retain the terms *dialectical* and *behavior therapy* in the name of this new treatment reflects the desire to acknowledge two of its fundamental roots, but the retention of these terms should not be taken to mean that they represent RO DBT's only roots. Also influential in RO DBT's development has been a wide range of philosophical, etiological, and treatment models and approaches, most notably dialectical philosophy and dialectical behavior therapy, mindfulness-based approaches, cognitive behavioral therapy, Gestalt therapy, motivational interviewing, basic emotion theory, affective neuroscience, personality and developmental theories, evolutionary theory, and Malâmati Sufism.

The core tenets of RO DBT are as follows:

- We are tribal by nature. The survival of our species required us to develop our capacities to form long-lasting social bonds, share valuable resources, and work together in tribes or groups.

- Psychological well-being involves the confluence of three factors: openness (receptivity), flexibility, and social connectedness. The term *radical openness* represents the confluence of these three capacities, and radical openness itself is the core philosophical principle and core skill in RO DBT.

- Social signaling matters. In disorders of overcontrol, deficits in prosocial signaling are posited to be the core source of OC clients' loneliness.

- Core genotypic and phenotypic differences between groups of disorders necessitate different treatment approaches.[1]

- Overcontrol is a multifaceted paradigm involving complex transactions among biology, environment, and individual styles of coping.

- In people with disorders of overcontrol, biotemperamental deficits and excesses make behavioral responses more rigid and thus less capable of flexible adaptation to changing environmental conditions.

- It takes willpower to turn off (that is, *downregulate*) willpower!

- Radical openness assumes that we don't see things as they are but rather as we are.

- One secret of healthy living is the cultivation of healthy self-doubt.

- Radical openness and self-enquiry are experiential and cannot be grasped on an exclusively intellectual basis. Therapists need to practice radical openness themselves in order to model it for their clients.

Overview of the Book's Contents

Chapter 1 poses the question of whether there can be such a thing as too much self-control, and it describes maladaptive overcontrol as well as its association with chronic and treatment-resistant psychopathologies. The chapter then establishes RO DBT's links to older evolutionary theory and more recent basic brain/behavioral research. It concludes with an overview of completed and ongoing clinical trials testing the efficacy of RO DBT.

Chapter 2 covers the rationale and basic science supporting the neurobiological theory of OC disorders.

Chapter 3 presents a step-by-step process for diagnosing disorders of overcontrol and includes relevant measures for establishing a diagnosis.

Chapter 4 gives an overview of RO DBT's treatment structure, therapeutic stance, and global targets and includes a section on the assessment and management of suicidal behavior in OC clients.

Chapter 5 offers guidance on maximizing OC clients' engagement by addressing (1) physical and environmental factors in the treatment setting, (2) strategies and protocols for orienting clients to treatment and gaining their commitment, and (3) the timing and sequencing of interventions.

Chapter 6 provides a detailed overview of core RO DBT principles that involve social signaling. The chapter includes information about how the therapist can use nonverbal social signals during treatment sessions as a way to maximize the client's engagement and improve treatment outcomes.

Chapter 7, in addition to presenting an overview of core RO and self-enquiry principles and strategies, discusses structural protocols for integrating RO principles into supervision or consultation and offers concrete illustrations of an ongoing self-enquiry practice.

Chapter 8 gives a detailed description of RO DBT's protocols for repairing ruptures in the therapeutic alliance. The chapter also discusses strategies for preventing clients from dropping out of treatment.

Chapter 9 presents a step-by-step protocol for using OC themes to create individualized treatment targets that are linked to clients' valued goals.[2] The chapter includes a clinical example of OC theme–based targeting to illustrate how much social signaling occurs during a session and to show how the therapist can use his or her own nonverbal social signals to block the client's maladaptive behavior and enhance the client's engagement.

Chapter 10 offers detailed descriptions of how RO DBT uses dialectical thinking to guide the therapist's behavior and facilitate new ways for the therapist to behave with clients. Specifically, the chapter discusses the core dialectic in RO DBT: the juxtaposition of compassionate gravity with playful irreverence. The chapter also presents an overview of core behavioral strategies in RO DBT, including information about using informal principles of behavioral exposure and using a detailed behavioral chain analysis.

Chapter 11, with the aim of stimulating further research and dialogue, outlines some future directions and implications of radical openness, both as a therapeutic concept and as a way of being. The chapter also includes commonly asked questions that therapists can use to assess whether they are providing RO DBT–adherent treatment. (Appendix 8 offers a formal checklist to be used for the same purpose. It, like all the appendices in this book, is available for download from www.newharbinger .com/39287.)

In RO DBT, Silliness Is No Laughing Matter[*]

We take silliness very seriously in RO DBT because OC clients take life too seriously. For an OC client, relaxation and play can feel like hard work. Indeed, laughing and frivolity are seen as staged performances for lost travelers on midnight ghost trains speeding through… [Editor's note: Stop! Cease! Desist! That is *quite* enough silliness for one page. We apologize for the author's undignified ramble and assure the reader that we requested—nay, *demanded*—a rewrite of this section and have carefully monitored the author's use of silly language throughout the remainder of the text. We urge the reader not to squander any more valuable time perusing the paragraphs that follow and instead to get right down to work, starting with chapter 1. As the saying goes, business and hard work before pleasure and silliness—and we mean business!]

In RO DBT, silliness is no laughing matter. Our OC clients are already too serious. They compulsively work and strive to achieve long-term goals yet have forgotten how to relax, play, or join in with others. For an OC client, socializing can feel like hard work. [Author's query: How am I doing so far?] [Editor's reply: I've seen better.]

The question is, why would silliness be therapeutic, especially since most adults work hard to avoid appearing silly in front of other people? The quick answer is that our avoidance stems from our deep-seated fear of being socially humiliated or ostracized. Yet if silliness is so feared, then why is it so common? Plus, why do so many people enjoy behaving in a silly manner, particularly when around friends? What is interesting, when you take a moment to think about it, is that we make funny faces, use silly voices, and exaggerate our gestures when interacting with young children, not so much because *we* feel safe but because we intuitively recognize that acting silly with kids helps *them* feel safe, which also makes it easier for them to learn, explore, and grow.

Thus, regardless of your age, your silly behavior around another person, especially when that person is in a power-down relationship with you—in a more vulnerable state, for example, like a client in therapy—is an act of kindness and a powerful signal of nondominance, equality, and friendship. However, the best silly behavior—as any parent knows—is the kind that stems from the heart and is as much fun for the sender of a silly social signal as it is for the receiver. The problem for those of us who are no longer seven years old or younger is that having fun while being silly can sometimes be hard to do. The good news is that even cranky adults can learn to enjoy being silly—it's all about giving yourself permission, throwing yourself into the deep end, and then practicing again and again and again.

---

[*]   …or, On the Importance of Being Absolutely, Positively, Indubitably, Superlatively, Incorrigibly, Unapologetically, Side-Splittingly, Over-the-Top, Spew-Coffee-Out-Your-Nose, Damn-the-Torpedoes *SILLY*

It's the same for our OC clients. They will not believe it is socially acceptable for them to play, relax, or openly express emotions unless they see their therapists model that behavior first. That's why, from time to time, you'll see in the chapters ahead some unusual language and text recommended by the association known as Writers Airing Silly Sayings Attributed to Unknown People (WASSA UP) that serves as the best way to remind you—repeatedly, of course—of just how silly life can be. So watch out for WASSA UP! [Editor's note: Heaven help us.]

CHAPTER 1

Radical Openness and Disorders of Overcontrol

Self-control—the ability to inhibit competing urges, impulses, behaviors, or desires, and to delay gratification in order to pursue distal goals—is often equated with success and happiness. Indeed, failures in self-control characterize many of the personal and social problems afflicting modern civilization. Deficient self-control has been linked cross-sectionally and longitudinally with a broad spectrum of problems, including substance abuse, criminal activities, domestic violence, financial difficulties, teen pregnancy, smoking, and obesity (Baumeister, Heatherton, & Tice, 1994; Moffitt et al., 2011), and significant portions of governmental spending and scientific research focus on understanding, preventing, and treating deficits in self-control.

Self-Control: Can You Have Too Much of a Good Thing?

However, research shows that too much self-control can be as problematic as too little. Excessive self-control is associated with social isolation, poor interpersonal functioning, and severe and difficult-to-treat mental health problems, such as anorexia nervosa, chronic depression, and obsessive-compulsive personality disorder (T. R. Lynch & Cheavens, 2008; Zucker et al., 2007). Because of the high value that most societies place on delaying gratification and inhibiting overt or public displays of potentially destructive emotions and impulses, the problems linked with excessive inhibitory control, or overcontrol, have either received little attention or been misunderstood, making recognition difficult for clinicians.

Maladaptive overcontrol is expressed discreetly. Even though OC individuals experience high defensive arousal (anxiety, depression, and resentment, for example), they are likely to downplay their personal distress when queried ("I'm fine"). As a consequence, they are less likely to seek mental health treatment. Oftentimes no one outside the immediate family is aware of OC individuals' inner psychological distress. Therefore, they can come to convince themselves and others that their constricted, rigid, rule-governed behavior and aloof interpersonal style are normal or even ideal. They tend to be serious about life, set high personal standards, work hard, and behave appropriately, and they frequently sacrifice their personal needs in order to achieve desired goals or help others. Inwardly, however, they often feel clueless about how to join with others or form intimate relationships. Overcontrol works well for sitting quietly in a monastery or building a rocket, but it creates problems when it comes to social connectedness.

Defining Overcontrol

Maladaptive overcontrol is characterized by four core deficits:

1. Low receptivity and openness, manifested by low openness to novel, unexpected, or disconfirming feedback; avoidance of uncertainty or unplanned risks; suspiciousness; hypervigilance regarding potential threats; and marked tendencies to discount or dismiss critical feedback

2. Low flexible control, manifested by compulsive needs for structure and order; hyperperfectionism; high social obligation and dutifulness; compulsive rehearsal, premeditation, and planning; compulsive fixing and approach coping; rigid rule-governed behavior; and high moral certitude (the conviction that there is only one "right" way of doing something)

3. Pervasive inhibited emotional expression and low emotional awareness, manifested by context-inappropriate inhibition of emotional expression (for example, presentation of a flat face in response to a compliment) or by insincere or incongruent expressions of emotion (for example, a smile in response to distress, or a show of concern when no concern is actually felt); consistent underreporting of distress; and low awareness of bodily sensations

4. Low social connectedness and intimacy with others, manifested by aloof and distant relationships; a feeling of being different from other people; frequent social comparisons; high envy and bitterness; and reduced empathy

Overcontrol Is Associated with Personality Dysfunction

A quick examination of the ten personality disorders (PDs) listed as being on Axis II in the fifth edition of the *Diagnostic and Statistical Manual of Mental Disorders*, or DSM-5 (American Psychiatric Association, 2013), reveals that they all involve some form of pervasive and long-standing difficulty with emotion or impulse control and with interpersonal relationships. What may be less obvious, however, is that it is possible to further demarcate these features into two superordinate classes or domains, which overlap with the well-established division between the internalizing and externalizing disorders (Achenbach, 1966; Crijnen, Achenbach, & Verhulst, 1997). This premise is based on remarkable consistency in outcomes reported from large-scale studies of comorbidity, revealing two broad styles of coping—overcontrol and undercontrol (UC)—as being associated, respectively, with the development of chronic forms of internalizing and externalizing problems. According to the DSM-5, PDs of undercontrol (borderline PD, histrionic PD, antisocial PD, and narcissistic PD) are characterized by low inhibitory control and chaotic or dramatic relationships, whereas PDs of overcontrol (obsessive-compulsive PD, avoidant PD, paranoid PD, and schizoid PD) are characterized by excessive inhibitory control and an aloof or distant interpersonal style (T. R. Lynch, Hempel, & Clark, 2015).

The vast majority of published research on personality disorders has focused on those that the DSM-5 places in Cluster B, most prominently borderline PD and antisocial PD (Clark, 2005b), but there has been a dearth of research examining the PDs of overcontrol that are placed in Cluster A and Cluster C, despite evidence that they are highly prevalent (Coid, Yang, Tyrer, Roberts, & Ullrich, 2006) and associated with impaired functioning and increased use of health care services (Maclean, Xu, French, & Ettner, 2014). Indeed, obsessive-compulsive PD, a prototypical disorder of overcontrol, is the most prevalent personality disorder in community as well as clinical samples (Lenzenweger, 2008; Zimmerman, Rothschild, & Chelminski, 2005).

Interestingly, research shows that PDs of undercontrol remit or recede with age (Zanarini, Frankenburg, Reich, & Fitzmaurice, 2010; Abrams & Horowitz, 1996), whereas PDs of overcontrol appear either to remain stable or to intensify with age (Abrams & Horowitz, 1996). A PD of undercontrol may be more likely to remit over time because dramatic displays and overtly reckless behavior attract attention, which in turn makes it more likely for someone with this type of PD to receive corrective feedback and psychological help. By contrast, a PD of overcontrol may be less likely to remit over time because OC individuals' innate capacity to tolerate distress, delay gratification, and avoid public displays of emotion makes it less likely

> Individuals with disorders of overcontrol are often quietly suffering, even though their suffering may not be apparent.

for their problems to be noticed and thus reduces opportunities for corrective feedback and psychological help (Morse & Lynch, 2004; T. R. Lynch & Aspnes, 2001). As a result, individuals with disorders of overcontrol are often quietly suffering, even though their suffering may not be apparent.

For Chronic Conditions, Personality Matters

A major underlying premise of this book is that *personality matters* when intervening with treatment-resistant and chronic conditions, signaling that broad-based personality dimensions and overlearned perceptual and regulatory biases are interfering with psychological change. For example, an estimated 40 to 60 percent of unipolar depressed clients meet the criteria for comorbid personality disorder (Riso et al., 2003), and PDs of overcontrol are at once the most common PDs and the ones least likely to respond to treatment (Fournier et al., 2009). Similarly, PDs of overcontrol (especially obsessive-compulsive PD) are the most prevalent PDs found among people suffering from chronic pain, with rates now up to 62 percent (see the review by Dixon-Gordon, Whalen, Layden, & Chapman, 2015).

RO DBT posits that biotemperament may be the driving force behind this phenomenon (T. R. Lynch et al., 2015; see also Clark, 2005b, for similar conclusions). What makes an individual's biotemperament so powerful is that it can influence his perception, learning, and overt behavior at the sensory receptor (or preconscious) level of responding as well as at the central cognitive (or conscious) level of responding. For example, an OC individual walking into a party and seeing a group of people laughing together is biologically more predisposed to see the potential for harm in the situation than to see the potential for reward; in a matter of milliseconds (L. M. Williams et al., 2004), his defensive arousal and urges to flee are triggered at the preconscious level. Before he even knows it, the OC individual has perceived a threat—his brain has already made up its mind, so to speak—and this threat perception may be quickly followed by conscious thoughts like *I'm an outsider* or *I'm no good at telling jokes, and I'll look stupid if I join them.* By contrast, a person without biotemperamentally heightened threat sensitivity—someone who also has normal reward sensitivity—is likely to walk into the same party and think *They look like they're having a good time. I'm going to join them.*

It is important to understand that undercontrol and overcontrol are not one-dimensional personality constructs; that is, they do not simply represent opposite ends of a self-control continuum. Each is a multifaceted construct reflecting core genotypic (related to biology) and phenotypic (related to behavioral expression) differences between spectrums of disorders. As such, these two multifaceted constructs give rise to two important treatment implications:

1. Treatment needs to account for individual differences in biotemperament that may bias perception and impair learning and flexible responding.

2. Treatments targeting problems of undercontrol should emphasize interventions that enhance inhibitory control and reduce mood-dependent behavior, whereas treatments targeting problems of overcontrol require interventions designed to relax inhibitory control and increase emotional expressiveness, receptivity, and flexibility.

Examples of disorders characterized by maladaptive undercontrol and maladaptive overcontrol are listed in table 1.1.

Table 1.1. Difficult-to-Treat Disorders with Characteristics of Undercontrol and Overcontrol

Disorders of Undercontrol (Emotionally Dysregulated and Impulsive)	Disorders of Overcontrol (Emotionally Constricted and Risk-Averse)
Borderline personality disorder	Obsessive-compulsive personality disorder
Antisocial personality disorder	Paranoid personality disorder
Binge-purge eating disorders	Avoidant personality disorder
Narcissistic personality disorder	Anorexia nervosa
Histrionic personality disorder	Schizoid and schizotypal personality disorders
Conduct disorders	Autism spectrum disorders
Bipolar disorder	Treatment-resistant anxiety
Externalizing disorders	Internalizing disorders

Basic Postulates of RO DBT

The Importance of Defining Psychological Well-Being

A central tenet of RO DBT is that self-control is highly and perhaps universally valued in most societies, and that the value placed on self-control influences how a society defines deviant or abnormal behavior.[3] Deviance from social norms involves formal violations of explicit rules (as in criminal activity) as well as informal violations of social customs or expectations that are less well defined, and that involve social etiquette (as in transgressions with respect to cultural expectations around eye contact).[4] Societal values and norms also influence treatment values and goals because, arguably, treatment equates by definition to the reestablishment of "normal" functioning.

For overcontrolled clients, societal veneration of self-control is both a blessing (these clients' capacity for self-control is often admired) and a curse (their personal suffering, linked as it is to overcontrol, often goes unrecognized). Indeed, OC clients set high personal standards for themselves (and others) and are expert at not appearing deviant on the outside (that is, in public). They are not the people fomenting riots or robbing convenience stores on a whim. They are not the ones you see yelling at each other from across the street. They are perfectionists who tend to see mistakes everywhere (including in themselves), and they tend to work harder than most others to prevent future problems. They don't need to learn how to take life more seriously, or try harder, or plan ahead, or behave more appropriately in public. They have too much of a good thing—their self-control is out of control, and they suffer as a result. Therefore, RO DBT, instead of highlighting what's "wrong" with an individual client, starts from observations about what's healthy *in all of us* and then uses these observations to guide treatment interventions.

Psychological health or well-being in RO DBT is hypothesized to involve three core transacting features:

1. Receptivity and openness to new experience and disconfirming feedback, so that learning can occur

2. Flexible control, so that adaptation to changing environmental conditions can occur

3. Intimacy and social connectedness with at least one other person, based on the premise that our survival as a species depended on our ability to form long-lasting bonds and work together in tribes or groups

The core idea is that hyperperfectionist OC clients are most likely to benefit from treatment approaches that teach them how to actively seek well-being.

Self-Control as a Precursor for Community

If too much self-control generates so much individual suffering, then why is excessive self-control so rarely linked with abnormal or deviant behavior? I contend that the answer lies in the essential role played by self-control in the creation of society itself—in other words, that the answer lies in our tribal nature, a premise whose rationale originates in ideas influenced by evolutionary theory.

Humans, compared to other species, are not particularly robust, at least when it comes to pure physicality—we lack sharp claws, horns, thick hides, and protective fur. And yet because we have survived (and thrived), it seems plausible that our physical frailty is itself proof that our species' survival depended on something more than individual strength, speed, or toughness. From the perspective of RO DBT, we survived because we developed the capacity to work together in tribes and share valuable resources with others in our tribe who were not in our immediate nuclear family. These developments required the discovery of a way to bind genetically diverse individuals together in such a way that survival of the tribe could override older, more selfish tendencies linked to survival of the individual (see Buck, 1999, for similar observations). RO DBT posits that the end product of this evolutionary challenge required us to find a way to bind genetically diverse individuals together in such a way that "survival of the tribe" could override older, selfish tendencies linked to the survival of the individual, including:

1. The ability to inhibit our propensities for action: This means that we developed capacities to regulate the outward expression of emotion-based action tendencies or impulses (for example, the urge to attack or run away). Not acting on every impulse allowed us to live in close proximity to each other because we could trust our fellow tribe members not to automatically express a potentially damaging action urge (for example, a desire to hit).

2. The ability to regulate how we signal our intentions and personal observations about the world: This means that we developed a highly sophisticated social signaling system that allowed us to communicate intentions and feelings (for example, an angry glare linked to a desire to attack), without having to fully express the actual propensity itself (for example, hitting someone). *Signaling our intentions* from afar (for example, via facial expressions, gestures, or vocalizations) reduced unnecessary expenditures of energy and provided us a safer means of resolving conflict and initiating collaborations with others, without having to fully commit ourselves. Plus, revealing intentions and emotions to other members of our species was essential to creating the type of strong social bonds that are the cornerstone of human tribes. *Communicating our observations* involved nonverbal behaviors, such as gaze direction and pointing, as well as with verbal observations. Revealing to others our observations about nature (for example, "I see a cow") and then receiving verification (or not) about our perception by another member of our species (for example, "No, I see a tiger—let's run!") provided a huge evolutionary advantage because our individual survival no longer depended solely on our personal perception. This helps explain why we are so concerned about the opinions of others.

3. The ability to persist and to plan for the future: The evolution of persistence and planning likely involved the development of areas of the brain associated with evaluating nonimmediate contingencies, as when we imagine a potential future consequence. But persistence and planning differ in that planning involves considering the consequences of taking a future action, whereas persistence involves considering the consequences of ceasing to do what one is already doing (Smith et al., 2007).

These evolutionary developments facilitated the ability of our species to survive in increasingly diverse and inhospitable environments. For example, our enhanced capacities for planning ahead allowed us to remember that in the past food availability had depended on the season, and to use this knowledge to make plans for the future. At the same time, our ability to inhibit our excitatory response tendencies (for example, by not immediately consuming every valuable resource) and downregulate defensive response tendencies (for example, by not immediately attacking someone who stepped on our toe) allowed us not only to work together in groups, without fear of being attacked, but also to save valuable resources for a future time of need.[5] Thus the capacity for inhibitory control was the basis for community; combined with persistence, it allowed us to actualize our long-term goals and plans. For example, even though we may have been tired, we continued to pick apples over many weeks instead of simply lying back and feasting on the fruits of summer.[6] And, as we've seen, the capacities for social signaling and communication helped save those nearsighted members of our tribe who tended to mistake tigers for cows, which meant that the tribe continued to benefit from the efforts of its myopic members throughout the apple-picking season.

The Hidden Costs of Self-Control

Lacking command over oneself and acting against one's better judgment have been contemplated as core sources of human suffering since at least 380 BCE, when Plato's *Protagoras* is thought to have first seen the light of day. But if self-control was so important to the survival of the individual and the species, then why do so many individuals with high self-control suffer from loneliness and chronic mental health problems?

Current psychological theories regarding self-control consider the resolution of this conundrum to involve two sequential stages: a person must first identify the presence of a conflict involving self-control and then take steps to actively resolve the conflict by reinstating efforts toward self-control (Neal, Wood, & Drolet, 2013). The core idea is that competing motivations—such as the motivation to give into temptation (for example, by watching television) and the motivation to stay the course and achieve a long-term goal (for example, by going running in order to stay healthy)—create dissonance in a person. We generally understand that acting against one's better judgment means being deficient in self-control, and so it's fair to wonder how habitual self-control could be against anyone's better judgment. But what counts for an OC individual as acting against his better judgment is not being *deficient* in self-control—it's having *excessive* self-control.

It appears that the innate biological advantage of high self-control becomes an OC individual's worst enemy. Self-control is often equated with approach coping. Traditionally, approach coping has been assumed to be the healthiest and most beneficial way of reducing stress, whereas avoidance coping has been associated with negative personality traits, potentially harmful activities, and generally poorer outcomes. In fact, the beneficial effects of approach coping have led to the development of a wide range of therapies that highlight an increase in approach coping as a core component of effective treatment (Hayes, Wilson, Gifford, Follette, & Strosahl, 1996; Linehan, 1993a; Kohlenberg & Tsai, 1991).

However, individuals characterized by excessive self-control tend to use approach coping *compulsively*, even when they may cause themselves harm by doing so. For example, an OC individual is unlikely to put off performing an important task simply because it's unpleasant; on the contrary, she's likely to work obsessively at completing the task, regardless of other life circumstances (for example, she may stay late at work and miss the regular social gathering of her colleagues at a local restaurant). Similarly, an OC individual, rather than avoiding a social event in order to escape the anxiety it inspires, is likely to force himself to attend, even when avoidance would be more adaptive (for example, he may feel compelled to go ahead and attend a book club luncheon even though he just got mugged on the subway). The problem for OC individuals is that they engage in *too much* active problem solving, whereas many therapies focus on correcting clients' deficits in precisely this area. What is perhaps perplexing, often as much for OC clients as for their therapists, is that the OC individual's superior capacity for approach coping does not necessarily translate into superior outcomes in all contexts. It's true that, in general, people scoring high on measures of approach coping are good at getting things done. Trains run on time, projects are completed, resources are properly saved, and important goals are achieved. But this kind of OC mastery appears to fall apart when it comes to relationships. The dilemma for the OC individual seeking an intimate relationship is that, by definition, intimacy will require her to relinquish control and reveal vulnerability to the other person—or, in other words, go opposite to her natural inclinations to mask inner feelings and avoid appearing incompetent. Plus, simply encouraging her to approach a potentially rewarding social encounter is likely to backfire, since she cannot simply do, think, or accept her way out of a brain-based behavioral problem.

When Good Habits Go Bad

The motto of an overcontrolled client is "When in doubt, apply more self-control," irrespective of circumstances or potential consequences. Thus overcontrol is both a habit and hard work. It requires the client to exert effortful control over emotion-based action urges, and to delay gratification.

But if excessive self-control is causing so many problems for overcontrolled clients, then why don't they just use their superior capacity for self-control to inhibit their *maladaptive* self-control? The problem is that too much self-control appears to deplete the very resources needed to override habitual self-control when the immediate environmental cues suggest that doing so would be adaptive; research shows that willpower depletes energy resources, in the form of glucose, and that this depletion can negatively impact coping afterward (see Gailliot et al., 2007). Thus excessive self-control is habitually exhausting. When our energy resources are depleted, our capacity for self-control tends to go as well, and it becomes more likely for habitual responses to become dominant (Neal et al., 2013; Muraven & Baumeister, 2000). Habitual responses are most likely to be cued when current environmental stimuli are familiar. The advantage for the individual is that a habit can often be at least as effective as a deliberate effort, but the habit also demands fewer cognitive resources (for example, driving my car doesn't require a great deal of cognitive effort because I am an experienced driver, and I probably drive better when I don't think too much about what I'm doing).

Why Are Social Situations So Exhausting for an OC Individual?

OC clients almost universally report mental exhaustion in response to social events, very often the very events that others report having experienced as rewarding, exciting, or invigorating. After a social event, it is not uncommon for OC clients to yearn for down time and sensory deprivation (for example, by lowering all the window shades, putting in earplugs, advising family members to leave them alone, swallowing an aspirin, and retiring to bed). It doesn't cost much energy for an OC individual to take a difficult exam or complete a tax form, whereas an unplanned party can be overwhelming. (This response represents a fundamental difference between overcontrolled individuals and other people.)

But *why* does an OC individual find social situations so exhausting? One explanation is that social interactions are highly unpredictable—we can never know for certain how other people will respond to us. This inherent lack of predictability is compounded by OC individuals' biotemperament-based high threat sensitivity, which makes it more likely for them to perceive social interactions as potentially hostile. Interestingly, OC clients usually report that a social interaction involving a set agenda, clearly defined goals, or preassigned roles—for example, a business meeting, a class, or a choir rehearsal—is less anxiety-provoking and preferable to a social interaction like a picnic, a group celebration, or a team-building activity, where conversation flows freely and there are no assigned roles. OC individuals participating in unstructured social events often feel clueless about how to behave or what to say. Though their strong desire to do the right thing, behave properly, and exert control over situations is fundamentally prosocial, when these same attributes are applied rigidly and compulsively, regardless of context, they function to undermine social connectedness.

Broadly speaking, OC individuals don't know how to party hearty, whoop it up, throw down, paint the town, get in the groove, put on their dancing shoes, cut a rug, kick out the jams, or go off the hook. [Editor's note: Oh dear.] Ask an undercontrolled client why he went to a party, and he's likely to say, "Because I felt like going." Ask an overcontrolled client, and she's likely to say, "Because I thought it was the right thing to do." In this way, much of an OC individual's behavior is excessively rule-governed rather than driven by moods. This kind of behavior—combined with a biological predisposition for high threat sensitivity, low reward sensitivity, and high inhibitory control—leads to an overly serious attitude toward life and makes it hard to know how to celebrate with others, without feeling self-conscious. After all, an OC individual cannot simply leave her biotemperament at home every time she attends a social event. It's this pattern that is posited to be a key factor underlying the loneliness of OC individuals.

16

It's important to note that when a person's willpower is depleted, environmental cues trigger not just bad habits, such as overeating, alcohol abuse, and overspending, but also good habits, such as exercise, planning, and studying hard (Hofmann, Rauch, & Gawronski, 2007). Good habits are good precisely because they promote the attainment of long-term goals; bad habits are bad because they promote short-term pleasure or relief and impede long-term goal attainment (Neal et al., 2013). Not surprisingly, good habits characterize overcontrolled coping, and bad habits characterize undercontrolled coping.

Unfortunately for OC clients, being good all the time leads to trouble. OC clients are likely to believe that it's imperative not to reveal weakness or vulnerability. Therefore, even though they're highly anxious on the inside, they work hard not to let others see it on the outside, thus placing an additional burden on their already exhausted self-control system. A type of catch-22 emerges, with excessive self-control exhausting the resources needed to control excessive self-control, thereby making it harder to turn to alternative ways of coping (for example, taking a nap or asking for help). The OC client may feel inside like a prisoner of self-control, but his natural tendency to inhibit (control) the expression of his emotions makes it harder for others to know he is distressed and be able to offer assistance.

Using Neuroregulatory Theory to Target Biotemperament

How does one find the energy to change a habit that perpetually depletes one's energy? RO DBT's answer to this conundrum is to take advantage of basic emotion research demonstrating neuroinhibitory relationships between the parasympathetic nervous system (PNS) and the sympathetic nervous system (SNS; see Berntson, Cacioppo, & Quigley, 1991; Porges, 1995), and to teach the OC client bottom-up regulatory techniques designed to get him back to a state where the influences of biotemperament are less powerful, and where his top-down regulatory capacities are consequently less depleted (see the skills training manual, chapter 5, lesson 3). These techniques not only do not require much effort to produce beneficial effects, they also provide the executive control areas of an OC client's brain a much-needed minibreak to replenish central cognitive energy reserves, thereby making it easier for the client to learn and apply new RO skills.

A Novel Mechanism of Change: Social Signaling Matters

None of the preceding discussions has addressed a core issue regarding the development of self-control in our species. To be specific, why did *Homo sapiens* thrive while rival humanoids (for example, the Neanderthals in Western Europe) failed, despite presumably possessing inhibitory and tribal tendencies similar to our own? The answer may lie in our development of a unique way to enhance our group strength, whereby individual tribe members were able to viscerally experience others as themselves. It's this premise that underlies the core mechanism of change in RO DBT.

Ever since the publication of Charles Darwin's seminal *The Expression of the Emotions in Man and Animals* (Darwin, 1872/1998), a number of theorists and researchers have similarly argued that our emotions evolved for the purpose of communication. Nevertheless, as science became increasingly sophisticated at investigating internal experience (such as cognition, physiology, attention, and neurobiology), treatment approaches increasingly tended to overlook this argument. RO DBT, by linking *neuroregulatory theory* and the *communicative functions of emotional expression* to the *formation of close social bonds*, introduces a unique thesis regarding the mechanism by which overcontrolled behavior leads to psychological distress.

A central notion of this thesis is that biotemperamentally heightened OC threat sensitivity makes it more difficult for an OC client to enter into his or her neurobiologically based social safety system (T. R. Lynch et al., 2013; T. R. Lynch, Hempel, & Dunkley, 2015). The experience of feeling safe activates an area of the brain—the PNS ventral vagal complex (see chapter 2), associated with contentment, friendliness, and social engagement—that innervates social engagement muscles involved in modulating tone of voice, facial expressions, listening to human speech, and maintaining eye contact (Porges, 1995, 2001). When we feel safe, we naturally desire to affiliate with others, and our facial and vocal expressions are more relaxed, variable, and playful. However, when the environment is perceived as threatening, another area of the brain associated with mobilization behavior—that is, the SNS fight-or-flight response—becomes dominant, increasing heart rate and downregulating the activation of the striated muscles of the face and head, thus reducing the individual's ability to engage with the social world (Porges, 2001).

Robust research shows that *context-inappropriate suppression* of emotional expression or *incongruent* emotional expression (that is, a mismatch between outward expression and inner experience) will make it more likely for others to perceive one as untrustworthy or inauthentic (Boone & Buck, 2003; English & John, 2013; Kernis & Goldman, 2006), thereby reducing social connectedness and exacerbating psychological distress (see Mauss et al., 2011). In this way, OC biotemperamentally based threat sensitivity *and* SNS-mediated withdrawal of social safety responses, *combined with* overlearned tendencies to mask inner feelings, are hypothesized to engender social ostracism and loneliness, thus exacerbating psychological distress.

Uniquely, RO DBT posits that emotions evolved in humans not only to *motivate* actions (for example, the fight-or-flight response) and *communicate* intentions (via facial expressions, for instance) but also to *facilitate* close social bonds and altruistic behavior among genetically dissimilar individuals, through micromimicry and proprioceptive feedback. This process is posited to have provided our species with a huge evolutionary advantage and to be a core element of developing empathy and altruism. Through the ability to join viscerally with another person, we become more likely to treat other people as we would like to be treated ourselves (for example, we may be willing to risk serious injury or even death to save someone we hardly know).

There are three ways in which RO DBT incorporates these theoretical observations into treatment interventions:

1. It teaches clients context-appropriate emotional expression and the use of nonverbal social signaling strategies that have been shown to enhance social connectedness.

2. It targets biotemperament-based OC deficits and excesses by teaching skills designed to activate areas of the brain associated with the social safety system, and it encourages clients to use these skills prior to engaging in social interactions. This approach enables an overcontrolled client to naturally relax the facial muscles and send nonverbal signals of friendliness, thereby facilitating reciprocal cooperative responses from others as well as fluid social interactions.

> RO DBT, instead of highlighting what's "wrong" with an individual client, starts from observations about what's healthy *in all of us* and then uses these observations to guide treatment interventions.

3. It teaches therapists how to use the mirror neuron system and proprioceptive feedback to enhance OC clients' engagement and learning by deliberately employing gestures, postures, and facial expressions that universally signal openness, nondominance, and friendly intentions. This aspect of RO DBT highlights the need for therapists to practice radical openness skills in their personal lives, since overcontrolled clients are unlikely to believe that it's socially acceptable to play, relax, admit fallibility, or openly express emotions unless they see their therapists model such behavior first.[7]

Treatment Development and Efficacy Research

This book is the end product of a translational research process that focused on understanding and treating maladaptive overcontrol. Treatment development in RO DBT began nearly twenty-five years before this book's publication, when standard dialectical behavior therapy, or DBT (Linehan, 1993a), was applied to treatment-resistant and chronic forms of depression. At the time, I had yet to fully comprehend the difficulties that might arise when a treatment targeting poor self-control was applied to people characterized by excessive self-control, high tolerance of distress, and interpersonal aloofness—in other words, people who were essentially the dialectical opposite of the population that DBT had originally been designed to treat (that is, people with borderline PD). Standard DBT had clear protocols for improving self-control, but it offered less clarity about what might be needed to help individuals characterized by excessive self-control.

I had long seen high self-control as invariably adaptive. But when it came to treating people whose self-control was out of control, what I observed about the limitations of standard DBT presented a challenge to my thinking, and that challenge was the impetus for the development of what eventually became RO DBT. As my understanding of OC disorders became more sophisticated, so did the theory and interventions underlying the new treatment. Indeed, such modifications and changes are considered a core part of effective treatment development (Carroll & Nuro, 2002; Waltz, Addis, Koerner, & Jacobson, 1993). The iterative nature of this modification process is reflected in the changing acronyms—adapted DBT, DBT-D, DBTD+PD, DBT for EOC, and MED + DBT—that were used to describe the treatment during its early phases of development.

Despite the difficulty of settling on a name, the pilot randomized control trials in our developmental years produced some key outcomes, including the creation of core RO concepts and skills, the development of the first version of our biosocial theory of overcontrol, and the creation of the first RO DBT treatment manual. Moreover, the strength of our preliminary findings (T. R. Lynch, Morse, Mendelson, & Robins, 2003) and growing clinical experience encouraged us to continue refining the manual.

The transdiagnostic nature of the nascent RO DBT approach also spurred new thinking and new research targeting a broader range of disorders and treatment settings. Thus, at the time of this writing, current RO DBT research, training, and clinical work have been extended to different age groups (young children, adolescents, young adults, older adults), different disorders (anorexia nervosa, chronic depression, autism, OC personality disorders, treatment-resistant anxiety), different cultures and countries in Europe and North America, and different settings (forensic, inpatient, outpatient). In addition, training has been extended to a wide range of providers (psychologists, nurses, social workers, psychiatrists, family therapists, occupational therapists), with research examining components of RO DBT already showing promise (for example, skills training alone; see Keogh, Booth, Baird, & Davenport, 2016) and adaptations of the manual in progress (for multifamily RO skills training and RO couples therapy). More than three hundred patients have received RO DBT treatment in research trials around the world, and many more have been treated in clinical settings. Thus the feasibility, acceptability, and efficacy of RO DBT are evidence-based and informed by the findings from five published clinical trials and one recently completed multicenter trial. The remainder of this chapter provides an overview of this efficacy research, with brief descriptions of completed and ongoing studies, along with some notes on future directions.

Randomized Controlled Trials Targeting Treatment-Resistant Depression and Maladaptive Overcontrol

To date, there have been three randomized controlled trials (RCTs) examining the feasibility, acceptability, and efficacy of RO DBT (and its earlier versions) for the treatment of maladaptive overcontrol and chronic depression. Our first two RCTs (T. R. Lynch et al., 2003; T. R. Lynch & Cheavens, 2007) were pilot studies using adapted versions of standard DBT (Linehan, 1993a), which we modified to target depression and features linked to maladaptive overcontrol, with the aim of producing a comprehensive RO DBT treatment manual. Both trials purposefully recruited samples of middle-aged and older depressed adults, on the basis of research showing that this age group was more likely to be characterized by overcontrolled coping (rigidity, cognitive inflexibility, low openness, and diminished expression of emotion; see Morse & Lynch, 2000; T. R. Lynch, Cheavens, Morse, & Rosenthal, 2004; Schaie, Willis, & Caskie, 2004). Our third study in this area—a large multicenter RCT, with three independent sites—was designed to extend the generalizability of the treatment by recruiting adults of all ages with refractory depression. Each of these trials is described in detail in the sections that follow.

First Randomized Controlled Trial

The main objective of our first RCT (T. R. Lynch et al., 2003) was to explore the feasibility and utility of adapting standard DBT (Linehan, 1993a) for refractory depression and problems of overcontrol (T. R. Lynch et al., 2003; T. R. Lynch & Cheavens, 2008).[8] Given that the problems associated with OC depression are essentially opposite to the problems found in borderline personality disorder (BPD), the skills used in this initial RCT, although they were based on standard DBT, were modified in order to address the unique problems associated with OC disorders. For example, very early on we recognized rigidity, low openness to new experience, and emotion inhibition as important mediators or moderators in middle-aged and older depressed samples (Morse & Lynch, 2000; T. R. Lynch, Robins, Morse, & Krause, 2001), and these observations strongly influenced treatment targeting and the development of the new skills and interventions that were incorporated into the first trial.

The experimental condition consisted of two presentations of a fourteen-week sequence of an adapted version of standard DBT skills training, modified to target depression and problems of overcontrol (RODBT-Early, or RODBT-E), plus weekly thirty-minute telephone contact with an individual therapist, followed by three months of phone contact every two weeks and then three months of contact every three weeks. Treatment targets linked to OC problems were developed, including inhibition of emotional expression, bitterness and resentment, hyperserious coping, rigid rule-governed behavior, and fatalistic thinking. Dialectical dilemmas specific to OC problems (for example, bitter attachment versus mindless acquiescence; see C. Reynolds, Arean, Lynch, & Frank, 2004) were also developed and incorporated into the manual. The global aim of treatment was to help clients learn how to respond more flexibly and let go of habitual rigid responding (T. R. Lynch, 2000).

Thirty-four chronically depressed individuals who were sixty years old or older were randomized to either antidepressant medication (MED) alone or antidepressant medication plus RODBT-E (using an early version of what was then the current RO

21

DBT manual). To be included in the study, participants were required to meet the criteria for a current episode of unipolar major depressive disorder according to the Duke Depression Evaluation Schedule (see George, Blazer, Hughes, & Fowler, 1989) and to score 18 or more on the seventeen-item Hamilton Rating Scale for Depression (HAM-D; see Hamilton, 1960) or 19 or more on the Beck Depression Inventory (BDI; see A. T. Beck, Rush, Shaw, & Emery, 1979). Diagnoses based on the fourth edition of the *Diagnostic and Statistical Manual of Mental Disorders*, or DSM-4 (American Psychiatric Association, 2000), were assigned in a consensus diagnostic conference that included a board-certified or board-eligible psychiatrist and used the longitudinal, expert, all data (LEAD) standard (Spitzer, 1983). Of those participants randomized to the RODBT-E condition, 45 percent met the Structured Clinical Interview for DSM-IV Axis II Disorders (SCID-II) criteria for at least one personality disorder, whereas only 18 percent of those randomized to the MED-only condition met strict criteria for at least one personality disorder. Attempts were made to keep assessors blind to the variable of treatment condition, although this was not always possible. The majority of the participants reported an average of more than eight previous episodes of depression in their lives. Randomization was successful—the groups did not differ on measures at pretreatment assessment. Two-tailed tests ($p \leq 0.05$) were used for all between-group comparisons; within-group comparisons used Bonferroni corrections, with p values considered significant if they were less than or equal to 0.006. Depression remission was defined as a HAM-D score of less than 8 (E. Frank et al., 1991).

Findings revealed that at post-treatment assessment, 71 percent of the RODBT-E participants were in remission, in contrast to 47 percent of the MED-only participants. At six-month follow-up, 75 percent of the RODBT-E participants were in remission, compared with only 31 percent of the MED-only participants—a significant difference (T. R. Lynch et al., 2003). The RODBT-E group showed significantly decreased self-reported depression scores on the BDI from pretreatment to post-treatment, a change maintained at follow-up, but change on this dimension was not significant for the MED-only group. Only the RODBT-E participants demonstrated significant improvement in a maladaptive personality style that is associated with fears related to being liked by others. In addition, the RODBT-E participants showed significant improvement in adaptive coping after stressful events, and these changes were maintained at six-month follow-up. Improvements in total coping were associated with feeling less overpowered, being more likely to seek social support, and being less likely to take frustrations out on others.

Secondary analyses of these data showed that higher levels of thought suppression were associated with higher depressive symptoms six months after treatment, a finding that provided preliminary support for hypotheses linking poorer outcomes to inhibition of emotional experience and expression (Rosenthal, Cheavens, Lejuez, & Lynch, 2005). The major limitation of our first RCT was its small sample size, with only seventeen participants randomized to each condition. The new RO skills that were piloted in this study were developed in part from weekly meetings of the treatment team.[9] These meetings included discussion of how patients were responding to

RODBT-E, discussions about relevant literature, and discussion of research findings that had to do with potential moderators and mediators of outcomes (T. R. Lynch et al., 2004; Rosenthal et al., 2005). In addition, as the treatment developer, I conducted focus group meetings as well as individual interviews with participants who had completed treatment. The purpose of the meetings and interviews was to gain a better understanding of OC problems and a sense of the modified interventions' acceptability and credibility. Information garnered from these meetings and interviews helped us further refine RODBT-E, and it provided the clinical foundation for our next RCT.

Second Randomized Controlled Trial

Our second RCT (T. R. Lynch & Cheavens, 2007) was designed to further test the newly developed RO skills and treatment targets piloted in the first trial, with the aim of creating an even more comprehensive RO DBT treatment manual targeting OC problems and treatment-refractory depression.[10] To be included in the study, participants had to be at least fifty-five years old and meet the Structured Clinical Interview for DSM-IV Axis I Disorders (SCID-I) criteria for a current episode of major depressive disorder, the SCID-II criteria for a personality disorder, and score 18 or more on the seventeen-item HAM-D. In our sample, 78 percent met the criteria for a personality disorder of overcontrol; the most common Axis II disorders were obsessive-compulsive PD, paranoid PD, and avoidant PD. All the assessors were blind to the variable of treatment condition, and the primary outcome measure was the seventeen-item HAM-D. Depression remission was defined as a HAM-D score of less than 10.

To prospectively ensure that the experimental sample would include only individuals with treatment-resistant depression and comorbid PD, the study design had two treatment phases. In phase 1, participants (N = 65) met regularly with a research psychiatrist who prescribed and monitored eight weeks of antidepressant medication at dosages recommended by best-practice guidelines. Only 14 percent of the participants in this initial phase demonstrated at least a 50 percent reduction in their interviewer-rated depressive symptoms, with the result that 85 percent of the sample met the criteria for treatment-resistant depression.

In phase 2 of the study, those individuals who did not adequately respond to antidepressant medication, and who consented to continue participation (n = 37, or about 57 percent of the original group), were then randomized to either twenty-four weeks of RODBT-E2 (that is, RODBT-Early, manual 2) or a control group that received general psychiatric care plus antidepressant medication (MED).[11] Participants in both conditions were prescribed antidepressant medication by a board-certified psychiatrist.

The RODBT-E2 condition consisted of weekly two-hour skills training classes, with the addition of one hour per week of in-person individual therapy plus antidepressant medication. Telephone consultation with an RODBT-E2 therapist was available to participants outside of therapy hours (although this resource was rarely used), and RODBT-E2 research therapists came together weekly for a ninety-minute consultation team meeting. The general psychiatric care–MED condition included regularly scheduled meetings (at least monthly) with a research psychiatrist who provided general psychiatric care consisting of counseling, as needed, and who monitored antidepressant medication. Research psychiatrists were encouraged to adjust dosages or change the type or class of prescribed medication in order to ensure optimal dosage and treatment.

Results showed that 71 percent of the RODBT-E2 participants were in remission at the post-treatment evaluation, compared with 50 percent of the participants in the control condition, a trend that was maintained at three-month follow-up but leveled off at six-month follow-up. The RODBT-E2 participants demonstrated significant improvement in personality dysfunction (interpersonal aggression and interpersonal sensitivity) compared to the control group in the general psychiatric care–MED condition, and these advantages were maintained at six-month follow-up.

The major limitation of both of our first two RCTs was that neither study had enough statistical power to detect between-group differences. Nevertheless, major and significant advantages were found for the RODBT-E participants, as represented by their having achieved and maintained high rates of depression remission, compared to the control condition (see T. R. Lynch et al., 2003), and RODBT-E2 demonstrated significantly better outcomes on measures of personality, compared to the control condition. Both studies included the most difficult-to-treat clients: they were older, had personality disorders, were suicidal, and suffered from chronic conditions. Dropout rates for the experimental conditions (RODBT-E and RODBT-E2) were low—6 percent and 28 percent, respectively. The higher dropout rate for the second study may reflect the more severe nature of the sample (a diagnosed personality disorder was a requirement for participation). In addition, the participants in the first study were concurrently taking part in a larger longitudinal study, and that may have been a protective factor against dropout. Results from both trials provided preliminary support for our earliest versions of RO DBT, including support for its feasibility, its acceptability, and its clinical utility.

Our second trial also allowed us to further develop the new treatment manual (T. R. Lynch & Cheavens, 2008). A novel biosocial theory for OC disorders was developed, and new RO skills emerged that were designed to maximize openness, increase flexible responding, and reduce rigid, rule-governed behavior.[12]

Third Randomized Controlled Trial

Notwithstanding the advances achieved in our first two RCTs, the development of RO DBT for treatment-resistant and chronic depression could have ended after the second trial. One reason was that we had received feedback from several independent US and UK grant reviewers that the data from our first two RCTs were sufficiently strong for us to publish the RO DBT manual as it was, without further modification or research. Yet I remained skeptical. My clinical experience suggested that we had only begun to scratch the surface of knowing our OC clients. Moreover, I had decided to relocate our research lab from Duke University to the University of Exeter and, eventually, to the University of Southampton, in the United Kingdom, and these moves brought a wave of new opportunities, ideas, and collaborations, which helped RO DBT mature into its current form. Our third RCT—studying refractory depression and overcontrol, and known as Project RefraMED (for Refractory Depression: Mechanisms and Efficacy of RO DBT)—emerged from this.

Project RefraMED was a multicenter randomized trial in which we randomized participants to receive either seven months of RO DBT plus treatment as usual (TAU) or TAU alone. RO DBT comprised twenty-nine weekly individual sessions lasting one hour plus twenty-seven weekly skills classes lasting two and a half hours. We permitted patients allocated to TAU to access any treatment offered to them by the National Health Service (NHS) or by private providers. We recruited participants from three centers in the United Kingdom—Dorset, Hampshire, and North Wales. Patients were eligible if they were eighteen years or older; had a score of at least 15 on the HAM-D; had a current diagnosis of major depressive disorder on the SCID-I; were suffering either refractory or chronic depression; and, in the current episode, had taken an adequate dose of antidepressant medication for at least six weeks, without relief. However, we excluded patients who met criteria for dramatic-erratic personality disorder (Cluster B), had bipolar disorder or psychosis, or had a primary diagnosis of substance dependence or abuse.

We used an adaptive algorithm to allocate participants at random between treatments and therapists, using three stratifying variables to ensure balance between groups:

1. Early or late onset of depression

2. HAM-D score above or below 25

3. Presence or absence of a personality disorder

Trained assessors blind to these allocations assessed participants seven, twelve, and eighteen months after randomization. Our primary outcome measure was severity of depressive symptoms on the HAM-D, measured at these three points. We allocated 250 participants by adaptive randomization, 162 to RO DBT and 88 to TAU. Patients reported substantial comorbidity: 86 percent reported at least one comorbid Axis I disorder, and 78 percent reported at least one comorbid Axis II disorder. In addition, the RO DBT adherence self-assessment scale (see appendix 8) and new measures to facilitate identification of OC clients (see chapter 3) emerged from this trial.

RO DBT for Anorexia Nervosa

RO DBT has also been used in the treatment of anorexia nervosa (AN), a serious psychiatric illness characterized by low body weight and intense fear of gaining weight

(American Psychiatric Association, 2000). For adults with AN, no specific treatment has been shown to be superior (H. J. Watson & Bulik, 2013). British and US guidelines (National Collaborating Centre for Mental Health, 2004; American Psychiatric Association, 2006) make no specific recommendations for the treatment of AN in adults, a fact suggesting the need for new theoretical and treatment approaches to this disorder.

AN has long been conceptualized as a disorder of overcontrol, as manifested by propensities for aloofness and social withdrawal, cognitive rigidity, insistence on sameness, low novelty-seeking behavior, strong personal needs for structure and symmetry, heightened threat sensitivity, and hyperperfectionism (Fairburn, 2005; T. R. Lynch, Hempel, Titley, Burford, & Gray, 2012; Safer & Chen, 2011; Zucker et al., 2007). Deficits in emotional functioning in AN include impaired recognition of emotion in others and reduced emotional expression, particularly when it comes to the expression of negative emotions (Geller, Cockell, Hewitt, Goldner, & Flett, 2000). Thus AN fits well within the biosocial theory of overcontrol, since a number of researchers have found it to be associated with the following OC characteristics:

- Sensitivity to threat (Harrison, Tchanturia, & Treasure, 2010)

- Insensitivity to rewards (for a review, see Harrison, O'Brien, Lopez, & Treasure, 2010)

- An invalidating and critical childhood environment (Kyriacou, Treasure, & Schmidt, 2008; Mountford, Corstorphine, Tomlinson, & Waller, 2007)

- Inhibited emotional expression (Geller et al., 2000)

- Low sensation-seeking behavior (Rossier, Bolognini, Plancherel, & Halfon, 2000)

- Perfectionism (Franco-Paredes, Mancilla-Díaz, Vázquez-Arévalo, López-Aguilar, & Álvarez-Rayón, 2005)

- Aloof or distant relationships (for a review, see Zucker et al., 2007)

RO DBT offers an original perspective on the etiology and treatment of anorexia nervosa (T. R. Lynch et al., 2013) by conceptualizing restrictive and ritualized eating as symptoms or consequences stemming from rigid maladaptive overcontrolled coping, based in part on research showing that OC coping preceded the development of the eating disorder. Plus, the neuroregulatory theory that underlies RO DBT provides a novel means of understanding compulsive self-starvation, based on neuro-inhibitory relationships between the parasympathetic and sympathetic nervous systems. Specifically, according to the RO DBT model, after periods of intense restrictive eating, the client's neuroregulatory system "perceives" the body's depleted metabolic state as life-threatening, thereby triggering the dorsal vagal complex of the evolutionarily older parasympathetic nervous system (the PNS-DVC), which inhibits energy-depleting action tendencies (urges to flee or fight) mediated by the sympathetic nervous system while reducing sensitivity to pain and increasing emotional numbing (as seen, for example, in the client's flat affect). Thus the client's restrictive eating develops as a means of downregulating anxious arousal—but with a hidden price, RO DBT posits, because the flattened affect secondary to PNS-DVC activation increases the likelihood that the client will be socially ostracized (J. J. Gross & John, 2003; T. R. Lynch et al., 2013).

Unlike most other approaches targeting eating disorders, RO DBT considers it essential for therapists treating AN to identify clients' goals and values that are not solely linked to food, weight, body shape, or other, similar issues related to eating disorders. From the outset, the RO DBT–adherent therapist will smuggle the idea that the client is much more than an eating disorder. This approach is purposefully designed to let the therapist attend to the client's psychological issues while also preventing therapy from possibly reinforcing the client's maladaptive AN behavior by making it the top treatment priority (for more on this point, see "Overview of Treatment Structure and Targets," chapter 4).

In RO DBT, mindfulness-based approaches to anorexia nervosa focus on teaching clients the practice of urge-surfing their food-averse response tendencies (for example, sensations of bloating, nausea, urges to vomit, and catastrophizing thoughts). In this practice, the goal is not the client's mindful enjoyment of food; on the contrary, the focus is on the client's noticing aversive sensations, emotions, and thoughts associated with food ingestion but not responding as if such a sensation, emotion, or thought were a crisis. Instead, the client is encouraged to dispassionately observe food-averse response tendencies and is reminded that this practice is similar to the techniques used by sailors to overcome seasickness, or by jet pilots to overcome severe nausea.[13]

Research by T. R. Lynch et al. (2013) has tested the feasibility and outcomes of using a modification of RO DBT for the treatment of restrictive-type anorexia nervosa (AN-R) in an inpatient setting.[14] In this study, forty-seven individuals diagnosed with AN-R (the mean admission body mass index, or BMI, was 14.43) received inpatient RO DBT (the mean length of treatment was 21.7 weeks). Intent-to-treat (ITT) analyses demonstrated significant improvements in weight, despite the fact that RO DBT does not emphasize weight gain and focuses instead on the client's gaining a life worth sharing. The increase in BMI demonstrated in the ITT analyses was equivalent to a large effect size of 1.71, by contrast with an effect size of $d = 1.2$ reported for other inpatient programs (see Hartmann, Weber, Herpertz, & Zeeck, 2011). Of those who completed treatment, 35 percent achieved full remission, and an additional 55 percent achieved partial remission, for an overall response rate of 90 percent. The same individuals demonstrated significant and large improvements in ED-related psychopathology symptoms ($d = 1.17$), ED-related quality-of-life issues ($d = 1.03$), and psychological distress ($d = 1.34$). These rates of remission are encouraging, since the literature on AN recovery has demonstrated that attainment of a higher BMI during treatment predicts better relapse prevention (Carter et al., 2012; Commerford, Licinio, & Halmi, 1997). Furthermore, these rates of remission are comparable to those achieved in outpatient settings and are noteworthy because they were achieved in a more severely underweight and more chronic population.

Also promising are the results of a small case-series pilot study in which standard individual DBT was augmented by an average of thirty-two weeks of RO skills training that addressed overcontrol (E. Y. Chen et al., 2015). The participants were nine adult female AN outpatients, ranging in age from nineteen to fifty-one, with an average baseline BMI of 18.7.[15] Of this sample, 75 percent met either subclinical or full criteria for the binge-purge subtype of AN. At baseline, the majority (88 percent) had a comorbid DSM-4 Axis I disorder (such as depression), and 63 percent had a comorbid DSM-4 Axis II disorder (such as obsessive-compulsive personality disorder), with 25 percent reporting histories of suicidal or nonsuicidal self-injury. Independent assessors conducted standardized clinical interviews both before and after treatment. ITT analyses demonstrated significant rates of weight gain and menses resumption for 62 percent of the sample by the end of treatment. Results demonstrated large effect sizes for increased BMI ($d = 1.12$), and these were sustained both at six-month follow-up ($d = 0.87$) and at twelve-month follow-up ($d = 1.21$). Furthermore, improvements in total Eating Disorder Examination scores at the end of treatment yielded an effect size of $d = 0.46$, which was sustained at six-month follow-up ($d = 0.45$) but declined at twelve-month follow-up ($d = 0.34$).

Research on using RO DBT with adult AN clients continues, in collaboration with colleagues at Sweden's Uppsala University, with a special emphasis on hypothesized mechanisms of change. Preliminary research examining the efficacy of using RO DBT with treatment-resistant adolescent AN clients is also under way, in collaboration with the South London and Maudsley NHS Foundation Trust and the Institute of Psychiatry in London. This research includes a novel multifamily RO skills training program.

RO Skills Training for Treatment-Resistant Disorders of Overcontrol

An important issue for multicomponent treatments like RO DBT is to determine the extent to which structural components of the treatment are also essential components. For example, how effective is RO skills training alone in achieving important clinical outcomes? To address this question, an independent research team (Keogh et al., 2016) used a nonrandomized controlled design to investigate, without our involvement, the effectiveness of RO skills training alone in the treatment of overcontrolled personality dysfunction as compared to TAU.

In this study involving treatment-resistant adult subjects ($N = 117$), participants were recruited to an RO skills training group ($n = 58$) or, if that group was full, were placed on a waiting list and given TAU ($n = 59$). The TAU participants went on to attend RO skills training sessions as space became available.[16]

On sociodemographic and clinical measures there were no statistically significant differences at baseline between the RO skills training group and the TAU group. Participants in both groups completed a battery of measures at pretreatment and again at post-treatment. In addition, participants in the RO skills training group completed measures at three-month follow-up as well as measures of therapeutic alliance and group processes at the sixth and eighteenth sessions of the training.

Of the fifty-eight people in the RO skills training condition, six dropped out, for a treatment dropout rate of 10 percent; five did not complete postgroup measures; and forty-seven did complete postgroup measures, for a response rate of 81.5 percent. There were no significant differences between dropouts and treatment completers. Of the fifty-nine TAU participants, twenty-two did not return post-treatment questionnaires; thirty-seven did complete post-treatment questionnaires, for a response rate of 62.7 percent.

The results of this study showed significantly greater improvement in global severity of psychological symptoms, with medium effects post-treatment, for RO skills training alone than for TAU.[17] This study is important, not only because it was conducted without the clinical involvement or supervision of the treatment developer but also because it provides preliminary evidence for the utility of RO skills training alone for treatment-resistant OC adults.

RO DBT with Forensic Populations

More recently, RO DBT has been applied in forensic settings, on the basis of research identifying two broad classes of violent offenders characterized as either overcontrolled or undercontrolled (Megargee, 1966; Megargee & Bohn, 1979). In comparison to undercontrolled offenders, overcontrolled offenders have been shown to be more introverted, shy, timid, tense, and apprehensive as well as and more likely to plan, act responsibly, and deny hostility toward others (Robins, John, Caspi, Moffitt, & Stouthamer-Loeber, 1996; Du Toit & Duckitt, 1990; M. Henderson, 1983a, 1983b; Hershorn & Rosenbaum, 1991). Early theories posited OC violence as stemming from an accumulation of repressed anger that, with repeated provocation, eventually overwhelmed an OC offender's capacity for self-control and erupted in extreme displays of rage (and acts of violence), quickly followed by the offender's humiliation and despair (Tsytsarev & Grodnitzky, 1995). More recent models, based on research showing that acts of OC violence can be driven by other than emotional factors (Chambers, 2010), have demarcated two subtypes of the violent overcontrolled personality: the inhibited subtype (characterized by reactive violence) and the controlled subtype (characterized by planned violence). Indeed, extensive research (see, for example, Bandura, 1973; Polaschek & Collie, 2004) has shown that anger is neither necessary nor sufficient for violence to occur.

To date, however, the majority of research in forensic settings has been dominated by theory and treatment interventions relevant to undercontrolled offenders (Novaco 1997; Davey, Day, & Howells, 2005), with offense-related programs aiming to improve self-control, typically through cognitive behavioral therapy (CBT), especially anger-management interventions (Hanson, Bourgon, Helmus, & Hodgson, 2009; Hollin, Palmer, & Hatcher, 2013; Tew, Harkins, & Dixon, 2013; Wong & Gordon, 2013). Although CBT anger-management treatment with general

29

populations suggests at least moderate effect sizes (DiGiuseppe & Tafrate, 2003; Gansle, 2005; Sukhodolsky, Kassinove, & Gorman, 2004), studies with offender populations have been more mixed. Moreover, in a study of 131 violent male offenders participating in anger-reduction treatment (Low & Day, 2015), a group of offenders characterized by undercontrol were the only ones to benefit from treatment.[18] The Peaks Unit at Rampton Hospital in the United Kingdom is in the process of testing a model of treatment (RO DBT for OC offenders, and standard DBT for UC offenders) that accounts for both overcontrolled and undercontrolled coping.

RO DBT for Treatment-Refractory Anxiety

RO DBT is posited to have utility for treatment of resistant-anxiety disorders, although research to date is in its early stages. Effective, empirically validated treatments for anxiety have been developed, but only 60 percent of clients respond to them to any significant degree. Many clients are left with residual symptoms or stay treatment-refractory. Interestingly, research suggests that the clients who may be most resistant to treatment are those with the temperamental and personality traits characteristic of overcontrol. For example, obsessive-compulsive disorder (OCD) and obsessive-compulsive personality disorder (OCPD) share a number of classic OC coping problems, such as extremely rigid patterns of thinking (obsessions and mental rituals in the case of OCD) and difficulty tolerating change or uncertainty (Gallagher, South, & Oltmanns, 2003; A. T. Beck, Freeman, & Davis, 2004). In addition, both OCD and OCPD often involve forms of maladaptive hoarding, such as an inability to discard worn-out or worthless things (Steketee & Frost, 2003).[19]

RO DBT for Autism Spectrum Disorders

In the transdiagnostic model underlying RO DBT, autism spectrum disorders (ASD) are also considered to represent classic problems of overcontrol, including behavioral-cognitive rigidity, lack of emotional expression, and interpersonal aloofness. Research shows that individuals with ASD seek order and predictability, use rule-based methods of coping, exhibit a constricted range of expression, and have poor social cognitive abilities (see Baron-Cohen & Wheelwright, 2003; Lawson, Baron-Cohen, & Wheelwright, 2004). High-functioning ASD individuals are not only aloof and socially withdrawn but also focused on details; they fail to integrate the context or understand the gist of a situation (see Zucker et al., 2007). Preference for detail over global configurations has been repeatedly documented in ASD (for a review, see Happé & Frith, 2006); and, although research is limited, similar information-processing biases appear to characterize AN and OCPD (Zucker et al., 2007). Thus, although research applying RO DBT to ASD has yet to be systematically conducted, the clinical appropriateness of RO DBT for ASD appears to have face validity.

Now You Know...

▶ Too much self-control can be as problematic as too little.

▶ Biotemperamental factors may be the driving force behind excessive self-control because these factors can influence and interfere with perception, learning, and overt behavior at the preconscious level.

▶ Research using RO DBT, alone or in combination with RO skills training and standard DBT, has demonstrated promising results in the treatment of chronic and treatment-resistant disorders.

CHAPTER 2

A Neurobiosocial Theory for Disorders of Overcontrol

The aim of this chapter is to provide an overview of the theory and science that underpin treatment interventions in RO DBT. Two distinct yet interrelated theories will be outlined. The first is a broad-based neuroregulatory model of socioemotional functioning applicable to all humans. It accounts for both bottom-up and top-down processing of emotional stimuli and transacting cyclical processes between the central nervous system (CNS) and the autonomic nervous system (ANS) that (ideally) facilitate an individual's ability to flexibly respond to changing environmental conditions. The second refers to a neurobiosocial theory that describes how maladaptive OC coping develops and is maintained over time. Both models provide the foundation for RO DBT interventions, treatment targeting, and hypothesized mechanisms of change.

A Novel Neuroregulatory Model of Socioemotional Functioning

The RO DBT neuroregulatory model defines emotions as evolutionarily prepared and learned response tendencies triggered by unconditioned or conditioned stimuli that function to motivate actions, communicate intentions, and, at least in humans, facilitate the formation of close social bonds essential for individual and species survival. Similar to vertical-integrative views on emotion (see Panksepp, 2005; Tucker, Derryberry, & Luu, 2005), regulatory functions are posited to be processed from evolutionarily older to evolutionarily newer brain systems (for example, brain stem to limbic to cortical areas of the brain).

RO DBT highlights the importance of the autonomic nervous system and its associated neural substrates when it comes to understanding socioemotional behavior, primarily because the visceral and physiological changes occurring during an emotional response are mostly generated by this system. The ANS is part of the peripheral nervous system, defined as any nervous tissue lying outside of the brain and spinal cord (Sequeira, Hot, Silvert, & Delplanque, 2009), and it controls the viscera, glands, and sensory systems of the body, whereas the brain and spinal cord together form the central nervous system, which is responsible for processing signals sent to and from the rest of the body. The CNS can control, inhibit, or bypass lower reflex mechanisms of the ANS via activity in areas such as the hypothalamus, amygdala, and prefrontal cortex (Jessell, 1995). Because of the ANS, the human body is able to quickly alter its internal state to meet the demands of the external environment. This is extremely important when survival relies on the ability to quickly identify and appropriately respond to environmental threats or rewards (Darwin, 1872/1998; Porges, 2009). The visceral or bodily role played by the ANS also influences social signaling (for example, facial expressivity, voice tone, and body posture). Finally, the ANS innervates every organ in the body and has two divisions, the sympathetic branch and the parasympathetic branch.

The ANS Sympathetic Nervous System

The sympathetic nervous system (SNS) in the ANS is generally a catabolic system that expends energy and prepares the body for action (for example, fight-or-flight behaviors resulting in changes such as increased heart rate, increased sweating, and increased blood flow to skeletal muscle as well as the inhibition of the digestive system). According to our model, this system is activated whenever a stimulus is appraised as either a potential threat or a potential reward. Innervation of the adrenal medulla by the SNS releases the catecholamines adrenaline and noradrenaline into the bloodstream. Therefore, the SNS tends to have a diffuse effect throughout the body.

The ANS Parasympathetic Nervous System

The parasympathetic nervous system (PNS) is generally anabolic and promotes tissue growth, the conservation of energy, and a state of rest or digestion. Most of the PNS nerve fibers originate in the cranial or sacral regions of the spinal cord (that is, the very top and bottom regions of the spine), including the vagus nerve, which originates from nuclei in the brain stem and plays a major role in the PNS. Unlike in the SNS, parasympathetic ganglia tend to be found in or near the muscle or organ being regulated, thereby allowing the activity of the PNS to be localized and specific. Interestingly, the PNS-dominated vagus nerve, also known as the *tenth cranial nerve*, can be traced back to two origins within the brain stem: the nucleus ambiguous and the dorsal vagal motor nucleus (DVNX). These form parts of the ventral vagal complex (VVC; new vagus) and dorsal vagal complex (DVC; old vagus), respectively (Porges, 1995). Both of these vagal branches function to slow heart rate, yet their broader effects are qualitatively and quantitatively different (Porges, 1995, 2001). The PNS-VVC (new vagus) is associated with social safety, affiliation, and exploration, whereas the PNS-DVC (old vagus) is associated with shutdown, immobilization, and pain numbing (see Porges, 2001).

In order to account for these complexities, our model parses emotion regulation into three broad transacting elements:

1. Perceptual encoding regulation

2. Internal cognitive regulation

3. External expressive regulation

Perceptual encoding factors account for automatic preconscious regulatory processes, while separating internal from external regulation helps explain how a person can feel anxious on the inside yet show no overt signs of anxiety on the outside. *Arousal*, in our model, pertains to the intensity of an inner experience of emotion, involving ANS-mediated visceral responses and bodily sensations that most people refer to as "feelings," whereas *valence* represents the hedonic value assigned to an evocative stimulus (that is, positive or negative). Both arousal and valence moderate metabolic processes linked to expenditures of energy (such as the amount of effort employed in order to avoid a noxious stimulus) and influence the type and strength of internal action urges and response tendencies (such as an urge to affiliate).

The Human Response

The ideal set point for humans is posited to be a state of safety, or calm readiness, that involves a sense of receptivity and low-level processing of both internal and environmental stimuli. However, when sensory inputs are evocative (meaning discrepant from expectations based on stored representations; see L. Gross, 2006), *or* when a substantial change in sensory neuron firing occurs, a typically unconscious evaluative process ensues that quickly assigns valence (positive or negative) more specifically, to classify them according to five broad classes of emotionally relevant phenomena:

1. Safety (valence positive, arousal low)

2. Novelty (valence ambiguous)

3. Reward (valence positive, arousal high)

4. Threat (valence negative, arousal high)

5. Overwhelming threat or reward (valence irrelevant, arousal low)

Each class of stimuli reflects the end result of a natural selection process that equipped humans to automatically attend and respond to certain types of environmental stimuli (such as spiders or human facial expressions) linked to species survival (see Adolphs, 2008; Davis et al., 2011; Mineka & Öhman, 2002). Each class of stimuli is also associated with its own unique neural substrate and pattern of bodily responses, which influence our desire for affiliation with others as well as our nonverbal social signaling (such as our facial expressivity, voice tone, and body posture). These species-specific unconditioned stimuli elicit unconditioned responses that, at least initially, are unalterable, although they are subject to epigenetic modulation over the course of a person's life, as a function of learning and brain maturation (Bendesky & Bargmann, 2011; McEwen, Eiland, Hunter, & Miller, 2012). Emotional responses can be triggered by an internal cue (such as a bodily sensation or a memory), an external cue (such as a barking dog), or a temporal cue (as when a particular time of day triggers the urge to smoke a cigarette).

Initial evaluations or primary appraisals of evocative stimuli occur at the sensory receptor or preconscious level. For example, research suggests that we need at least seventeen to twenty milliseconds (recall that one second is equal to one thousand milliseconds) to become consciously aware of a face expressing emotion, and yet our brain-body begins physiologically reacting to that facial expression after as short a time as four milliseconds (L. M. Williams et al., 2004, 2006). Perceptual encoding factors function to screen out the vast array of incoming sensory stimuli that would otherwise overwhelm the brain's capacity to attend to relevant stimuli essential for survival and individual well-being. If a stimulus is of low intensity, repetitive, or both, then the generalized arousal systems fails to excite or activate higher brain areas, thereby providing an important preconscious regulatory function. Thus the initially annoying sound of a ticking clock, for most individuals, will habituate or fade from awareness over time, due to its low intensity and repetitive nature. Without this, we would likely be overwhelmed by the vast array of incoming stimuli, since a great deal of information entering the central nervous system is irrelevant (for example, the color of the wall in front of my computer as I write this).

> We need at least seventeen to twenty milliseconds to become consciously aware of a face expressing emotion, and yet our brain-body begins physiologically reacting to that face after as short a time as four milliseconds.

Neuroceptive tendencies also involve innate reactions to unconditioned stimuli (such as the sight of a snake) or learned reactions to conditioned stimuli (to an infant, for example, a gun is not emotionally evocative, whereas for an older child guns are highly evocative). Plus, the influence of biotemperament may be most powerful at the sensory receptor level of emotional processing because it functions to bias perception and regulation preconsciously. Fortunately, primary appraisals can be reappraised at the central cognitive level via top-down regulatory processes. For example, a runner sighting a curvy stick on a woodland trail is likely to exhibit a startle response, followed quickly by the word "Snake!" and a brief heightening of defensive arousal, yet most often the curvy shape is quickly recognized or reappraised as a stick, whereupon autonomic defensive arousal is downregulated and the runner is returned to his prior positive mood state. Reappraisals at the central cognitive level are also strongly influenced by individual differences in experience. For example, children and their parents have different reactions to seeing that a deep snow has fallen overnight, which vary further depending on whether it is a weekday or weekend. Plus, the urging component of an internal response tendency is a propensity for action, not the action itself—that is, feeling like hitting someone does not mean one will automatically engage in a boxing match. Whether or not a person actually hits another person depends greatly on his innate capacity for self-control as well as the situation he is in, his prior learning, and his biotemperamental predispositions. As already alluded to, our model contends that our brains are evolutionarily hardwired to detect and react to five broad classes of emotionally relevant stimuli, described next.

Social Safety Cues

Social safety cues are stimuli associated with the feeling of being included in a tribe. For our very early ancestors living in harsh environments, belonging to a tribe was essential to individual survival. Nonhuman primates isolated from their community will die of exposure, from lack of nourishment, or from predation in a matter of days or weeks (Steklis & Kling, 1985); for our human ancestors, social isolation from the tribe meant almost certain death from starvation or predation. When we feel included in a tribe, we feel safe, protected, secure, loved, fulfilled, and cared for.

> For our human ancestors, social isolation from the tribe meant almost certain death from starvation or predation.

The social safety system promotes social connectedness: when it is activated, we experience a sense of calm readiness and a desire to affiliate with others; we are naturally more open, playful, and curious about the world. Our social safety system contains nerves that govern the muscles in our body needed to communicate and form close social bonds (Porges, 2007). These social safety muscles help us hear better what others are saying by tuning into the higher-frequency sound vibrations associated with human speech (middle ear muscles), communicate warmth and friendliness to others via a musical tone of voice (laryngeal and pharyngeal, or voice box, muscles), and signal authenticity and trustworthiness by openly revealing (rather than hiding) facial expressions of emotion (facial muscles). The source nuclei of these responses are located in the special visceral efferent column of the brain stem and are anatomically linked to the cardiac vagal fibers projecting from the nucleus ambiguous. Consequently, the motor nerves that control the muscles of the face and head communicate directly with the inhibitory neural system that slows heart rate, lowers blood pressure, and reduces arousal in order to produce calm states (Porges, 2003a). Porges hypothesizes that, due to this heart–face link in the brain stem, successful social engagement is contingent on a calm and self-soothing physiological state, which is determined by activation of the PNS-VVC (Porges, 2003b, 2009; Porges & Lewis, 2009). According to our model, social safety responses trigger social engagement signals, reductions in metabolic expenditures of energy, and free operant behaviors. Our body is relaxed, our heart rate slows, and our breathing slows and deepens; our facial expressions match our inner experience; we are able to effortlessly make eye contact, accurately listen, and desire to reach out and touch someone. Yet when social safety cues are withdrawn or not present, PNS-VVC regulation of the striated muscles of the face and head is downregulated, thereby automatically impairing empathic perception and prosocial signaling. Heightened biotemperamental threat sensitivity makes it less likely for OC clients to experience mood states linked to social safety. Fortunately, however, the neurobiology-based social safety system can be consciously evoked simply by the way in which the facial muscles are moved and the way in which the body is positioned. The treatment implications of these points will become clear in later chapters.

> The neurobiology-based social safety system can be consciously evoked simply by the way in which the facial muscles are moved and the way in which the body is positioned.

Novelty Cues

Novelty cues are discrepant or unexpected stimuli that trigger an automatic evaluative process designed to determine whether the cue is important for our well-being. When something unexpected occurs, our PNS-VVC social safety system is briefly withdrawn, without SNS activation. We are alert but not aroused. Our body is immobile but prepared to move (Bracha, 2004; Schauer & Elbert 2010); we freeze, hold our breath, and orient our attention toward the novel cue in order to evaluate its potential significance (in milliseconds), a process known as an "orienting response" (Bradley & Lang, 2007; Porges, 1995). The end result is the assignment of valence (safe, threatening, rewarding, or overwhelming). If the novel stimulus is evaluated as safe, then we return to our set point of calm readiness and are likely to signal safety to nearby others via facial affect, body posture, and vocalizations. However, if the novel stimulus is evaluated to be rewarding or threatening, then SNS activation occurs. Biotemperamentally heightened detail-focused processing may make it more likely for an OC client to notice minor discrepancies in the environment, thereby triggering more frequent orienting responses relative to less detail-focused others, while heightened OC threat sensitivity may bias interpretations of ambiguous stimuli toward the negative. Interestingly, across all humans, ambiguous stimuli are rated as more unpleasant and are associated with longer reaction times relative to unambiguous stimuli (Hock & Krohne, 2004). According the RO model of emotions, our brains are evolutionarily hardwired to appraise ambiguous stimuli at the sensory receptor level (for example, a blank facial expression or an unfamiliar sound) as a potential threat (since the cost of not detecting a true threat stimulus for our ancestors living in harsh environments was too high to ignore), whereas evolutionarily newer evaluative processes involving logic and language are needed when primary appraisal processes at the sensory receptor level are unable to assign valence, resulting in slower reaction times but, hopefully, more accurate appraisals and more effective behavior in the long run. Thus OC heightened threat sensitivity is hypothesized to make automatic assignment of negative valence to ambiguous stimuli in the present moment more likely and top-down evaluations less likely, a process that is posited to reverse when it comes to the evaluation of future contingencies.

Evolution and Facial Expression of Emotion

Among humans and nonhuman primates alike, fearful and aggressive facial expressions have been shown to trigger automatic defensive responses (Adolphs, 2008; Davis et al., 2011). The unconditioned and contagious nature of a facial expression as a stimulus is posited to influence perception of subsequent stimuli as well. For example, subliminally brief views of happy facial expressions have elicited higher subjective ratings of the attractiveness, pleasantness, and monetary value of a fruit drink, without conscious awareness of these subliminal visual stimuli (Berridge & Winkielman, 2003). Thus the embodiment of affect in facial expression appears to have evolved in humans as a means of communicating with and influencing others—as a means, that is, of signaling intentions and triggering emotional reactions in those to whom such signals are directed.

Rewarding Cues

Rewarding cues are stimuli appraised as potentially gratifying or pleasurable; our sympathetic nervous system excitatory approach system is activated. We experience a sense of anticipation that something pleasurable is about to occur. We feel excited and elated; our heart rate goes up and we breathe faster. Reward sensitivity is the neuroceptive tendency to detect signals of positive reinforcement from our surroundings. It is conceptually related to the constructs of the behavioral activation system (Gray, 1987; Gray & McNaughton, 2000; Smillie & Jackson, 2005) and positive affectivity (Brenner, Beauchaine, & Sylvers, 2005; D. Watson & Naragon, 2009). Signals of reward motivate excitatory approach and goal-directed activity, which lead to increased activation of the SNS (Brenner et al., 2005), referred to in our model as SNS *appetitive reward*. Individuals with high reward sensitivity are posited to exhibit heightened excitatory responses to lower-level rewarding stimuli in comparison with lower reward sensitivity. Mania vulnerability is an example of heightened reward sensitivity (Depue & Iacono, 1989; Depue, Krauss, & Spoont, 1987; Meyer, Johnson, & Carver, 1999; Salavert et al., 2007), whereas depression has been consistently linked with low reward sensitivity (Henriques & Davidson, 2000) as well as deficits in approach motivation (Shankman, Klein, Tenke, & Bruder, 2007). When strongly activated, SNS appetitive reward response tendencies are posited to reduce PNS-VVC empathic responding, manifested by reductions in facial affect and social cue sensitivity (for example, one may overlook important vocal cues or facial expressions exhibited by others). Hyper-goal-focused behavior secondary to SNS appetitive reward activation can negatively impact the social environment (imagine someone talking over or dominating a conversation because she is so excited by what she is thinking about or doing). The predominant overt behavioral responses during SNS appetitive reward activation involve two general overt behavioral responses:

1. Excitatory approach (for example, reaching for a delicious-looking red apple)

2. Pursuing, which involves hyper-goal-focused appetitive behavior (imagine a fox in a henhouse)

Our model differentiates between anticipatory reward and consummatory reward. The term *anticipatory reward* refers to approach/pursuit responses and SNS excitatory arousal (chasing and catching the rabbit), whereas the term *consummatory reward* refers to reward attainment (consuming and digesting), PNS activation, hedonic pleasure, rest, digestion, and contentment.

Threatening Cues

Threatening cues are stimuli appraised as potentially dangerous or harmful. Detection of threat is related to the activation of the fight-or-flight system (Gray, 1987) and is somewhat related to the activation of the behavioral inhibition system (Gray, 1987; Gray & McNaughton, 2000). When we feel threatened we experience a sense of anticipation that something bad may happen or that desired goals may be blocked. Our sympathetic nervous system is activated, triggering feelings of anxiety, irritation, and an urge to flee or attack. Both our social safety (PNS-VVC) empathic perception and prosocial signaling become impaired. Our body feels tense; our breath is fast and shallow and our heart rate speeds up as we prepare to fight or take flight. For example, we can only force a fake smile, our facial expressions are constricted, our voice tone becomes monotonic, our gestures are tight and nonexpansive, and we are more likely to avert our gaze or stare with hostility and misinterpret what another person says. If the level of threat arousal continues to increase without the threat being removed, a state of fright or panic may occur; the balance between SNS and PNS dominance may tip toward the older evolutionary system (that is, the old vagus or PNS-DVC; see Porges, 2007), causing tonic immobility, yet the organism is still able to escape should an opportunity arise (that is, the SNS can be reactivated).

Overwhelming Threat or Reward Cues

Overwhelming cues trigger an evolutionarily older emergency shutdown system (Porges, 2007) whenever threatening or rewarding stimuli continue unabated or increase in intensity and SNS behavioral coping responses (for example, flight, fight, or excitatory approach) are ineffective or blocked. For example, people with extreme fears of flying are more likely to faint (a shutdown response) after the plane's cabin doors are secured; that is, the locked door blocks escape while the eliciting cues not only remain present but also gradually increase in intensity as takeoff becomes imminent. Thus, when SNS-based responses are ineffective or overwhelmed (for example, it looks like we are going to be dinner for a bear), our brain-body copes by turning off our flight/fight/approach behaviors in order to conserve energy and maximize survival. (For an example of an overwhelming reward cue, see "So Close and Yet So Far Away" in the skills training manual, chapter 5, lesson 2.) Shutdown responses upregulate the old vagus (PNS-DVC; see Porges, 2007), an unmyelinated pathway innervating the gut that, under less onerous circumstances, functions to regulate digestion. Heightened activation of the PNS-DVC usually results in downregulation of PNS-VVC social safety responses, SNS excitatory arousal, and SNS defensive arousal. PNS-DVC shutdown triggers bradycardia (reduced heart rate), apnea (suspension of breathing), increased gastric motility, and increased pain thresholds (Porges, 2007). Our heart rate, breathing, and body movements slow because both our social safety system and our fight-or-flight systems are deactivated; we lose all facial expression, become immobilized, numb out, may faint, and are less able to feel pain.

Animal research investigating the role of the DVC in sickness-induced behaviors has suggested that activation of the DVC may underlie behaviors that parallel symptoms seen in clinical depression; for example, loss of interest, lethargy, and social withdrawal have been linked to DVC activation (Marvel, Chen, Badr, Gaykema, & Goehler, 2004). Indeed, chronically depressed individuals may alternate between high SNS defensive arousal and high PNS-DVC numbing. Specifically, intense periods of anxious worry or rumination may be neuroceptively perceived as overwhelming, leading to PNS-DVC-mediated immobilization and numbing (that is, anhedonia) that turns off or inhibits SNS defensive arousal. This may explain why it is extremely difficult to motivate chronically depressed overcontrolled individuals to change some of their maladaptive behaviors because they are intermittently reinforced via reductions in autonomic arousal. Self-induced starvation (anorexia nervosa) may be similarly reinforced via PNS-DVC shutdown responses since the brain-body interprets extreme food deprivation as life-threatening. The unfortunate consequence is that although the individual with anorexia nervosa may feel calmer when in the PNS-DVC (that is, she is not eating), her regulation strategy is literally killing her. Plus, her flattened affect secondary to PNS-DVC activation makes it harder to flexibly signal genuine desires for social connectedness, leading to an increasing sense of social isolation (T. R. Lynch et al., 2013). Similarly, nonsuicidal self-injury may be partially reinforced via activation of the PNS-DVC. Even when self-injury is preplanned, the very act of cutting oneself to the extent that blood is clearly visible may trigger PNS-DVC-mediated shutdown responses that turn off SNS-anxiety/arousal, thereby intermittently reinforcing cutting behavior. Regardless, research testing these hypotheses is sorely needed in humans.

In our model, it is important to note, a person is never completely free of perceptual and regulatory biases (that is, personal history and biotemperamental predispositions) when it comes to neuroception. Individual differences in learning and experience as well as in biotemperament make misappraisal of an evocative stimulus a relatively common event (as when a genuine offer of help is misinterpreted as a manipulative ploy). Most of the time, however, our neuroregulatory system works well, allowing us to quickly respond to changing environmental conditions and adjust our behavior to match the demands of the moment, as in the following story:

> After a pleasant evening meal, Mr. Bean decides to take a leisurely stroll in his neighborhood. (*High social safety: PNS-VVC is dominant; Mr. Bean is relaxed and sociable.*) However, on this particular night, his street seems unusually quiet—traffic is nonexistent. (*Mild novelty cue: PNS-VVC is slightly withdrawn; Mr. Bean is curious and slightly alert.*) Suddenly a white van appears at the end of the street. It loudly accelerates toward Mr. Bean. His body freezes, he holds his breath, and he stares intently. (*High novelty cue: PNS-VVC social safety system is further withdrawn; Mr. Bean is highly attentive and focused.*) The van screeches to a halt, and three burly men jump out, all wearing identical white uniforms and masks. They run toward Mr. Bean. (*Moderately high threat cue: SNS defensive arousal is activated.*) As they run they chant, "Teeth! Teeth! Glorious teeth!"
>
> Mr. Bean decides to make a run for it. (*SNS flight response is activated: Mr. Bean wants to escape and flee.*) But his pursuers are too fast. They grab him, and he tries to hit them. (*SNS fight response is activated: Mr. Bean launches a defensive attack.*) But they are too strong. They throw him into the back of the van and tie him to a reclining chair with a bright light overhead.
>
> Mr. Bean freezes in terror but continues to seek a means of escape. (*SNS fright response: Mr. Bean is panicked but still able to move.*) Unfortunately, the bonds are too tight, and there appears to be no means of escape. He feels helpless. (*PNS-DVC flag response: Mr. Bean feels the urge to give up.*) And, to make matters worse, the villains force his mouth open and begin poking and prodding at his teeth with pointy objects and tubes, their efforts accompanied by low-level whirring and gurgling sounds. Mr. Bean feels increasingly detached from the situation and can barely hear what his abductors are saying. (*PNS-DVC shutdown is fully activated: Mr. Bean is dissociating and fainting.*)

When Mr. Bean comes to, he's sitting in a police car next to a kindly officer who tells him what happened. It seems that Mr. Bean is the latest victim of the Order of Maleficent Flossing Gurus (OMFG), a reprobate cabal of dental hygienists gone rogue. [Editor's note: OMFG, indeed.] Mr. Bean smiles weakly and takes a deep breath. He's a bit worn out but pleasantly surprised that his teeth feel so exceptionally clean and his breath is so minty fresh. *(Mr. Bean's PNS-VVC social safety system is starting to reengage.)*

Summary of Basic Postulates

Our neuroregulatory model represents an integrative (as opposed to reductionist) theory of socioemotional functioning. It integrates centralized top-down models (Thayer & Lane, 2000, 2009) with peripheral bottom-up models of emotional functioning (Porges, 1995, 2007) by separating sensory receptor, central cognitive, and response-selection regulatory factors. It accounts for a range of potential moderating influences, including those listed here:

- Biotemperamental (threat and reward sensitivity)

- Sociobiographical (trauma history, culture or family, reinforcement history)

- Temporal (quick and automatic versus slow and effortful)

- Arousal (stimulus intensity)

- Valence (hedonic or positive and negative appraisals)

- Internal motivational (urges to rest, affiliate, explore, freeze, approach, pursue, flee, fight, flag, or faint)

The model accounts for stable and context-independent patterns of responding (also known as personality, habits, and moods) and introduces a mechanism by which rigid habitual responses (and biotemperamental biases) can be modified via use of skills that capitalize on neuroinhibitory relationships between the PNS and SNS (Berntson et al., 1991; T. R. Lynch et al., 2015). It also contends that we are evolutionarily hardwired to constantly scan the environment for the presence of safety, novelty, reward, threat, or overwhelming reward or threat and, as a consequence, emotional experience is ever present, albeit often at a low level of intensity that precludes conscious awareness. Finally, the model strongly influences RO DBT treatment strategies via its emphasis on social signaling, social safety, and the communicative and facilitative functions of emotion, asserting that species survival and individual well-being are strongly dependent on our ability to form long-lasting bonds and work together in tribes. Table 2.1 provides a graphical overview of the core ANS components of our neuroregulatory model and how each is hypothesized to impact social signaling.

Table 2.1. The RO DBT Neuroregulatory Model of Emotions

	Neuroception[a] of Evocative Cues[b]				
	Safety Cue	Novelty Cue	Rewarding Cue	Threatening Cue	Overwhelming Cue
Primary neural substrate response	PNS[c]-VVC[d] engaged	PNS-VVC withdrawn without SNS[e] activation	SNS-E[f] (excitatory) engaged	SNS-D[g] (defensive) engaged	PNS-DVC[h] engaged
ANS system triggered	Social safety engagement system (*adaptive function*: enhances intraspecies communication, facilitates social connectedness)	Orienting and primary appraisal system (*adaptive function*: provides a quick means to identify and appropriately respond to environmental threats or rewards)	Excitatory approach system (*adaptive function*: promotes goal-pursuit behaviors that maximize goal attainment)	Defensive avoidance system (*adaptive function*: promotes defensive fight and flight behaviors that maximize harm avoidance)	Emergency shutdown systems (*adaptive function*: conserve vital energy reserves needed for survival when SNS fight/flight/approach responses are ineffective)
Primary action urge	Socialize	Stand still	Approach or pursue	Flee or attack	Give up
Autonomic responses	Body is relaxed Breathing is slow and deep Heart rate is reduced	Body is frozen Breath is suspended Orientation is toward cue	Body is animated and vivacious Breathing is faster Heart rate is fast	Body is tense and agitated Breathing is fast, shallow Heart rate is fast Sweating	Body is immobile Heart rate and breathing is slowed Increased pain threshold
Emotion words associated with interoceptive experience[i]	Relaxed, sociable, contented, open, playful	Alert but not aroused; curious, focused, evaluative	Excited, elated, passionate, goal-driven	Anxious or irritated, defensively aroused	Numb, unresponsive, trancelike, nonreactive, apathetic, insensitive to pain

	Social signaling enhanced	Social signaling capacities momentarily suspended	Empathic perception impaired; individual still expressive	Empathic perception capacities and prosocial signaling capacities both impaired	SNS approach, fight, and flight responses withdrawn; social signaling irrelevant
Impact on social signaling					
Action or expression (*overt behavior or social signal*)	Effortless eye contact and facial expressions Listening to and touching others Appearing approachable, sociable, receptive, open to exploration	Orienting response ("What is it?") Stopping, looking, listening	Excitatory approach Goal-driven behavior Expansive gestures Insensitivity to others' facial expressions and subtle social cues	Constrained facial expressions, tight gestures Monotonic voice Averted gaze or hostile stare Fight-or-flight response	Flat, unexpressive face Monotonic voice Slow speech Dissociation, swooning, fainting

a   The term *neuroception* denotes how a person appraises or assesses evocative stimuli. Primary appraisals are quick evaluations, elicited without conscious awareness and originating at the sensory receptor level. Secondary appraisals are slower, top-down reappraisals of primary evaluations; they involve evolutionarily newer central cognitive and conscious levels of emotional processing.

b   A cue is an emotionally evocative stimulus that occurs inside the body (a happy memory, for example), outside the body (an unexpected loud noise), or as a function of context (the time of day).

c   PNS = parasympathetic nervous system.

d   PNS-VVC = ventral vagal complex ("new" vagus) of the parasympathetic nervous system; social safety system.

e   SNS = sympathetic nervous system; activating system.

f   SNS-E = SNS excitatory approach system.

g   SNS-D = SNS defensive avoidance system.

h   PNS-DVC = dorsal vagal complex ("old" vagus) of the parasympathetic nervous system; shutdown system.

i   The term *interoceptive* refers to emotion based phenomena and sensations occurring inside the body.

Next, I review the RO DBT biosocial theory specific for disorders of overcontrol that emerged from our neuroregulatory model. Both are essential for treatment of maladaptive overcontrol. Our neuroregulatory model provides the basis for interventions targeting specific OC difficulties, whereas the biosocial theory helps clinicians' and clients' empathic understanding of how OC developed and was maintained over time.

A Biosocial Theory for Disorders of Overcontrol

Maladaptive overcontrol is posited to result from a convergence of three broad factors:

1. Nature (biotemperamental and genetic influences)

2. Nurture (influences having to do with the family, cultural and environmental factors, and learning)

3. Coping (tendencies to exert excessive self-control under stress, to compulsively fix problems, and to have deficits in prosocial signaling)

The theory also posits that maladaptive OC involves both perceptual deficits (in receptivity to change, for example) and regulatory deficits (context-inappropriate inhibited or disingenuous expressions of emotion). Specifically, biotemperamental predispositions for heightened threat sensitivity, diminished reward sensitivity, high inhibitory control, and heightened detail-focused processing are posited to transact with early family, environmental, and cultural experiences valuing correctness, performance, and self-control to result in a risk-avoidant, emotionally constrained, and aloof/vigilant style of socioemotional coping that limits opportunities to learn new skills and exploit positive social reinforcers. The theory emphasizes the importance of openness and social signaling as well as the idea that optimal well-being requires the following three elements:

1. Receptivity to novel or discrepant feedback, for the sake of learning

2. Flexible adaptation to changing circumstances

3. Social connectedness with at least one other person

A graphic representation of the theory is shown in figure 2.1.

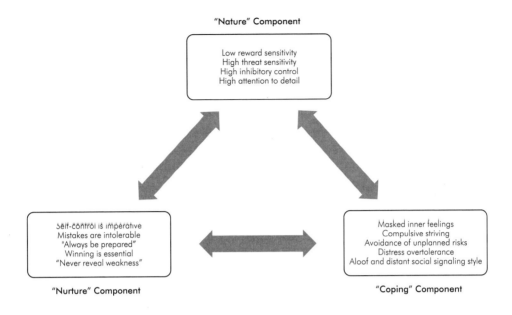

Figure 2.1. Biosocial Theory for Disorders of Overcontrol

The "Nature" Component

The "nature" component of the theory has to do with biogenetic and biotemperamental predispositions that function to exacerbate overcontrolled coping. OC clients are posited to be biologically predisposed to four specific biotemperamental deficits or excesses, which are in turn posited to underlie disorders of overcontrol:

1. Heightened states of defensive arousal and anxiety (secondary to high biotemperamental threat sensitivity)

2. Diminished experiences of spontaneous pleasure and excitatory arousal (secondary to low biotemperamental reward sensitivity)

3. Superior capacities for self-control, distress tolerance, and delay of gratification (secondary to high biotemperamental inhibitory control)

4. Prioritized attention to detail over more global processing (secondary to high biotemperamental detail-focused processing)

Biotemperamental predispositions are powerful because they can impact perception and regulation at the sensory receptor (preconscious) level of emotional responding and, as a consequence, indirectly influence central cognitive functioning (such as language-based reappraisals) and response selection (such as overt actions and social signals), without the person being influenced ever knowing it. When extreme, they are posited to make overt behavioral responding more rigid and less adaptive to changing environmental contingencies.[20] For example, biotemperamental predispositions for high threat sensitivity and constraint make it more likely for an OC client to feel and appear uptight pervasively and regardless of context—at work, at home, at the gym, or when at a party—whereas individuals with fewer biotemperamental biases can more easily modify their behavior in order to match the context they are in (constrained at work but able to dance with abandon at an office party).

High Inhibitory Control

The term *high inhibitory control* refers to superior capacities in being able to inhibit emotion-based action or expressive tendencies (for example, by masking inner feelings), delay gratification (for example, by resisting temptation), attend to nonimmediate future contingencies (for example, by planning ahead) and persist in nonrewarding behavior in the short term in order to achieve a long-term goal (for example, by tolerating distress). Inhibitory control becomes a problem when an individual is unable to voluntarily disinhibit or relinquish control in situations that call for flexibility, humor, unrehearsed responses, and open expression of emotion (for example, when the individual is at a party, or dancing in the rain, or on a romantic date, or at a holiday meal with her family, or listening to feedback from her teenage son). Individuals characterized by excessive inhibitory control are overreliant on strategic rather than hedonic means of achieving desired goals. Much of their behavior, rather than mood-driven, is excessively rule-governed. Thus an OC client is likely to report having attended a party because of a sense of duty or obligation rather than because of anticipatory pleasure. This point cannot be overstated in the treatment of OC clients, because what it means is that their actions, rather than driven by current mood or dysregulated emotions, are often the consequences of nonemotional executive processes involving reasoning, logic, prediction, and rules.

Research examining individuals high in the trait of needing structure and control has collectively revealed that they are more likely to attempt to quickly fix uncertainties and look for set solutions when they are stressed (that is, they are likely to prioritize the use of past solutions over new ones). This type of response style often leads to more errors because the individual finds it difficult to let go of set solutions, or rules, even when environmental changes indicate that a prior solution no longer applies (Brand, Schneider, & Arntz, 1995; Neuberg & Newsom, 1993; Thompson, Naccarato, Parker, & Moskowitz, 2001). Rigid rule-governed behavior and set-shifting problems characterize OC disorders and are suggestive of an information-processing bias and a problem-solving style that favor reason and logic over emotion and intuition.

Research suggests the existence of two biotemperamentally driven yet qualitatively different responses to threat. The first involves *avoidance coping*, or automatic tendencies to turn away from threat-related cues in order to reduce aversive arousal;

the second involves *vigilance coping*, or automatic tendencies to turn toward or approach threat-related cues in order to prevent future occurrences (Hock & Krohne, 2004). Traditionally, approach coping (or vigilant coping) has been considered the healthiest and most beneficial way to reduce stress (Kohlenberg & Tsai, 1991; Hayes et al., 1996), yet more recent research suggests that problems can occur when either the approach or vigilant style of coping becomes rigid or habitual (Hock & Krohne, 2004). For OC clients this distinction may be particularly salient, since they are more likely to compulsively use vigilant and approach coping styles when under stress.

Compulsive striving and excessive approach coping may reflect the influence of biotemperamental blends. For example, research suggests that not only people who are repressors but also people who are sensitizers (Hock, Krohne, & Kaiser, 1996) are hypersensitive to threat, although with some important differences. Repressors quickly respond to a threat cue but then also quickly avoid or distract their attention away from the cue, a strategy that leaves them with an impoverished memory of the threat. Sensitizers also quickly react to a threat cue, but instead of turning their attention away, they intensify their processing of the threat in an attempt to control or prevent future negative occurrences. Repressors' early sensitivity is inhibited by top-down executive control processes (Hock & Krohne, 2004). From our perspective, this may reflect high biotemperamental threat sensitivity combined with high temperamental inhibitory control (a core feature of OC), a combination that may instigate a process whereby low-level threats are detected at the sensory receptor level but quickly downregulated via superior inhibitory control.

Excessive inhibitory control and self-restraint have also been repeatedly linked with a repressive coping style. Repressors value logic and a nonemotional approach to life. Weinberger, Schwartz, and Davidson (1979, p. 338) describe repressors as individuals who fail to recognize their own emotional responses and, in order to appear more socially desirable, "seem actively engaged in keeping themselves (rather than just other people) convinced that they are not prone to negative affect." By contrast, defensive, high-anxiety individuals do admit to their anxious feelings but appear uncomfortable or embarrassed when doing so.[21]

According to Derakshan and Eysenck (1999), individuals high in the repressive coping style, or high repressors, generally believe what they are reporting—namely, that they are not experiencing any emotion—and they attempt to behave accordingly. Yet, despite reporting low anxiety, they respond to threat with high physiological arousal (for a review, see Weinberger, Tublin, Ford, & Feldman, 1990) as well as with decreased heart rate variability by comparison with individuals who actually are low in anxiety (Pauls & Stemmler, 2003). In addition, repressors have been shown to exhibit attentional and encoding strategies that are highly sensitive to threatening or negative stimuli (Bonanno, Davis, Singer, & Schwartz, 1991; Fox, 1993; Furnham, Petrides, Sisterson, & Baluch, 2003). For instance, across four experimental studies that required processing of threat stimuli, Calvo and Eysenck (2000) showed that repressors demonstrated early vigilance followed by avoidance, which manifested later for them than it did for individuals who were low in anxiety.

Repressors are also characterized by high impression management (for example, excessively agreeable or conforming behaviors during conflict), which is hypothesized to help them avoid negative affect and prevent loss of self-esteem from anticipated social rejection (Kiecolt-Glaser & Murray, 1980; Weinberger, 1995). High repressors also appear to exhibit responses that vary with the context and the content of an interaction. For example, multiple studies suggest that repressors tend to downplay the negative rather than overstate the positive (for a review, see Myers, 2010). In addition, when high repressors receive feedback privately, they appear to prefer an avoidant, self-deceptive strategy, whereas when feedback is public they may pay close attention to it, ruminate about how others perceive them, and engage in impression-management activities (Baumeister & Cairns, 1992; Pauls & Stemmler, 2003). What is perhaps most important is that all the findings just cited appear to apply equally to the patterns of behavior that are commonly observed in maladaptive overcontrol, and that are targeted for change in RO DBT.

Detail-Focused Processing

OC clients are posited to exhibit a preference for details (such as hyperawareness of small discrepancies) and high pattern recognition (such as hyperawareness of asymmetry) over more global patterns of processing (for example, broad perspective taking, or taking into account the big picture). Research examining individuals diagnosed with anorexia nervosa and autism spectrum disorders (two core OC disorders) reveals poorer performance on tasks demanding global processing (Happé & Frith, 2006; Lang, Lopez, Stahl, Tchanturia, & Treasure, 2014; Lang & Tchanturia, 2014) and superior capacities for detail-focused or local processing (Aloi et al., 2015; Lopez, Tchanturia, Stahl, & Treasure, 2008, 2009; Losh et al., 2009). Detail-focused processing is posited to represent a nonemotional biotemperamental attribute initiated at the sensory receptor or subcortical level of processing (that is, preconsciously). As a consequence, OC clients may be more inclined than others to notice the trees but miss the forest. It is posited to be nonemotional because it involves basic perceptual processes pertaining to pattern recognition (for example, a misaligned book) that can quickly become emotional. For example, noticing a book out of alignment on a bookshelf may trigger an urge to straighten or realign the book, an urging tendency that if blocked may lead to frustration or trigger anxiety. High detail-focused processing combined with OC superior inhibitory control may strongly influence career, relationship, and recreational choices. For example, OC individuals tend to engage in recreational/career activities requiring detailed analysis (such as chess, map reading, data analysis, or accounting), persistence, rehearsal, and self-discipline (such as ballet dancing, skydiving, scuba diving, or mountain climbing), and they often favor solitary activities that allow greater personal control (such as marathon running or computer gaming) over team and interpersonal activities in which success is measured in terms of prosocial cohesion and mutual striving.

High Threat Sensitivity

High OC detail-focused processing may increase the possibility for noticing minor changes in the environment (that is, novelty), whereas high OC threat sensitivity makes it more likely that these minor discrepancies are appraised as potentially dangerous. In a longitudinal study of two cohorts of children selected in their second or third year of life for being extremely cautious and shy (inhibited) or fearless and outgoing (uninhibited) in the context of unfamiliar events, these characteristics were shown to endure to the sixth year of life; at six years, the more inhibited children showed signs of activation in one or more of the physiological areas that normally respond to novelty and challenge—namely, the hypothalamic-pituitary-adrenal axis, the reticular activating system, and the sympathetic nervous system (Kagan, Reznick, & Snidman, 1987a). This finding suggests that for shy and inhibited children, the threshold of response is lower in those parts of the nervous system that contribute to states of uncertainty and physiological arousal.

Low Reward Sensitivity

Risk aversion and reward insensitivity are crucially related to low approach motivation and heightened behavioral inhibition (Kasch, Rottenberg, Arnow, & Gotlib, 2002; Smoski et al., 2008). Reward responses can be differentiated into three components (for a review, see Dillon et al., 2014):

1. Anticipatory (incentive) reward responses

2. Consummatory reward responses

3. Reward learning

Anticipatory or incentive reward responses involve appetitive-positive affect systems and expectancy processes linked to reward seeking, wanting, and foraging, and brain substrates associated with the ventral striatal dopamine system. Consummatory reward responses also are linked to positive affectivity and brain systems associated with hedonic tastes and pleasurable touch and opiate and gamma-aminobutyric acid (GABA) systems in the ventral striatum and orbital frontal cortex (Berridge & Robinson, 2003; Ikemoto and Panksepp, 1999; Panksepp, 1981, 1982, 1986, 1998). Not surprisingly, chronic stress reduces both anticipatory and consummatory reward responses (see Kumar et al., 2014). Reward learning refers to changes in behavioral responses secondary to positive reinforcement. For example, individuals with anhedonia have been shown to exhibit deficits in reward learning following delivery of a positive reinforcer (see Dillon et al., 2014).

Anticipatory Reward

The term *anticipatory reward* refers to appetitive or incentive motivations that in humans are associated with feelings of desire, wanting, excitement, elation, energy, enthusiasm, and potency (for a review, see Depue & Morrone-Strupinsky, 2005) as well as sympathetic nervous system activation, excitatory approach behaviors, and dopamine release. Anticipatory reward responses are also an important part of social bonding and affiliation in humans and have been linked to unconditioned social stimuli, such as facial features (for example, attractive faces), smiles, friendly vocalizations, and gestures (Porges, 1998). When applied to social interactions, the term refers to the degree to which a person desires social intimacy or seeks social engagement.

OC individuals are posited to be biotemperamentally predisposed to be less sensitive to rewarding stimuli relative to others. Reward sensitivity is defined as the threshold or set point whereby a particular stimulus in the immediate surroundings is evaluated as potentially rewarding or signals the possibility of positive reinforcement. Diminished reward sensitivity makes it less likely for OC individuals to report feeling enthusiastic or joyful and to exhibit excitatory approach behaviors. For example, a recent review of anticipatory reward factors and related brain regions in eating disorders (Kaye, Wierenga, Bailer, Simmons, & Bischoff-Grethe, 2013) concluded that dopamine-mediated anticipatory reward is found to be higher in binge-purge (that is, an undercontrolled disorder in our model) and lower in anorexia (that is, an overcontrolled disorder).[22]

Consummatory Reward

The term *consummatory reward* refers to the feelings of pleasure associated with consuming or achieving a desired reward, experiences that have been shown to be linked with endogenous μ-opiate release, PNS ventral vagal activation, and PNS rest/digest behaviors. In humans, consummatory reward experiences are associated with feelings of increased interpersonal warmth, social connectedness, contentment, an experience of satiation, and feelings of euphoria and well-being. It is important to note that μ-opiate-mediated and μ-opiate-moderated reward experiences are posited to be essential for humans to desire intimacy with others in the first place; that is, the desire to socially engage with others in the present (anticipatory reward) is highly influenced by the magnitude of pleasure experienced during social encounters in the past (see Depue & Morrone-Strupinsky, 2005). Thus an individual with a high temperamental μ-opiate reward system is more likely to encode neutral, low-level prosocial or ambiguous encounters as rewarding (for example, a relatively low-intensity interaction with a store clerk may be experienced as highly pleasurable) compared to someone with a low temperamental μ-opiate reward system. Those with high temperamental μ-opiate reward systems would be expected to approach socially ambiguous situations because their prior experience suggests that they will find them pleasurable. Thus low anticipatory reward–sensitive individuals (that is, OC individuals) are predicted to require a higher level of prosocial safety signals, not only in order to activate their anticipatory reward system and associated excitatory approach behaviors but also in order to experience consummatory reward or pleasure during the social interaction itself. RO DBT posits that OC individuals exhibit *low* anticipatory reward responses (low reward sensitivity), *normal* consummatory reward responses to nonsocial rewards, and *low* consummatory reward responses to social or affiliative rewards.[23]

Interestingly, most research examining reward fails to distinguish between positive emotional experience and physiological quiescence. Our neuroregulatory model contends that calm quiescence can be distinguished from excitatory reward states in part by observing how they impact social signaling (refer to table 2.1). For humans at least, physiological quiescence is posited to mean social quiescence; that is, when we feel part of a tribe we feel safe, and concomitant social safety activation (see PNS-VVC) enhances empathic responding and prosocial signaling. In contrast, excitatory reward states are characterized by expansive social signals and lowered empathy (via downregulation of the PNS-VVC social safety system and upregulation of SNS excitatory reward). Plus, anticipatory reward has been linked with mental imagery and reward approach and responsiveness, whereas consummatory reward has been linked to openness to experience and positive affect (Gard, Gard, Kring, & John, 2006). RO DBT posits that OC clients are less likely to experience PNS-VVC social safety, partly as a function of high biotemperamental threat sensitivity; that is, it's hard to have a good time at a party when your sensory receptor system is hyperalert for potential danger.

The conundrum that OC presents for affiliative or social reward theory is that the amount of hedonic pleasure OC clients experience from nonsocial rewards is predicted to be the same as for other people (for a review, see Dillon et al., 2014), yet they are predicted to experience diminished hedonic pleasure from social interactions and be less responsive to positive social stimuli compared to other people. These hypotheses have yet to be investigated. Moreover, similar to observations made by McAdams (1982), models examining reward responses would benefit from separating affiliation needs (for example, fears of being alone, desires to be around others but not necessarily intimate) from intimacy needs (for example, need for close intimate social bonds, recognition that periods of social isolation may be necessary). Desires to affiliate or be around other people may represent lower-order or older evolutionary responses associated with safety in numbers, whereas desires for intimacy may represent higher-order or new evolutionary responses associated with the facilitative function of emotional expressions and our core tribal nature. Finally, I consider it plausible that our models would benefit if we expand the concept of reward to include nonhedonic motivations, particularly when attempting to understand human social interactions. For example, as noted earlier, OC individuals are posited to be motivated to approach social interactions out of obligation or sense of duty (nonaffective approach coping), not because they anticipate or experience them as rewarding or pleasurable.

Reward Learning

Reward learning among OC clients is also posited to be negatively impacted by their habitual avoidance of novelty or unpredictable situations. Current theories of reward learning posit that learning occurs when prediction fails—that is, new learning is possible only when there is a discrepancy between what was predicted to occur (based on past experience) and what actually occurred. Learning is most robust when expectations are disrupted (that is, unpredicted), whereas learning slows and eventually stops as outcomes become increasingly predictable (Hollerman & Schultz, 1998). Similar to concepts articulated in RO principles of self-enquiry (see chapter 7), it appears that learning is only possible when we encounter our "personal unknown."

The relevance of the preceding observations when it comes to understanding OC clients is clear; that is, their obsessive use of routine and their structured, controlled existence may make life predictable and keep anxiety at bay but have a hidden cost when it comes to enjoying life. Research suggests that dopamine neurons in the *substantia nigra* and *ventral tegmental* areas of the brain are most likely to be activated by unpredictable rewarding stimuli, a process that "then slows down as outcomes become increasingly predicted and ends when outcomes are fully predicted" (Hollerman & Schultz, 1998, p. 304). Thus it appears that rewarding experiences and subsequent learning depend on variety, unpredictability, and exposure to the unknown. Thus the obsessive desire to predict all possible future outcomes and plan ahead that characterizes most OC clients may not only prevent new learning but increase stagnation and resignation. Relatedly, OC positive mood states are often linked to a sense of accomplishment (for example, resisting temptation, detecting an error that others missed) rather than luck, chance, or current mood (for example, winning the lottery). From an OC perspective, happiness must be earned and leisure time must be self-improving. Unfortunately, OC biotemperamental capacities for superior self-control often make it seem possible to control others and the world similarly. Next, I describe the "nurture" component of the RO DBT biosocial theory of OC and the impact of the sociobiographical environment on the development and maintenance of maladaptive OC.

The "Nurture" Component

The "nature" component of our OC biosocial theory is hypothesized to transact with the "nurture" or sociobiographical component of the model (family, cultural, environmental) in ways that function to reinforce, maintain, or exacerbate OC coping. Sociobiographical influences can be historical (childhood trauma, past learning) or contemporary (present living conditions, new learning) and transactions are posited to be iterative and bidirectional; that is, nature influences nurture, and vice versa. For example, research examining behavioral inhibition among children has shown that anxious solitary children (that is, shy, timid, standoffish, verbally inhibited) may be temperamentally hypersensitive to social rejection (London, Downey, Bonica, & Paltin, 2007). Anxious solitary excluded children have been shown to display greater social helplessness (for example, failure to take the initiative in a social exchange or giving up easily when socially challenged) both before and after a socially rejecting experience (Gazelle & Druhen, 2009). They also report higher feelings of rejection both prior to and during a behavioral rejection task, including excessive suppression of vagal tone and sustained increases in heart rate relative to controls (Gazelle & Druhen, 2009). Low resting respiratory sinus arrhythmia (RSA), a measure of PNS-vagal tone, has been shown to be linked to anxiety (Beauchaine, 2001) and to children high in behavioral inhibition (Rubin, Hastings, Stewart, Henderson, & Chen, 1997), findings that, according to our model, suggest deficits in social safety system activation (that is, PNS-VVC). According to Downey, Lebolt, Rincón, & Freitas (1998), anxious expectations of social exclusion increase the likelihood that ambiguous social stimuli may be perceived by the anxious solitary child as rejecting. Social exclusion is a painful form of rejection involving peer ostracism (for example, not being approached by peers during school recesses or deliberate ignoring or refusals to allow the child to participate in peer games). Of particular relevance for understanding OC coping, anxious solitary excluded children (eight to nine years old) exhibited significantly greater observable behavioral "upset" compared to a normative control during an experimental manipulation of peer rejection; however, interestingly, they demonstrated a significantly steeper reduction in observable upset, to such an extent that within minutes they were indistinguishable from the normative group (Gazelle & Druhen, 2009). The quick inhibitory control of observable upset (for example, distressed facial expressions) displayed by anxious solitary excluded children following peer rejection parallels a similar process commonly observed in OC clients—that is, experiences of rejection are hidden or masked publicly. This biobehavioral pattern of responding represents an example of the types of nature-nurture transactions that are posited to underlie the development of OC coping.

A vast amount of research has examined the effects childhood trauma and familial psychopathology exert on socioemotional well-being (Cheavens et al., 2005; Cloitre, Miranda, Stovall-McClough, & Han, 2005; Cloitre, Stovall-McClough, Zorbas, & Charuvastra, 2008; White, Gunderson, Zanarini, & Hudson, 2003), including the development and maintenance of problems linked with maladaptive OC. For example, longitudinal research using a community-based sample found emotionally distant mothers (for example, endorsing "I do not praise my child") to be associated with an increased risk of OC personality disorder symptomatology (avoidant and paranoid) among their offspring, even after controlling for physical or sexual trauma, physical neglect, and other PD symptoms (Johnson, Smailes, Cohen, Brown, & Bernstein, 2000). Likewise, longitudinal studies suggest that emotional neglect and maltreatment experienced early in life (infancy, toddlerhood) result in the development of internalizing disorders (Keiley, Howe, Dodge, Bates, & Pettit, 2001; Kim, Cicchetti, Rogosch, & Manly, 2009; Manly, Kim, Rogosch, & Cicchetti, 2001), whereas children experiencing a broader range of maltreatment, especially physical or sexual abuse as opposed to emotional neglect, appear to be more likely to develop externalizing problems (Kim et al., 2009).

Family and cultural influences valuing performance and high achievement over social connectedness may further exacerbate maladaptive OC coping. High performance values trigger frequent social comparisons, primarily in order to confirm that one's performance is at least adequate (and hopefully better) than similar others, making unhelpful envy a likely consequence when social comparisons are unfavorable. Family and cultural values for high performance can reinforce notions that the child already is or should be special, different, or superior, compared to his peers (for example, more intelligent, more compliant, more responsible, more diligent, more skillful). Turkat (1985) contends that early childhood experiences emphasizing the importance of being special, unique, or high-achieving increase the probabilities of a child feeling socially anxious and behaving in awkward or "different" ways relative to less anxious peers. The specific type of disorder that may develop from this point forward largely depends on the behaviors that the child adopts to manage anxiety. For example, the pre-paranoid-PD child adopts a guarded stance and covertly blames others for his isolation (Turkat, 1985), and the pre-obsessive-compulsive-PD or anorexic child becomes increasingly perfectionistic and restrained in order to maximize positive evaluations, whereas the pre-avoidant-PD child avoids evaluative contexts (that is, reduces contact with others and situations where judgment is likely) and adopts a compliant or appeasing manner. These styles of interacting are posited to become intermittently reinforced over time and to interfere with normal developmental processes.

In addition, repeated family and cultural messages stressing mistakes as intolerable or unacceptable may inadvertently communicate to a child that she is never good enough (because life is full of mistakes), thereby exacerbating the development of maladaptive perfectionism. Consequently, the child learns to avoid taking risks in order to prevent the possibility of making a mistake; she becomes highly sensitive to perceived criticism and considers her self-worth to be based on how well she is performing relative to others. This can masquerade as fierce independence, nonchalance, indifference, boredom, dogged determinism, aloofness, or exaggerated prosocial behavior. Table 2.2 and table 2.3 list a range of behavior for which OC individuals are hypothesized to have been punished and rewarded.

Table 2.2. Behavior Punished by the Environment

Types of Behavior Eliciting Punishment	Relevant Examples
Making a mistake	Describing something in a vague manner
	Using an incorrect word
	Being unprepared for an exam or a meeting
	Not having an immediate answer to a question or a problem
Taking the initiative Calling attention to oneself Boasting	Trying something risky
	Taking a nap or a break
	Playing
	Being inquisitive
	Stating an unpopular or unique opinion
	Standing out in a crowd
Displaying emotion Showing vulnerability or weakness	Crying or moaning
	Getting angry
	Talking excitedly
	Dancing with abandon
	Being too direct or candid about inner feelings
	Being dependent
	Trusting someone too much
Requesting or desiring nurturance, love, or understanding	Asking for a hug
	Asking for help when injured
	Searching for romance or "true love"
	Caring about what others think

Table 2.3. Behavior Rewarded by the Environment

Types of Behavior Eliciting Rewards	Relevant Examples
Achieving great things Delaying gratification Appearing competent Making social comparisons Winning at all costs	Working or studying hard Planning, practicing, and rehearsing Saving for retirement or a rainy day Basing self-worth on how well one is doing in relation to peers Lying or cheating to achieve a goal or prevent humiliation Being right, vanquishing rivals, and never admitting defeat
Being orderly and following rules Being dutiful and diligent Making sacrifices	Approaching problems in a logical, unemotional way Never missing a deadline Always being polite and doing the right thing Taking care of others even when one is exhausted
Tolerating pain Showing persistence and perseverance Displaying self-control	Enduring a brutal training regimen at the gym Carrying on against all odds Pretending to oneself or others that all is well Always being patient Never displaying distress, overt anger, or pain
Expressing emotions or intentions indirectly	Giving someone the silent treatment Being secretive Plotting and taking revenge

In the following anecdote, an OC client describes the powerful impact of socio-biographical feedback:

> My mother always thought of herself as musically inclined, and she complained that she'd never had the opportunity to play a musical instrument when she was young. She bought me my first violin when I was five, and she arranged for a personal tutor. I had to practice for hours before I was allowed out to play.
>
> I actually got pretty good. Finally, when I was about nine, I was invited to perform a solo at a regional concert. I was really nervous, but I got a standing ovation.
>
> Afterward my mother came backstage, and I remember her being very cold. She said, "That might have been good if you hadn't been fidgeting so much."
>
> I realize now that she was trying to help me. But sometimes I wonder if her desire for me to do well somehow backfired.

Because overly controlled and emotionally constricted children are likely to be inhibited and avoid trouble, it would be reasonable to predict that caregiving adults would tend to view them as fairly well behaved, in contrast to children prone to high-intensity pleasure (high reward sensitivity), who are likely to be impulsive and behaviorally inappropriate (Rothbart, Ahadi, Hersey, & Fisher, 2001). Research has demonstrated that parents subtly reinforce (via attention) increases in children's submissive expressions of emotion over time (defined as sad-anxious expressions or mixed sad-anxious and happiness) but not disharmonious expressions (for example, anger; see Chaplin, Cole, & Zahn-Waxler, 2005). Though parental responsiveness is likely influenced by child biotemperamental predispositions (Kagan, 1994; Lewis & Weinraub, 1979), longitudinal findings suggest that parental attention to submissive emotion predicted the level of submissive expression two years later, even after controlling for the child's tendency for submissive expression at preschool age, while this did not hold for disharmonious expressions (Chaplin et al., 2005). Parents have also been shown to reward their children for inhibition of excessive fear and discourage outward expression of anxious emotion (see Kagan, Reznick, & Snidman, 1987b). With this in mind, it appears that the giving or withholding of attention by parents may subtly function to reinforce submissive or inhibited emotional expression.

The preceding findings suggest that there are multiple sociobiographical influences that can reinforce or exacerbate the development and maintenance of OC coping. For example, some OC clients report growing up in chaotic and dramatic households or settings (for example, one or both parents severely alcoholic or drug-addicted, frequent unpredictable geographical moves and changes in living conditions, frequent primary caregiver changes). It is not uncommon for OC clients to report that they undertook a caregiving role for other siblings or incapacitated parents from a young age. In addition, maladaptive OC can also develop in healthy families or similar contexts. Developmental research (Eisenberg et al., 2003) suggests that warm, positive parents may inadvertently promote overcontrolled behavior in their children (Park, Belsky, Putnam, & Crnic, 1997; Rubin, Burgess, & Hastings, 2002). Kimbrel, Nelson-Gray, and Mitchell (2007) have suggested that overprotective parents may enhance behavioral inhibition sensitivity in their children by inadvertently teaching or modeling that the world is a dangerous place to be feared. For example, a five-year-old child with heightened threat sensitivity might beg a parent to accompany him to a schoolmate's birthday party, and when the parent does so, she notices that the child appears to cope better. Yet this same behavior when the child is fourteen years old may not be seen in such a positive light, especially by the adolescent's peer group. As such, well-intentioned parents may overtly intend to communicate that life isn't scary but inadvertently signal or communicate the opposite by how they behave toward the child (for example, saying, "It is important to protect yourself"). Overprotection prevents habituation or extinction from taking place by reducing opportunities for the child to experience normal anxiety-provoking situations. Therapists are not immune to exhibiting similar overprotective behaviors. For example, a therapist who believes it is essential first to reduce anticipatory anxiety before requiring a client to attend a skills training class may inadvertently communicate that skills training is dangerous. As one OC client observed, "If this class is so safe, then why is my therapist so intent on ensuring that I am calm before I attend?"

The "Coping" Component

The end result of transactions between the "nature" and "nurture" components is hypothesized to lead to the development of an OC maladaptive coping style. Specifically, the pre-OC individual learns that if he avoids unplanned risks, masks inner feelings, hyperfocuses on minor discrepancies, and remains aloof and distant from others, he can reduce the potential of making a mistake and appearing vulnerable or out of control. Maladaptive OC coping becomes increasingly rigid over time as a function of intermittent reinforcement (for example, avoiding personal self-disclosure in conversations to occasionally reduce anticipatory anxiety; receiving occasional praise or appreciation from others for being diligent or steadfast) leading to long-term negative consequences.

Masking Inner Feelings Negatively Impacts Social Connectedness

The negative impact of inhibited or disingenuous expressions is posited to be a major contributor to commonly reported experiences of social ostracism and social isolation among OC clients. Conscious inhibition or suppression of distressing internal experiences has been consistently linked to psychopathology (Bijttebier & Vertommen, 1999; Cheavens et al., 2005; Forsyth, Parker, & Finlay, 2003; J. J. Gross & Levenson, 1997; T. R. Lynch et al., 2004; T. R. Lynch et al., 2001; Petrie, Booth, & Pennebaker, 1998; Stewart, Zvolensky, & Eifert, 2002; Wegner & Gold, 1995) as well as increases in psychophysiological responses (Wegner & Gold, 1995). Individuals with current or past depressive episodes report high use of thought suppression in an attempt to keep these negative thoughts at bay (Wenzlaff & Bates, 1998; Beevers, Wenzlaff, Hayes, & Scott, 1999; Wenzlaff, Rude, & West, 2002).

Plus, the negative impact of pervasive masking, constraining, and inhibiting emotional expression can be observed at a young age. For example, male and female preschool children involved in a longitudinal study were assessed for facial expressivity during a series of negative-mood inductions (Cole, Zahn-Waxler, Fox, Usher, & Welsh, 1996), and the children who were identified as inexpressive reported significantly more symptoms of dysthymia and anxiety approximately two and a half years later, compared to moderately expressive and highly expressive children. These self-reports were corroborated by parental data, which showed that mothers of inexpressive children reported higher frequencies of depressive episodes and depressive moods in their children, compared to mothers of moderately or highly expressive children. Developmental researchers have posited that overcontrol of emotional expression can become so habitual or biotemperamentally strengthened that inhibited or disingenuous expressions occur even when a situation is safe (Eisenberg, Fabes, Guthrie, & Reiser, 2000). The habitual nature of this risk-avoidant and inhibited style of expression has been shown to lead to social withdrawal and lower peer status (Rubin, Bukowski, & Parker, 1998). What is more, children with overcontrolling parents, a history of illness or disability, or an inhibited temperament early in life have been shown to be more prone to bullying by their peers (Gladstone, Parker, & Malhi, 2006). Correlational research has demonstrated that exposure to bullying is especially predictive of higher levels of general-state anxiety, the tendency to express anxious arousal externally when under stress, and a greater likelihood to become an anxious and depressed adult (Gladstone et al., 2006; Olweus, 1992). In fact, early peer victimization experiences may exacerbate OC behaviors associated with avoidance, risk aversion, and aloof interpersonal styles of interacting. This may stem from a vicious cycle in which victimization leads to internalizing problems, which in turn contribute to greater victimization (Dill, Vernberg, Fonagy, Twemlow, & Gamm, 2004; Vernberg, 1990). A study of children five to seven years old using peer and teacher nominations showed that victims of bullying were more submissive; had fewer leadership skills; were more withdrawn, more isolated, less cooperative, and less sociable; and frequently had no playmates (Perren & Alsaker, 2006). Victims of bullying are not only aware of their poor social standing but appear unable to change their status (Gottheil & Dubow, 2001). Escalating transactions may occur over time in which victimized children's lack of friends might render them psychologically and socially vulnerable and thus more prone to becoming easy targets. Finally, it would seem that children's reputations as victims are stable and become increasingly solidified over time; indeed, their plight appears to worsen in the late elementary school years (Biggs et al., 2010).

In a series of studies examining individual differences in emotional expression, habitual suppressors of expression reported feeling less satisfied with life, lower self-esteem, less optimism, greater negative affect, and less positive emotion compared to nonsuppressors (J. J. Gross & John, 2003). They were also less clear about what emotion they were feeling and less successful at mood repair; viewed their emotions unfavorably; and reported ruminating about aversive emotional events to a greater extent relative to individuals who did not inhibit expression. Crucially, in comparison to nonsuppressors, suppressors reported experiencing themselves as inauthentic and misleading others about their true selves. In spite of their attempts to be covert in suppression attempts, their suppressed emotion was detectable by peers, suggesting that the greater negative affect experienced by suppressors may be due to their painful awareness of their own inauthenticity. Lastly, consistent with notions that reluctance to share emotion would be linked to being uncomfortable with and actively avoiding close relationships, habitual suppressors reported substantially greater discomfort with intimacy and sharing personal feelings when relating to others (J. J. Gross & John, 2003).

Experimental research has shown that suppressing emotional expression appears to disrupt communication, interfere with relationship development, and increase physiological arousal for both the suppressor and those with whom the individual interacts (J. J. Gross & John, 2003; Butler et al., 2003). Emily Butler and her colleagues (Butler et al., 2003) examined the physiological, experiential, and social impact of expressive suppression on suppressors and their interaction partners. In each study, participants were assigned an unknown interaction partner with whom they discussed a previously viewed war film. In the first study, one member of each dyad was instructed to suppress expressive behavior, was instructed to reappraise emotional experience, or was uninstructed. Participants were instructed to discuss their reactions to the film with the interaction partner, during which time the interaction was videorecorded and physiological data were collected from both participants. Following the discussion, each participant completed several self-report measures, including ratings of emotional experience and rapport with the interaction partner. Expressive suppressors were rated as less responsive to their partners, and the interaction partners of the expressive suppressors experienced significantly greater increases in physiological arousal than did partners of reappraisers or controls, a finding that could not be accounted for by physical activity or speaking time. Accordingly, it appears that interaction with a partner engaging in expressive suppression was physiologically stressful, a finding that may be related to the lower levels of responsiveness displayed by expressive suppressors. The authors conducted a second study in which unacquainted female dyads again discussed an emotionally arousing film (Butler et al., 2003). Findings demonstrated that expressive suppressors expressed less negative emotion, expressed less positive emotion, and were less responsive than controls, which served as a manipulation check for the ability to suppress on instruction. Personal consequences for the expressive suppressors included higher levels of distraction, reduced positive emotion, and increased negative emotion about their interaction partners as well as increased blood pressure during conversation, compared to controls. Moreover, the partners of expressive suppressors reported less rapport, less liking, and less willingness to form a friendship with the interaction partner than did controls, suggesting substantial social consequences for emotion inhibition. Finally, emerging experimental research suggests the importance of context-appropriate expression; that is, successful adaptation may involve the capacity to flexibly enhance or suppress emotional expression, depending on situational demands. For instance, using a within-subjects experimental paradigm, researchers have shown that the ability to enhance or suppress emotional expression upon demand predicts positive adjustment and less distress over periods of two to three years (Bonanno, Papa, Lalande, Westphal, & Coifman, 2004; Westphal, Seivert, & Bonanno, 2010).

Critically, research suggests that people who interact with individuals who rarely or inappropriately reciprocate social cues are more likely to report decreased liking of their social partners (Cappella, 1985). Individuals conversing with a distressed partner report reduced feelings of engagement and greater desires to restrain or limit the intensity of their personal disclosure (Furr & Funder, 1998; Joiner & Metalsky, 1995). Indeed, this process could become a self-fulfilling prophecy. For example, Heerey and Kring (2007) reported that socially anxious participants, despite a desire to execute a smooth social performance, were more likely to ask fewer questions, were more likely to engage in more self-focused talk, and sought more reassurance. Thus unbalanced interactions, where one or both partners fail to match the other's expression or disclosure, appear to be experienced as less rewarding. This type of interaction pattern, common among OC individuals, would be expected to reinforce OC self-constructs suggesting that they are different, awkward, or unlovable.

Plus, scoring high on measures of alexithymia (difficulties labeling and noticing emotion) and repressive coping (underreporting emotional experience) has consistently been shown to lead to less accuracy in the detection of both pleasant and unpleasant emotions (R. D. Lane, Sechrest, Riedel, Shapiro, & Kaszniak, 2000; Parker, Taylor, & Bagby, 1993). Individuals with avoidant PD (AVPD, an OC disorder) have been found to be significantly less accurate than healthy controls in identifying fear, but not other emotions. One potential explanation for this finding is the tendency for individuals with AVPD to direct attention away from difficult emotions, such as fearful emotional faces (Rosenthal et al., 2011). Fearful faces have been found to be specifically avoided in children with social phobia, a disorder considered to be on the same continuum as AVPD (Chambless, Fydrich, & Rodebaugh, 2008), and socially phobic individuals have been shown to avoid negative faces (T. R. Lynch et al., 2015; Y. P. Chen, Ehlers, Clark, & Mansell, 2002).

The aloof and distant style of relating that characterizes OC coping may be exacerbated by difficulties perceiving emotional expressions in others or a result of pervasive masking of inner feelings. Signaling vulnerability by revealing our inner feelings to others transmits two powerful social signals:

1. We trust them; when we don't trust someone, we hide our true intentions and mask our inner feelings.

2. We are the same because we share a common bond of human fallibility.

63

True friendship may begin when we are able to share not only the positive aspects of our lives but also our secret doubts, fears, and past mistakes. Thus maladaptive OC habitual masking of inner feelings may occasionally help protect OC individuals from social disapproval yet in the long run functions to create the very problem it was developed to prevent, leading to an increasing sense of loneliness and isolation.

Low Openness and Rigid Responding Negatively Impact New Learning

Research has robustly demonstrated that individuals favor information that confirms their self-views over other reinforcers, particularly if those self-views are extreme, and the individuals become anxious or withdrawn when they cannot dismiss disconfirming feedback (Giesler, Josephs, & Swann, 1996; Pelham & Swann, 1994; Ritts & Stein, 1995; Swann, 1997; Swann, de la Ronde, & Hixon, 1994). In addition, a study examining the impact of self-views on relationship quality revealed that the partner of a person holding a negative self-view experiences disenchantment regarding the relationship and yet avoids disclosing the disdain or masks feelings of dislike with words of approval (Swann, Stein-Seroussi, & McNulty, 1992). Interestingly, the partner's disdain was detectable (via voice tone) by objective observers. However, the individual with the negative self-view left the interactions with little insight into the partner's negative appraisal. Thus an overall reluctance by interaction partners to deliver direct negative feedback, coupled with poor recognition of nonverbal cues, implies that those holding negative self-views may frequently be deprived of corrective interpersonal feedback. This could create a vicious feedback loop in which lack of honest interpersonal feedback reduces awareness of areas needing change, thereby preserving negative interpersonal exchanges and increasing possibilities for social ostracism. Lack of corrective interpersonal feedback is posited to be one of the major factors maintaining maladaptive OC.

Low openness and rigid responding have been linked to poor treatment response (Ehrlich & Bauer, 1966; Ogrodniczuk, Piper, McCallum, Joyce, & Rosie, 2002; Ogrodniczuk, Piper, Joyce, McCallum, & Rosie, 2003). For instance, rigidity has been found to predict greater symptom severity, longer hospitalization, and poorer prognosis in a psychiatric inpatient population (Ehrlich & Bauer, 1966), and those low in openness have been reported to be cognitively, affectively, and behaviorally constricted (for a review, see McCrae & Costa, 1996). Individuals scoring high on measures of rigidity have been shown to be less creative and divergent in how they think (McCrae, 1987), less likely to become absorbed in pleasurable experiences (Glisky, Tataryn, Tobias, Kihlstrom, & McConkey, 1991), and less aware of their emotions (R. D. Lane, Quinlan, Schwartz, Walker, & Zeitlin, 1990).

Rigidity is posited to be frequently expressed as maladaptive perfectionism, a trait involving excessively high performance standards and hyperconcern over making mistakes (Dunkley, Zuroff, & Blankstein, 2003). Individuals high on maladaptive perfectionism are more likely to use coping strategies such as disengagement, denial, somatization, and blaming outward (Dunkley et al., 2003), all strategies common among OC clients. Conceptually similar to Sidney Blatt's concept of self-criticism or autonomy (Dunkley et al., 2003; Powers, Zuroff, & Topciu, 2004), maladaptive perfectionism consists of themes associated with inferiority, unworthiness, failure, and guilt. Self-critical individuals are more likely to avoid intimacy, resist self-disclosure, and experience difficulties resolving conflicts (Blatt, 1974; Blatt, D'Afflitti, & Quinlan, 1976; Zuroff & Fitzpatrick, 1995). Hawley, Ho, Zuroff, and Blatt (2006), using data from the Treatment of Depression Collaborative Research Program, showed that high perfectionism predicted the subsequent rate of change in depression throughout therapy; interestingly, improvements in depression were predicated on the development of a strong therapeutic alliance (a primary treatment focus in RO DBT), which then significantly predicted reductions in maladaptive perfectionism.

Plus, individuals characterized by overcontrol are posited to possess superior capacities for distress tolerance and abilities to ignore short-term pain in order to achieve long-term goals (T. R. Lynch & Mizon, 2011). Distress tolerance refers to the ability to tolerate negative affect or aversive psychological or physical states (Bernstein, Trafton, Ilgen, & Zvolensky, 2008). Individuals characterized by undercontrolled coping (for example, BPD) have been robustly shown to exhibit poor distress tolerance, manifested by a wide range of escape or avoidance behaviors that function to minimize short-term distress yet lead to long-term negative outcomes (R. A. Brown, Lejuez, Kahler, Strong, & Zvolensky, 2005; Daughters et al., 2005; Nock & Mendes, 2008). Yet too much distress tolerance is posited to be similarly unhealthy. Distress overtolerance is defined as rigid or compulsive engagement in energy-depleting or distressing activities despite evidence suggesting that the desired goal may be unobtainable or that continued persistence may be damaging (for example, exercising despite injury, restricting food despite being underweight; see T. R. Lynch & Mizon, 2011). Thus distress overtolerance is not the same as healthy task perseverance. Plus, it is unlikely that distress overtolerance is reinforced via reductions in arousal, because it is not an escape behavior. Instead, it is more likely to be reinforced by feelings of pride linked to achieving a long-term goal or success in avoiding temptation. Distress overtolerance is posited to be a core part of OC compulsive striving and secret pride in self-control (for example, eating only one square of chocolate, never complaining when under duress, and persevering despite all odds). Unfortunately, distress overtolerance is posited not only to be exhausting but also to lead to a wide range of negative socioemotional consequences.

Finally, pervasive avoidance of unplanned risks, common among OC clients, is posited both to reduce opportunities for new learning (that is, learning something new requires taking a risk) and to make life feel stale or bland when it becomes habitual (for example, eating the same thing every day can become boring). This also means that OC individuals' risk taking is likely to be instrumental (that is, to achieve a goal, to right a wrong, to stand up for what they believe is morally correct) rather than relational (that is, quitting a job so they can live closer to a girlfriend, sharing with someone their deepest fears or doubts).

Social Signaling: A Novel Mechanism of Change

The vast majority of emotion research focuses on internal regulatory processes (see Cromwell & Panksepp, 2011, for related observations), spurred by technological advancements allowing us to peek inside the body (for example, psychophysiological measurements, brain imaging, gene mapping, neurochemical assessments). Yet a major premise of this book and its accompanying skills training manual is that we have forgotten our tribal nature. Our species' survival depended on our being able to form close social bonds, share resources, and work together with genetically unrelated individuals. RO DBT interventions are informed by a unique neurobiosocial theory linking current brain-behavioral science to the development of close social bonds and altruistic behaviors. Broadly speaking, the theory hypothesizes a core mechanism underlying RO DBT and posits (1) that OC individuals are biologically hardwired to perceive new or unfamiliar situations as dangerous rather than rewarding; (2) that their natural tendency to mask their inner feelings makes it less likely for OC clients to form close social bonds with others; and (3) that OC clients consequently suffer increasing social isolation, loneliness, and psychological distress, as posited in the following five-step sequence:

1. An OC individual's heightened biotemperamental threat sensitivity increases his vigilance for threat, thus hyperactivating his SNS-mediated defensive arousal as well as his stress-response systems, such as the hypothalamic-pituitary-adrenal (HPA) axis and fight-or-flight emotional action urges.

2. The OC individual's hyperactivated defensive arousal simultaneously triggers withdrawal of the PNS-VVC, making it more difficult for him to enter into his neurobiology-based social safety system, which is associated with feelings of contentment and social engagement.[24] In addition, the OC individual's chronic inhibition and disingenuous expression of emotion are posited to have been reinforced by early family and environmental influences that overvalued correctness and an appearance of control. The end result is that the transmitting channel he needs for effective prosocial and flexible social exchanges becomes impaired. Thus the OC individual, without his conscious awareness, may exhibit a blank facial expression and may maintain prolonged silence on the outskirts of a conversational circle, or he may scowl during a party or perhaps force a smile and behave in a stilted, overly prosocial manner that does not make sense in his immediate social context.

3. The OC individual's inhibited or disingenuous expression of emotion influences not only his transmitting functions of social communication but also his receiving functions. Specifically, withdrawal of the PNS-VVC is posited to reduce his empathic response behaviors by making him less sensitive to others' facial and vocal expressions during social interactions.[25]

4. People interacting with the OC individual become anxiously aroused and prefer not to affiliate with him.[26] Thus the OC client's biotemperamental predispositions, combined with his sociobiographical influences, are posited to bring him repeated experiences of social ostracism, rejection, and exclusion from an early age, and to simultaneously reduce his opportunities for hedonic reward or pleasure during social exchanges.[27] In short, the OC client brings his biotemperamental and sociobiographical biases with him into social interactions, where they exert a negative impact on his social signaling as well as on his reception of communications from others and thus increase his social isolation and loneliness and raise his risk for repeated episodes of depression.

> We don't feel connected because we feel safe. We feel safe because we feel connected.

5. The OC individual's repeated aversive and unrewarding social interactions function to scar him—that is, they produce a kind of "kindling effect"—and make him more likely to appraise neutral or ambiguous social stimuli as threatening, since repeated negative appraisals tend to kindle a cycle of negativity by way of the effects that heightened defensive arousal and withdrawal of the social safety system have on his social signaling and on his reception of communications from others.[28] As the cycle repeats, and as the OC individual becomes increasingly avoidant, socially helpless, isolated, and demoralized, he reacts with despair, depression, and perhaps even suicidal behavior (see figure 2.2).

Now You Know…

► In RO DBT, feeling safe, contented, or relaxed is not in itself a necessary precursor of psychological health—but belonging to a tribe may be.

► The way we feel is less important than the way in which we signal our intentions to others.

► We don't feel connected because we feel safe. We feel safe because we feel connected.

► Overcontrolled individuals are biotemperamentally predisposed to behave in ways that leave them disconnected from their tribe and put them at high risk for social isolation, loneliness, and psychological distress.

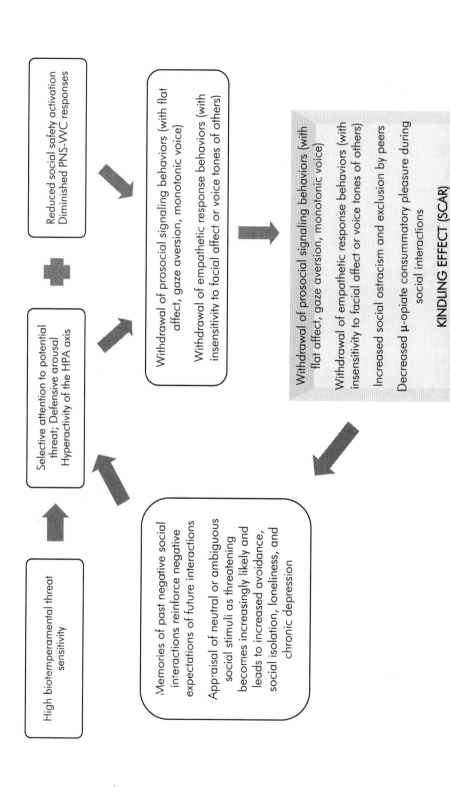

Figure 2.2. The Kindling Effect

CHAPTER 3

Assessment Strategies

This chapter is designed to provide clinicians (and researchers) an overview of assessment strategies and measures that can be used in determining the extent to which an individual matches prototypical features associated with maladaptive overcontrol. The chapter begins by briefly describing the basic tenets underlying RO DBT assessment approaches. Next comes a review of the most common assessment errors and assumptions that can make the identification of maladaptive overcontrol difficult. The RO DBT OC diagnostic protocol is then outlined, and the chapter ends with future directions and a full description of OC-specific measures and scoring guidelines.

Assessing Overcontrol: A Conceptual Framework

As noted previously, a major underlying premise of this book is that personality matters when intervening with treatment-resistant or chronic problems. Specifically, chronicity signifies the strong possibility of personality dysfunction—that is, habitual perceptual and regulatory biases that are either overcontrolled or undercontrolled in nature. Each of these superordinate personality factors, overcontrol (OC) and undercontrol (UC), is posited to consist of a number of domain-specific lower-order factors. This approach is consistent with research that has identified and described two similar superordinate personality or coping styles that have relevance for psychopathology more generally (see Clark, 2005a; Kendler, Prescott, Myers, & Neale, 2003; Krueger, 1999; Krueger, Caspi, Moffitt, & Silva, 1998; Vollebergh et al., 2001; Wright et al., 2012; Krueger & Markon, 2014):

1. Internalizing (problems of overcontrol)

2. Externalizing (problems of undercontrol)

Indeed, the DSM-5 (American Psychiatric Association, 2013, p. 13; see also National Institute of Mental Health, n.d.), in order to encourage further research into common factors, purposefully placed the section describing depressive disorders (internalizing problems) adjacent to the section describing anxiety disorders, whereas the section describing disruptive, impulse-control, and conduct disorders is adjacent to the section describing substance-related and addictive disorders (externalizing problems). Moreover, the personality domains reflected in the alternative DSM-5 model for personality disorders (see "Section III: Emerging Measures and Models," in American Psychiatric Association, 2013) have been further shown to comprise these higher-order factors (that is, externalizing and internalizing problems; see Krueger & Markon, 2014).

Yet, since RO DBT was developed for a spectrum of disorders sharing core phenotypic and genotypic features, rather than for an existing diagnostic category, we not only had to develop a treatment to address OC deficits but also had to develop a reliable and valid means for clinicians to identify maladaptive overcontrolled coping in their clients. Although aspects of the OC personality prototype have certainly been described before, in varying ways (see Haslam, 2011; Block & Block, 1980), our approach is distinct from most others in that it incorporates a wider range of potential determinants, including biotemperament, family and environmental influences, social connectedness, neuroregulatory factors, and style of self-control. Thus the RO DBT model for diagnosing maladaptive overcontrol combines dimensional models (designed to assess severity of dysfunction and biotemperament across multiple domains) with prototype models (which facilitate "low-cost" clinical decisions via assignment of a categorical diagnosis). It is founded on two core principles:

1. Clinical assessment should be guided, whenever possible, by empirical evidence.

2. Clinical assessment should serve to guide case formulation and facilitate decision making in clinical practice.

The measures and methods recommended in this chapter reflect these aims. However, before we begin this journey, it is important for clinician-assessors to be aware of the common errors and assumptions that occur when assessing problems of overcontrol.

Common Errors and Problematic Assumptions

Failure to Distinguish Private from Public Behavior

The idea of public as opposed to private behavior does not appear in any diagnostic system for mental disorders, such as the DSM-5 (American Psychiatric Association, 2013), or in any personality trait–based model of psychopathology (for a review of current models, see Krueger & Markon, 2014). Moreover, failure to account for whether a maladaptive behavior is expressed in public or in private is probably the most common factor underlying misdiagnosis of overcontrol (in my opinion). The word "public," broadly speaking, refers to any behavior expressed in the presence of another person who is not in one's immediate family (or similar social analogue), whereas the word "private" refers to any behavior expressed in a setting or situation in which we believe we are unidentifiable, anonymous, or alone. But what happens in private may be very different from what happens in public. For OC individuals, dramatic displays of emotion (such as temper tantrums and yelling, also known as *emotional leakage*) most often occur in private rather than public settings. OC individuals abhor public displays of emotion or behavior that may attract unwanted attention or criticism; they are highly capable of inhibiting an overt behavioral response in public, if they choose to do so. Indeed, assessors' failure to distinguish between public and private with respect to the setting in which a maladaptive behavior is expressed may be one of the core reasons why OC is so often misdiagnosed. Emotional leakage in public settings should be expected at least occasionally from OC individuals, especially in situations that feel anonymous (such as a political demonstration) or where strong displays of emotion are expected or socially sanctioned (such as a therapy session). Therefore, when an OC individual reports episodes of emotional leakage, it is important to explore the social signaling aspects of the behavior by determining the magnitude of the public exposure, for example, as well as its frequency, its intensity, and the extent to which an outside observer would consider the behavior abnormal or context-inappropriate (see "Assessing Emotional Leakage," page 72).

Assuming That Everything Is as It Seems

OC individuals, despite often feeling highly anxious, depressed, or distressed on the inside, work hard not to let others see it on the outside, a phenomenon strongly related to the public-versus-private issue just discussed. An OC individual is strongly motivated to create a public persona that signals competence, dutifulness, and restraint, as manifested in denial or minimization of distress, and this public persona makes it harder for another person (including an assessor) to know the true feelings or intentions of someone being assessed for a disorder of overcontrol. For example, when she says, "I was a bit disappointed," she may actually mean "I was really annoyed" or "That really hurt."

The assessor should also be prepared to broaden assessment questions if it appears that the individual is minimizing or is overly concerned about answering questions correctly or exactly. For example, if the person starts by saying, "I just want to answer this correctly," the assessor might reply, "I know this can feel important and tricky. But, really, there is no right or wrong answer. What's important is for you to tell me how you feel." Similarly, some OC individuals are so self-critical that they may repeatedly seek affirmation from an assessor that their problems are real or significant. The assessor should be alert for opportunities to validate the difficulty of reported problems when assessing potential OC clients, since doing so makes it more likely for these individuals to reveal their feelings.

Assessing Emotional Leakage

The following questions are designed to help assessors distinguish between public and private with respect to dramatic displays of emotion and other problematic behavior:

1. In what types of settings or situations does this problem behavior most often occur? For example, does it occur only when you are alone? Only when you are around immediate family members? Only in situations where you are certain of anonymity or of being unidentifiable?

   • Has this behavior ever occurred in public? If so, was it clearly observable to those present? How many people were present?

   • Can you show me, right now, what you actually did or said? What evidence do you have that others noticed?[a]

   • Does this type of public exposure of the behavior occur frequently? If so, how often?

2. To what extent do you strive to keep this behavior secret?

   • To what extent do you plan ahead or make preparations prior to engaging in this behavior, in order to ensure anonymity?

   • Are you careful to engage in this behavior only in situations or circumstances in which, if you were ever observed, you could plausibly deny the behavior?

   • Have you strived to inhibit the expression of the problem behavior in public but repeatedly failed to prevent it, despite good intentions on your part?[b]

Moreover, the assessor should be aware that many OC individuals in general, including OC clients, desire to please their assessors (or their therapists) and thus try to provide the answers they imagine their assessors or therapists want to hear. They also may feel a sense of moral obligation to report every possible difficulty they have ever experienced. For example, one OC individual who was asked about impulsivity reported that she was overly talkative and tactless, bought clothes she didn't need, and had impulsive bouts of drinking and smoking marijuana. However, upon further examination, she turned out to have smoked marijuana only once, and her supposed drunkenness had been limited to a few instances of mild intoxication when she was a university student. Furthermore, her talkative and tactless behavior had never been extreme; her description of it was a reflection of harsh self-criticism for any form of excited expression in public.

In addition, the assessor should expect OC individuals to respond to questions about their *emotional experience* with statements that reflect nonemotional *thoughts* about their *behavior*. For example, one woman, queried about her mood, said, "Do I

- How many people know about this problem behavior? Does anyone outside your immediate family know about this problem behavior?

- To what extent would the behavior in which you engaged be considered public knowledge? Would people who know you (outside your immediate family) be surprised or taken aback if they were to hear about you behaving in this way?

- How often have you discussed this problem behavior with another person? Who with? What type of relationship does this person have with you? Have you ever just randomly told someone you did not know, such as someone you'd just met on the bus or a casual acquaintance, about your problem behavior?[c]

- How often has this behavior required immediate medical or psychological intervention from outside agencies, such as a hospital emergency room, a crisis center, a police department, or other governmental agencies?[d]

[a] Often what an OC individual reports as loud or embarrassing behavior would not be considered so by other people.

[b] This would suggest undercontrolled behavior.

[c] OC individuals in general avoid talking about problems with other people, the primary exceptions being therapists, doctors, and immediate family members. They are unlikely to spontaneously reveal secrets or problems to people they have just met or do not know well.

[d] Most OC individuals are less likely to display crisis behavior that necessitates immediate outside intervention. Instead, when they need help, they are more likely to carefully plan their help-seeking behavior.

feel down or low? Well, I try to get past my depression, really. Try to get ahead of it. I get up earlier than I would like and get started with breakfast. Then I don't feel so down." In this instance, the individual did not directly answer the question; instead, she reported her thoughts about her low mood and her attempts to regulate or control it. In this situation, the assessor should redirect the client to the original question, all the while communicating that it is acceptable to feel down or depressed (in other words, that it's not wrong or socially undesirable to accurately report one's mood).

It is common for OC individuals to report mood changes or labile moods. After further examination, however, these are often found to be changes from a very low to a moderately low mood and not necessarily from a low to a high mood, or from a low to a normal mood. OC clients rarely experience highly positive mood states. Therefore, the assessor should ask potential OC clients to compare their current moods to their moods during periods when they felt more "normal," and to their moods during periods when they felt some joy. If they can't remember such periods, the assessor should ask them to imagine someone they know who seems to have normal moods (in terms of both sadness and happiness) and to use this person as a basis of comparison for how they think they are doing.

The assessor should avoid basing a diagnostic decision solely on the individual's verbal descriptions of his behavior. Obtaining additional information from family members or others who know the individual can be highly useful. Whenever possible, the assessor should ask the individual to demonstrate or show what his self-reported behavior actually looked like. For instance, one man reported explosive bouts of intense anger with his colleagues at work, and he described this behavior as "rages." When the assessor asked him to demonstrate what a rage looks like, he sat straight up in his chair, adopted a flat expression, and stated calmly, in a clipped tone, "I don't like what you are doing." In this case, the individual's use of the word "rage" was intended to accurately describe how he had behaved; without the demonstration, however, it is likely that the assessor would have been left with an entirely different impression. Thus it is important for the assessor not to assume that he and the person he is assessing speak the same emotional language. When an individual describes his behavior as highly dramatic, explosive, impulsive, risky, or outrageous, the behavior may not always match his words, and so, again, the assessor should try to get a demonstration of what the individual actually said or did.

It is important as well for the assessor to recognize that the therapeutic environment is a unique type of social setting, one that comes with its own set of rules, values, norms, and expectations regarding behavior. For example, an expression of extreme emotion during a therapy session (or a diagnostic assessment) is considered appropriate, whereas the same behavior would be frowned on if it were displayed on a bus. Thus an individual who is being assessed for a disorder of overcontrol may express extreme emotion (such as crying or suicidal ideation) during an assessment or therapy session but may rarely express similar emotions or sentiments outside the therapeutic context or outside his or her immediate family. Previous encounters with health care providers may also have reinforced such relevant maladaptive social signaling as hanging the head, covering the face, or displaying strong anger (some of these behaviors may be "pushback" or "don't hurt me" responses, as described in chapter 10).

Assuming That Self-Injury Is Always Impulsive

One of the most common assessment errors we have observed over the years pertains to clinical lore concerning nonsuicidal self-injurious (NSSI) behavior. Self-injury is commonly assumed to occur exclusively among individuals characterized by low self-control and high impulsive mood-dependent behavior, as in borderline personality disorder. However, growing empirical research suggests otherwise. Several studies have shown that intentional self-injury is a complex behavior serving a range of functions—most often regulation of negative affect and self-punishment—and should not be viewed solely as mood-dependent, impulsive, or attention- or sensation-seeking behavior (Klonsky, 2007; Nock, 2009). Indeed, self-harm is markedly frequent in disorders typifying overcontrol, such as dysthymia, depression, anorexia nervosa, and Cluster A personality disorders (Claes, Klonsky, Muehlenkamp, Kuppens, & Vandereycken, 2010; Ghaziuddin, Tsai, & Ghaziuddin, 1991; Hintikka et al., 2009; Klonsky, Oltmanns, & Turkheimer, 2003; Nock, Joiner, Gordon, Lloyd-Richardson, & Prinstein, 2006; Selby, Bender, Gordon, Nock, & Joiner, 2012). OC self-injurious behavior is typified by planning well in advance of the self-harming behavior. It occurs almost exclusively in private, and it rarely requires medical attention. In general, OC self-injury can be distinguished by its relatively non-mood-dependent, premeditated, private nature, meaning that OC self-injury is less likely to be motivated by a desire for attention.

Assuming That Everything Important Is Emotional

It is important for the assessor not to assume that all problematic behaviors are necessarily mood-dependent, or that they always represent some form of escape or avoidance coping. As discussed in chapter 1, OC individuals are more likely to engage in excessive approach coping than in excessive avoidance coping. Their brains are hardwired to ignore short-term pain for the sake of achieving long-term gain. For example, an OC individual is unlikely to put off an important task simply because it elicits discomfort, and he is more likely to work obsessively on completing the task even when it's clear that he would be better off resting or avoiding the task altogether. An important point to remember in assessing an individual for overcontrol is that a great deal of OC behavior may stem from rule-governed and sensory receptor processes that are relatively emotion-free.

> A great deal of OC behavior may stem from rule-governed and sensory receptor processes that are relatively emotion-free.

Judging a Book by Its Cover and Assuming All Risks Are the Same

Despite their pervasively overcontrolled style of coping, many OC individuals describe themselves as rebels or adopt an eccentric style of dress or manner of behaving that appears superficially unconventional, dramatic, or liberated. For example, they may hold passionate and unconventional political or philosophical views, may have tattoos or piercings, and may dismiss the need to follow societal rules. Nevertheless, despite the apparently undercontrolled nature of these social signals, an OC "rebel" can be differentiated by the extent to which planning is involved in her rebellious activities (as in a rehearsed speech or a scheduled protest) and also by the extent to which such activities depend on following rules, holding rigidly dogmatic views, or adhering blindly to an ideology.

For an OC individual, the need to appear competent and in control is pervasive and stable; it is not dependent on mood, state, or context. In contrast, the undercontrolled individual, such as the individual with borderline personality disorder, is *apparently* competent, meaning that his or her "impulse control in the therapist's office may not generalize to settings outside" (Linehan, 1993a, p. 81). The core difference lies in the *variability* of competence and self-control; that is, the undercontrolled individual is incapable of maintaining competent behavior and self-control over long periods of time, whereas the OC individual is biotemperamentally predisposed to be highly constrained and is intermittently reinforced to be self-controlled, regardless of how distressing a situation may seem. Therefore, when assessing a potential OC client, it is important to determine the extent to which a reported risky, rebellious, or impulsive behavior occurred spontaneously and without much forethought as opposed to having been planned and rehearsed in advance (skydiving, for example, is a carefully planned risk). Indeed, many OC individuals revel in their risk-taking abilities, quite rightly, and yet further analysis shows that the types of risks they tend to report have almost always involved some form of premeditation. In addition, OC risk-taking behavior, rather than being motivated by the desire to avoid distress or conflict, is often motivated by a desire to control or dominate resources or to gain power

> Risk-taking behavior in OC individuals tends to be instrumental rather than relational—it's about nailing something down rather than opening themselves up.

or status over others in order to achieve a long-term personal goal (as when the CEO of a company takes the risk of buying out a competitor). Thus OC individuals are also more likely to report taking risks that involve striving and winning as opposed to risks that involve the disclosure of genuine feelings or doubts in order to foster intimacy. In general, as explained in chapter 2, risk-taking behavior in OC individuals tends to be instrumental rather than relational—it's about nailing something down rather than opening themselves up.

The OC Diagnostic Protocol: Diagnosing Overcontrol, Step-by-Step

The diagnostic protocol for OC, organized into three sequential steps, is designed for easy integration into clinical practice. As mentioned earlier, it combines dimensional models with prototype models. Our approach shares features with the polythetic system used in the DSM-5 for assessing personality disorder (American Psychiatric Association, 2013). For example, according to the DSM-5, a client must meet five out of nine possible symptomatic criteria in order to be diagnosed with borderline personality disorder, an assessment approach whereby many combinations of symptoms lead to the same categorical label or diagnosis, and all nine criteria need not be met.

Similarly, the approach outlined in this section of the chapter is designed for the assessor to identify OC clients on the basis of various combinations of "symptoms," or behaviors, that surpass a cutoff point at which the OC diagnosis is considered clinically meaningful. This is important to keep in mind because a person can still be diagnosed as OC without meeting all the criteria; there are many combinations of behaviors or symptoms that can add up to a diagnosis of OC. Our approach, similar to the alternative DSM-5 model for personality disorders (see "Section III: Emerging Measures and Models," in American Psychiatric Association, 2013), also allows for empirically derived severity ratings on trait measures, an integral aspect of the assessment. It is important to remember, however, that there is no perfect assessment tool for any type of disorder.

Step 1

In step 1 of the OC diagnostic protocol, the potential OC client completes three short self-report measures that take approximately fifteen minutes to complete and can be part of a battery of self-report measures (involving, for example, demographics, ratings of distress, and measures of occupational or interpersonal functioning) that clients are routinely asked to complete prior to the first meeting with a therapist (for interested clinicians and researchers, our research team has also created a supplemental list of OC measures, which includes measures of both hypothesized mechanisms and outcomes):

1. Assessing Styles of Coping: Word-Pair Checklist (see appendix 1 for a copy of this measure and its scoring instructions)

2. Personal Need for Structure measure

3. Acceptance and Action Questionnaire–II

Assessing Styles of Coping: Word-Pair Checklist (ASC-WP)

The ASC-WP self-report measure uses paired words and phrases derived from research examining terms descriptive of personality (see Ashton, Lee, & Goldberg, 2004; Goldberg & Kilkowski, 1985). The ASC-WP should not be considered a measure of psychopathology but rather a measure of the extent to which a person leans toward an overcontrolled or undercontrolled personality style and style of coping. Someone can be content with her life and yet score extremely high on either overcontrol or undercontrol; therefore, the ASC-WP can be used in nonclinical settings.

For each set of paired words or phrases, the person completing the ASC-WP places a checkmark in the box next to the one that better describes him, and each pair on the completed measure should have only one of the boxes checked. This forced-choice approach is designed to mitigate the faking of supposedly good or socially desirable responding (it can be helpful to explain beforehand that there is no right answer or better style of behaving). It is also important to tell individuals completing the ASC-WP that they should base their choices on how they are right now, not on how they would like to be (that is, the choice of a word or phrase should reflect the individual's actual self, not an idealized or desired self). If someone has difficulty knowing whether a particular word or phrase describes him, ask him whether the other word or phrase in the pair would be a better fit. Some individuals also find it useful to consider how friends, peers, colleagues, or family members might see them in terms of a particular pair of words or phrases, especially when they are finding it difficult to make that assessment themselves.

Top Ten Prototypical Features of Overcontrolled Individuals

The following list of prototypical OC features can be used to guide clinical interviews as well as treatment planning:

1. Mood-independent action; high tolerance for distress; high capacity for perseverance; superior ability to delay gratification

2. High sense of social obligation and dutifulness; willingness to make sacrifices to care for others or do what is regarded as the right thing

3. Compulsive rehearsal, premeditation, and planning

4. Seriousness; unexcitability; constrained emotional expression; tendency not to be easily impressed

5. Focus on performance; frequent engagement in social comparisons; secret competitiveness

6. Aloof and distant manner; slowness to warm up; possible feeling of being different from others or detached from others; low social connectedness

7. Self-injurious behavior that tends to be planned well in advance, to occur in private, and to rarely require immediate medical attention

8. Superior capacity for detail-focused processing; high degree of moral certitude; belief that there is a right and a wrong way to do things

9. Positive mood states linked to sense of accomplishment (as in resisting temptation, detecting errors, or dominating circumstances)

10. Dislike of the limelight; great effort to avoid unplanned and unrehearsed public displays of emotion; outbursts of anger and displays of dysregulated emotion in private or among very familiar others

At the time of this writing, there is no cutoff score for determining whether a person leans more toward an overcontrolled or an undercontrolled style of coping. Instead, the ASC-WP should be seen as an opportunity for individual exploration of personality style. Most of the individuals who become OC clients will check the boxes next to words and phrases describing OC characteristics, and so clinicians will find interpretation of these individuals' ASC-WP scores straightforward.

The ASC-WP can also sometimes be used to generate discussion when a particular client appears to be struggling with knowing his style. However, most often this is not necessary—in our experience, most of the individuals who become OC clients easily identify themselves as overcontrolled (see "Enhancing Client Engagement via Orientation and Commitment," chapter 5).

Personal Need for Structure (PNS) Measure

The eleven-item PNS measure consists of two subscales, "Desire for Structure" and "Response to Lack of Structure," both reflecting core OC traits. Questions are answered via a Likert scale ranging from 1 ("strongly disagree") to 6 ("strongly agree").

The psychometric properties of the PNS measure have been shown to be excellent, and a free copy is provided by its authors (see Neuberg & Newsom, 1993); scoring instructions are also provided, with "high PNS" defined as an average score of 3.5 or higher. Individuals scoring high on the PNS measure have been shown to have several characteristics associated with overcontrolled coping:

- Less likelihood of changing beliefs in the face of new information (low openness)

- Greater likelihood of stereotyping

- Preference for structured rather than unstructured social events

- High focus on performance

In addition, a rigid desire for structure, as determined by the PNS measure, has been shown to improve as a function of RO DBT skills training (see Keogh et al., 2016).

Acceptance and Action Questionnaire–II (AAQ-II)

The AAQ-II (F. W. Bond et al., 2011) is a seven-item scale measuring psychological inflexibilty. Questions are answered via a Likert scale ranging from 1 ("never true") to 7 ("always true"). An AAQ-II score higher than 24 indicates the presence of maladaptive and inflexible coping and comorbid psychological distress.

The AAQ-II has been shown to have excellent psychometric properties in a range of differing samples. Higher levels of psychological inflexibility, as measured by the AAQ-II, are related to greater levels of depression, anxiety, and overall psychological distress and predict future maladaptive functioning.

Step 2

In step 2 of the OC diagnostic protocol, the clinical assessor (or therapist) conducts a structured or semistructured diagnostic interview—a standard clinical practice. In the event that an unstructured format is employed, the assessor should be attentive to statements suggesting the presence of an overcontrolled style of coping. For example, if an individual reports obsessive behaviors, the assessor should follow up with questions informed by the diagnostic criteria for obsessive-compulsive disorder and obsessive-compulsive personality disorder to ascertain whether either of these disorders is present. The following questions can facilitate this process:

- Do you believe it is important to do things properly or in the right way?

- Are you a perfectionist?

- Are you cautious and careful about how you do things?

- Do you prefer order and structure? Are you organized?

- Do you like to plan ahead? Do you think before acting?

- Are you able to delay gratification? Are you able to easily inhibit an impulse?

- Do you consider yourself conscientious? Are you dutiful?

- Are you quiet, restrained, or reserved by nature?

- Is it hard to impress you?

- Does it take time to get to know you?

- Are you likely not to reveal your opinion immediately but wait until you get to know someone better?

If the interview is structured, then the assessor can use such measures as the Structured Clinical Interview for DSM-5 (First, Williams, Karg, & Spitzer, 2015), the Structured Clinical Interview for DSM-IV Axis II Personality Disorders (First, Gibbon, Spitzer, Williams, & Benjamin, 1997), and the International Personality Disorder Examination (Loranger, Janca, & Sartorius, 1997). OC Axis II personality disorders are subsumed under DSM Cluster A (paranoid, schizoid, and schizotypal) personality disorders and Cluster C (obsessive-compulsive, avoidant, and possibly dependent) personality disorders. Core shared features among OC personality disorders are as follows:

- Strong desires to control one's environment

- Reserved emotional expression

- Limited social interactions and aloof or distant interactions

- Cognitive and behavioral rigidity

OC Axis I disorders in DSM-5 are represented by autism spectrum disorders, anorexia nervosa, treatment-resistant anxiety disorders (for example, generalized anxiety disorder not responding to treatment), chronic or treatment-resistant depressive disorders (for example, persistent depressive disorder or dysthymia not responding to treatment), chronic forms of rumination disorder, social anxiety disorder or social phobia, and somatic symptom disorder. Maladaptive overcontrol may also underlie disorders in adolescence that show poor adherence to standard treatment protocols, especially when they have very early onset (for example, early-onset obsessive-compulsive disorder, especially with tics, and early-onset somatoform disorders).

Step 2 of the diagnostic protocol is optional. It is included here because it is standard practice in most clinics and provides additional information that may aid the assessment process. It is important to emphasize, however, that OC can be reliably diagnosed without this step.

Step 3

Step 3 of the diagnostic protocol takes approximately seven minutes and occurs after the clinical interview has been completed and the potential OC client has left the room where the assessment took place. At this point, the clinician completes two measures:

1. The Clinician-Rated OC Trait Rating Scale, forms 3.1 and 3.2 (see appendix 2)

2. The Overcontrolled Global Prototype Rating Scale, forms 3.3 and 3.4 (see appendix 3)

The Clinician-Rated OC Trait Rating Scale (OC-TS), Forms 3.1 and 3.2

The OC-TS uses a seven-point global trait rating scale to assess eight personality traits that provide an estimate of "caseness," or the extent to which an individual is a close match for each of the eight OC traits. Form 3.1 provides scoring instructions and descriptions of the eight core OC traits, and form 3.2 provides a copy of the measure itself. A score of 6 or 7 denotes "caseness" for a particular trait, and a total score of 40 or higher on the instrument as a whole reflects greater global OC behavior. Research examining the psychometric properties of this scale is currently in progress. The scale can also be used also as an adjunct for purposes of treatment planning.

The Overcontrolled Global Prototype Rating Scale (OC-PRS), Forms 3.3 and 3.4

The OC-PRS is informed by prototype models of personality assessment (see Westen, DeFife, Bradley, & Hilsenroth, 2010). It was developed and based in part on person-centered approaches that focus on the configuration of personality traits within an individual (Chapman & Goldberg, 2011; Goldberg, 1993; McCrae & Costa, 1997; Westen et al., 2010; Asendorpf, 2006) and measurement templates developed by Drew Westen and his colleagues (Westen et al., 2010). The OC-PRS addresses the four core OC deficits discussed at length in chapter 1:

1. Deficits in deficits in receptivity and openness

2. Deficits in flexible responding

3. Deficits in emotional awareness and emotional expression

4. Deficits in forming intimate interpersonal relationships

The assessor who completes form 3.3 of the OC-PRS uses a 5-point key to rate the overall similarity between a potential OC client and each of eight OC prototypical descriptive paragraphs. As noted by Westen et al. (2010, p. 483), "For purposes of communication, ratings of 4 or 5 denote a categorical diagnosis ('caseness'), and a rating of 3 translates to 'features' or subthreshold." The idea is for the assessor to evaluate the potential OC client in terms of each descriptive paragraph as a whole instead of counting individual symptoms. This format has been shown to provide rich diagnostic data, and it avoids problems associated with memorized lists of symptoms and with arbitrary or variable cutoffs across disorders (Westen et al., 2010). The assessor checks the relevant box under each of the descriptive paragraphs and adds up the numbers; a total score of 17 or higher indicates OC. With practice, the instrument can be completed in five or six minutes, and it can be repeated over the course of treatment to monitor clinical improvement.

For an individual with an overall score of 17 or higher on form 3.3 of the OC-PRS, the assessor can use form 3.4 to determine whether the individual, now prototyped as OC, meets the criteria for two OC social signaling subtypes, the *overly disagreeable* subtype and the *overly agreeable* subtype, which differ primarily in terms of how the OC individual wants to be perceived by others—that is, form 3.4 addresses the OC individual's public persona. The scoring instructions are similar to those for form 3.3. Identifying a client's OC subtype can be highly useful in treatment planning and targeting. For example, OC individuals whose traits are a match with the overly agreeable subtype need to learn how to express anger directly instead of keeping it bottled up; by contrast, those whose traits are a match with the overly disagreeable subtype need to learn how to reveal their vulnerability to others instead of compulsively pretending to be unfazed or strong. For more about these two subtypes and effective treatment strategies regarding them, see chapter 9.

Future Directions

Obviously, one challenge our team encountered as we developed RO DBT for disorders of overcontrol was that there was a vast literature examining overcontrolled coping and similar constructs, but a comprehensive measure of overcontrolled coping that included all the elements in our model had yet to be developed. As such, our research team, in collaboration with like-minded colleagues (such as Lee Anna Clark), initiated a separate line of research aimed at developing and validating several new measures that captured how we conceptualized maladaptive overcontrol. For example, research examining the utility of a new self-report screening questionnaire for overcontrol is in progress, as is work on measures examining hypothesized mechanisms of change.

In addition, one new and exciting area of research pertains to the development of reliable and valid nonverbal coding schemes for evaluating the extent to which an individual naturally engages in prosocial signaling behaviors during interactions with others (for example, by smiling frequently, offering eyebrow wags, and using a warm tone of voice). It is hoped that such coding schemes can be used to augment diagnostic assessments as well as to assess hypothesized mechanisms of change linked to improved social signaling. To this end, our research team developed the Nonverbal Social Engagement Coding Scheme (Greville-Harris, Hempel, Karl, Dieppe, & Lynch, 2016), which is used to code eight nonverbal behaviors (eye gaze, smiling, frowning, laughing, and four differing patterns of head movements). Modifications of this instrument are in progress in our lab and include improved methods of coding RO-specific nonverbal prosocial behaviors taught in treatment.

Now You Know…

- ► Overcontrol is a multidimensional personality construct that can be assessed reliably in clinical settings and used as a basis for guiding treatment decisions.

- ► Traits associated with disorders of overcontrol are sometimes taken as evidence of other disorders, including disorders of undercontrol, because of assessors' errors and assumptions.

- ► A three-step protocol for diagnosing overcontrol is available. It combines dimensional models with prototype models, and it uses potential OC clients' self-report measures along with diagnostic interviewing and postinterview measures completed by an assessor.

CHAPTER 4

Overview of Therapy Assumptions, Structure, and Targets

After a client has been assessed with the protocol described in chapter 3, and after it has been determined that the client meets the criteria for maladaptive overcontrol, the next step is to initiate treatment. This chapter offers a brief overview of the therapeutic assumptions, structural components, and treatment targets used in RO DBT for disorders of overcontrol. The chapter begins by briefly describing the basic tenets underlying the RO DBT therapeutic stance and then outlines the core assumptions guiding treatment and provides an overview of the treatment structure. Specific strategies, protocols, or skills that are briefly touched on in this chapter are covered in detail in later chapters. It is important to note that the chapter focuses primarily on RO DBT outpatient treatment, but this should not be considered the only means of treatment delivery (for example, the evidence base supports both RO DBT for treatment of adult inpatients with anorexia nervosa and the use of RO skills training alone; see chapter 1).

Individuals who are able to delay gratification, make plans, persist in onerous activities to achieve long-term goals, and behave conscientiously are highly valued in most communities. They are the doers, the savers, the planners, and the fixers—the people you see working late at night and then rising early to ensure that things work properly. They strive for moderation in all aspects of their lives, and they are able to put money aside for their retirement in order to avoid being a burden on others. The therapeutic stance taken in RO DBT cannot be separated from these underlying, fundamentally prosocial features of self-control—indeed, overcontrol is posited to be prosocial at its core (see table 4.1)—and yet, as we've seen, OC individuals' greatest strength also turns out to be their greatest weakness. They feel exhausted by their habitual self-control but helpless to stop it.

Table 4.1. Overcontrol Is Fundamentally Prosocial

OC Characteristic	Prosocial Attribute
Ability to delay gratification	Enables resources to be saved for times of less abundance
Desire to be correct, exceed expectations, and perform well	Essential to communities' ability to thrive and grow
Valuing of duty, obligation, and self-sacrifice	Helps societies flourish and ensures that people in need are cared for
Valuing of rules and fairness	Helps societies remain balanced and enables resistance to powerful but unethical individuals or harmful societal pressures
Detail-focused processing and quick pattern recognition	Increases precision and thus the likelihood that problems will be detected and solved so that everything functions properly

RO DBT recognizes the prosocial nature of overcontrol by adopting a therapeutic stance that simultaneously acknowledges the client's sense of separation or difference from others. Despite desiring social connectedness, OC clients inwardly experience themselves as outsiders and are often clueless about how to join with others or form intimate relationships (although they are unlikely to tell anyone about this). They feel like strangers in a strange land, often even when around their family members, always watching but rarely ever fully participating. To help correct this, the role of the RO DBT therapist may be best described as that of a *tribal ambassador*—that is, someone who is able to appreciate the unique self-sacrifices OC individuals make to meet or exceed community expectations and perform well, and who warmly welcomes them back into the tribe.

RO DBT Core Assumptions

The metaphor of the therapist as tribal ambassador is designed to provide therapists a visceral sense of their fundamental role and goal in work with OC clients. It also serves as the basis of the core treatment assumptions in RO DBT:

- Psychological well-being involves the confluence of three factors: receptivity, flexibility, and social connectedness.

- RO DBT highlights our tribal nature. It prioritizes social connectedness as essential to individual well-being and species survival.

- Social signaling matters. Deficits (not excesses) in prosocial signaling are the core problem in disorders of overcontrol and are posited to be the source of OC clients' loneliness.

- Radical openness assumes that we don't see things as they are but rather as we are.

- Radical openness involves a willingness to question ourselves when we're challenged by asking ourselves. *What is it that I might need to learn?*

- RO DBT therapists practice radical openness and self-enquiry themselves, since RO is not something that can be grasped solely via intellectual means.

- RO DBT therapists model humility by taking responsibility for their perceptions and actions in a manner that avoids harsh blame of themselves, others, or the world, and they do this in order to encourage their OC clients to adopt a similar practice.

- RO DBT encourages clients to celebrate problems as opportunities for growth instead of seeing problems as obstacles.

- RO DBT therapists recognize the arrogance of assuming that they can ever fully understand their clients, but they continue striving to understand.

- RO DBT therapists recognize that the lives of their OC clients are often miserable, even though their clients' suffering isn't always evident.

- RO DBT therapists recognize that OC clients take life very seriously and that they need to learn how to chill out, laugh at their own foibles, and play.

> RO DBT encourages clients to celebrate problems as opportunities for growth instead of seeing problems as obstacles.

- RO DBT therapists believe in silliness. They recognize that OC clients will not believe it is socially acceptable for someone to openly play, relax, or disinhibit unless they see their therapists model such behavior.

- RO DBT therapists recognize that even though they may not have been the sole cause of an alliance rupture, they are still responsible for repairing it.

- RO DBT therapists, rather than telling their clients what is "wrong," encourage them to discover for themselves what ails them via regular practices of self-enquiry.

- RO DBT therapists encourage OC clients to actively engage in resolving an interpersonal conflict instead of automatically avoiding a situation or abandoning a relationship.

- In their work with OC clients, RO DBT therapists look for opportunities to reinforce candid disclosure and uninhibited expression of emotion.

- RO DBT therapists may be easygoing, but they are not necessarily calm. They recognize the value of equanimity but also the value of passionate participation in life.

It is important to understand that treatment assumptions are not truths. They help guide behavior, but if they're held too tightly, they can interfere with new learning.

Overview of Treatment Structure and Targets

The RO DBT outpatient treatment protocol consists of weekly one-hour individual therapy sessions and concurrent weekly RO skills training classes, with individual therapy and skills training taking place over a period of approximately thirty weeks. Clients normally start skills training during the third week of individual RO DBT.

Telephone consultation with therapists outside normal working hours is encouraged on an as-needed basis. Although this optional resource is not often used by OC clients, it has proved invaluable in creating a sense of connection with socially isolated or distant OC clients. Consultation by phone also provides important opportunities for aloof OC clients to practice asking for help and celebrating their successes.[29]

If a client needs extra help (to reach a desired goal, for example, or to manage the termination of a relationship), or if the therapist and the client agree that it would be beneficial to continue therapy, then they can schedule additional sessions of individual therapy, and particular lessons within the RO skills training module can be repeated. For more information about RO skills training, see the skills training manual, which includes the material needed for each of the thirty lessons along with notes for instructors and a variety of user-friendly handouts and worksheets keyed to each of the thirty lessons.

It is strongly recommended that any treatment program for OC clients include a means of supervision for therapists and, ideally, a supportive environment where therapists can practice RO skills together.[30] The best consultation arrangement would probably include a weekly team meeting, and so therapists without teams are encouraged to find a means of re-creating the function of an RO consultation team (a virtual team, for example, or outside supervision).[31]

Orientation and Commitment

In RO DBT, the stage of orientation and commitment takes up to four sessions and includes four key components:

1. Confirming the client's identification of overcontrol as the core problem

2. Obtaining a commitment from the client to discuss, in therapy sessions, any desire to drop out of treatment before dropping out

3. Orienting the client to the RO DBT neurobiosocial theory of overcontrol

4. Orienting the client to the RO DBT key mechanism of change, whereby open expression leads to increased trust, which in turn leads to social connectedness

A major aim of orientation and commitment is the therapist's and the client's collaborative identification of the social signaling deficits and related factors that are blocking the client from living according to his values and keeping him from actualizing his valued goals. Often this process also requires helping the client identify his values and goals, which then serve to guide treatment throughout the duration of therapy. Here, the term *value* denotes a principle or a standard, which a person considers important in life, and which guides behavior, whereas the term *goal* denotes some means by which that value is realized. For example, a person who holds passion as a value may realize this value by achieving the goal of forming a romantic partnership; another, who holds close family ties as a value, may realize this value by being a warm and helpful parent; still another, who holds financial independence and rewarding work as values, may realize these values by becoming gainfully and happily employed.

Hierarchy of Treatment Targets in Individual Therapy

The primary treatment targets in RO DBT are to decrease the client's OC social signaling deficits (posited to exacerbate the client's emotional loneliness) and to increase the client's openness, flexibility, and social connectedness so that the client can create a life worth sharing (see "Radically Open Living: Developing a Life Worth Sharing," chapter 9). RO DBT arranges the treatment targets of individual therapy according to the following hierarchy of importance (see figure 4.1):

1. Reducing life-threatening behaviors

2. Repairing alliance ruptures

3. Addressing social signaling deficits linked to common OC behavioral patterns or themes

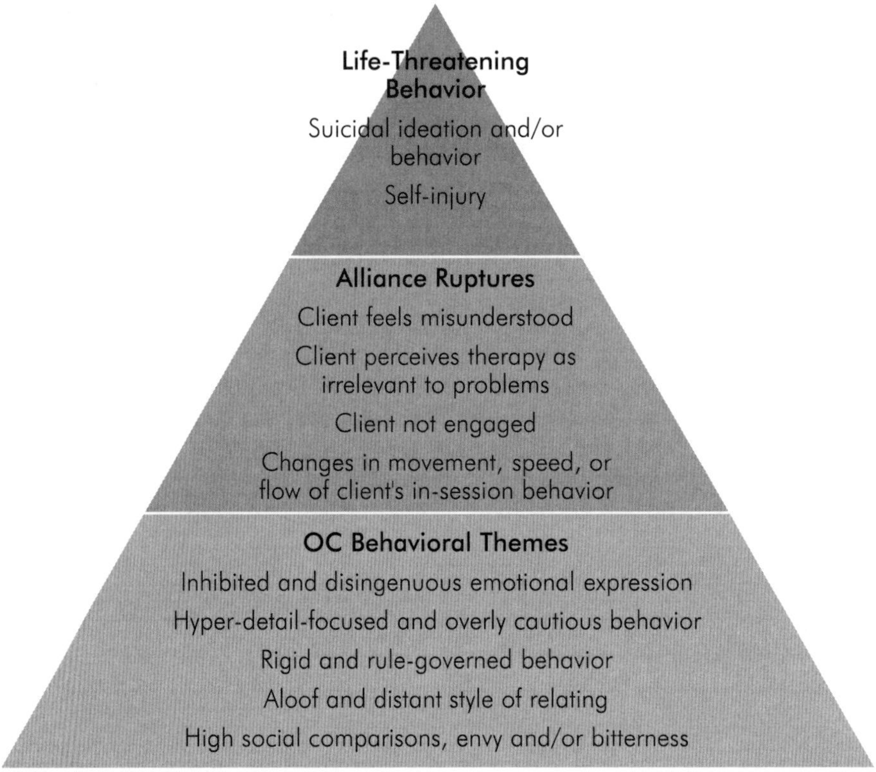

Figure 4.1. Individual Treatment Target Hierarchy for Disorders of Overcontrol

Reducing the Client's Life-Threatening Behaviors

The first priority in treating disorders of overcontrol is to bring about a reduction in the client's imminent life-threatening behaviors (if present), defined as follows:

- Engaging in intentional self-harm and suicidal actions, such as cutting, burning, and overdosing

- Exhibiting a sudden increase in suicidal ideation, urges, or plans aimed at intentionally caused tissue damage or death[32]

- Engaging in behaviors that are not aimed at intentionally caused tissue damage or death but that do constitute an imminent threat to life

For example, if a client maintains a condition of being severely underweight, eats restrictively, or purges, her behavior is seen as symptomatic of OC maladaptive responding *until the moment a physician declares the behavior to be imminently life-threatening.* It is at this point that the behavior also comes to be seen as life-threatening in RO DBT (even if the client's goal is not tissue damage or death), and reducing this behavior now trumps all other treatment targets. The key word here is "imminent."

This approach provides a coherent rationale for the therapist to avoid expressions of overconcern about medical risk when doing so might inadvertently reinforce dysfunctional behavior. For instance, the therapist's heightened concern about a low body weight might unintentionally reinforce a client's restrictive eating by conferring a special status on the client that excuses her from normal expectations or responsibilities (T. R. Lynch et al., 2013).[33]

Repairing Alliance Ruptures

The second treatment priority in RO DBT has to do with any rupture that appears in the alliance between the therapist and the OC client.[34] As defined in RO DBT, an alliance rupture involves one or both of two main themes:

1. The client feels misunderstood.

2. The client is experiencing the treatment as not relevant to his unique problems.

Both issues are the responsibility of the therapist to manage (that is, a client is not blamed for creating an alliance rupture). Although an alliance rupture represents a potential problem for the therapist (for example, it can lead to the client's premature dropout), in RO DBT an alliance rupture is also seen as an opportunity for the client's growth in that a successful repair can be instrumental in helping an OC client learn that conflict can enhance intimacy. Thus an alliance rupture and its subsequent repair can provide an important means for an OC client to practice the skills needed to resolve interpersonal conflicts and to learn that expressing feelings, including those that involve conflict or disagreement, is an important part of a normal, healthy relationship. In addition, a successfully repaired alliance rupture is considered strong evidence of a good working relationship between the therapist and the client. Since OC clients are expert at masking their feelings and, despite their inner suffering, giving the appearance that all is well, in RO DBT the therapeutic relationship is considered superficial if by the fourteenth of the thirty outpatient sessions there have not been multiple alliance ruptures and repairs (see chapter 8 for specifics).

> RO DBT therapists recognize that even though they may not have been the sole cause of an alliance rupture, they are still responsible for repairing it.

Addressing the Client's Social Signaling Deficits Linked to OC Behavioral Themes

Although life-threatening behavior and the repair of alliance ruptures both take precedence over therapeutic work that addresses an OC client's social signaling deficits, these deficits are considered to be the core problem underlying the loneliness, isolation, and psychological distress of OC clients. Ideally, then, the vast majority of time in RO DBT will be spent on social signaling deficits, which result from habitual maladaptive OC coping (see chapter 2). Five behavioral themes are posited to be uniquely influential in their development and maintenance:

1. Inhibited or disingenuous emotional expression

2. Extreme caution and excessive focus on details

3. Rigid, rule-governed behavior

4. An aloof, distant style of relating to others

5. Frequent use of social comparisons along with frequent feelings of envy or bitterness

These themes provide an evidence-based framework that allows therapists to introduce discussions of what may have been, for many OC clients, taboo or otherwise undisclosed topics, and such discussions can start the important process of helping socially isolated OC clients rejoin the tribe. Most important, these five behavioral themes function as the backdrop for the creation of individualized treatment targets, which are essential to OC clients' recovery (see chapter 9). Table 4.2 shows the themes in relation to specific deficits in social signaling.

Table 4.2. OC Behavioral Themes in Relation to Social Signaling Deficits

OC Behavioral Theme	Examples of Social Signaling Deficit
Inhibited and disingenuous emotional expression	Displaying one emotion to hide another (such as smiling when angry), indirect and ambiguous use of language, disguised demands, low use of emotionally valenced words, pervasive constraint of emotional expressions
Hyper-detail-focused, overly cautious behavior	Insistence on sameness, automatic rejection of critical feedback, rarely enthusiastic, compulsive correction of minor errors, lying to avoid novelty
Rigid, rule-governed behavior	Always circumspect, polite, and appear calm or in control; high social obligation and dutifulness, compulsive self-sacrifice, moral certitude

Aloof and distant style of relating	Rarely expressing desires for intimacy or feelings of love, walking away during conflict, low vulnerable self-disclosure, limited validation of others, lack of reciprocity during interactions—e.g. mutual smiling, laughing, or crying
Frequent social comparisons, with envy or bitterness	Secretly sabotaging, lying or cheating to get ahead, eye rolls, callous smiles, disgust reactions, dismissive gestures, silent treatment, harsh gossip, sarcasm

Using the Treatment Hierarchy to Structure Individual Therapy Sessions

In RO DBT, the successful conduct of individual therapy presents a dialectical dilemma—namely, the therapist must be able to model openness and flexibility within a highly structured format. The RO DBT hierarchy of treatment targets provides a means for the therapist to organize an individual session and make adjustments as needed.

In general, all individual sessions in RO DBT follow a similar structure (see "Individual Therapy Structure and Agenda," page 94). Within a session, however, the therapist on more than one occasion may deliberately move between levels of the hierarchy in order to address issues that emerge in the moment. For example, the therapist, after determining at the first level of the hierarchy that there is no indication of suicidal behavior or self-harm, would likely follow the regular structure of an RO DBT session, which typically involves conducting, at the third level of the hierarchy, a behavioral chain analysis regarding social signaling deficits linked to OC behavioral themes (see chapter 10). Nevertheless, if the client divulged severe and imminent suicidal urges during the chain analysis, the therapist would drop the focus on the behavioral theme, return to the first level of the hierarchy, and attend once again to the assessment and treatment of life-threatening behavior. With this assessment satisfactorily completed, the therapist could then return to the third level of the hierarchy and resume the chain analysis. Later in the session, however, a rupture in the therapeutic alliance might occur, in which case the therapist would leave the third level of the hierarchy and move to the second level, where the rupture could be repaired. Then, with the rupture repaired, the therapist could return yet again to the third level of the hierarchy and continue the chain analysis. In these ways, the RO DBT treatment hierarchy allows the therapist both to structure an individual therapy session and to modify its agenda according to what is happening in the moment.

Individual Therapy Structure and Agenda

The following list outlines the structure for what typically takes place from the fifth through the twenty-ninth sessions of individual therapy in RO DBT:

1. Welcoming and checking in with the client (about one minute). This involves greeting the client, welcoming the client back, and briefly checking in by asking how the client is doing. The therapist should be alert for signs of the client's nonengagement and for indications of a possible alliance rupture; as necessary, the therapist should address the nonengagement or repair the rupture before proceeding. The therapist should avoid prolonged discussion of the past week's events until the client's RO DBT diary card[a] has been reviewed and an agenda has been set for the session.

2. Reviewing the client's diary card and agreeing on the social signaling deficit or overt problem behavior that will be targeted for the session's chain analysis[b] (approximately six minutes). Social signaling deficits are superseded by the presence of imminent life-threatening behavior or by an alliance rupture.

3. Conducting a brief check-in about the client's attendance at and participation in RO skills training class (approximately one minute). As necessary, the therapist should then assess and address any problems.

4. Conducting a brief check-in about the client's completion of the homework assigned from the previous session (approximately three minutes). The therapist should identify any difficulty needing further attention and either do some quick problem solving or place the issue on the session's agenda as an item for discussion.

5. Finalizing the session's agenda and agreeing on the amount of time that will be spent on each agenda item (approximately three minutes). The therapist and the client will agree, for example, on how much time to spend on chain analysis and how much to spend on teaching and learning a new RO skill.

6. Conducting a behavioral chain and solution analysis targeting the problem behavior of the week, as identified from the diary card (approximately twenty to twenty-five minutes). Ideally, given core RO DBT principles that posit overcontrol as a problem of emotional loneliness, the majority of chain analyses in RO DBT will target the client's OC social signaling deficits and problems linked to the client's overt expression of emotion rather than the client's internal experiences (such as thoughts, emotions, and sensations).

7. Discussing other agenda items (approximately fifteen minutes). For example, the therapist may target non-OC problem behaviors (such as restrictive eating) or other kinds of problems (difficulties finding a job, legal difficulties). The therapist may also teach new skills (such as loving kindness meditation) already planned for the session, celebrate the client's successes, or define new treatment targets derived from OC themes.

8. Ending the session (approximately two minutes). The therapist should briefly summarize the session's events and any new skills that the client has learned. The therapist should also include a reminder of any specific homework that may have been assigned for the coming week (such as a specific self-enquiry practice or RO skill).

a   See chapters 5 and 9.

b   See chapter 10.

Now You Know...

▶ Before treatment can begin with OC clients, they must be willing to see their overcontrolled style of coping as a core problem.

▶ RO DBT therapists practice radical openness and self-enquiry themselves, since radical openness is not something that can be grasped solely via intellectual means.

▶ Rather than focusing solely on fixing, correcting, or improving hyperperfectionistic OC clients, RO DBT teaches therapists to model living a life worth sharing and to adopt the stance of tribal ambassador in order to encourage emotionally lonely and isolated OC clients to return to the tribe.

▶ The treatment priorities in RO DBT are, first, to reduce life-threatening behaviors; second, to repair ruptures in the therapeutic alliance; and, third, to address deficits in the client's social signaling, with reference to the five OC behavioral themes.

▶ The five OC behavioral themes are (1) inhibited or disingenuous emotional expression, (2) extreme caution and excessive focus on details, (3) rigid, rule-governed behavior, (4) an aloof, distant style of relating to others, and (5) frequent use of social comparisons along with frequent feelings of envy or bitterness.

CHAPTER 5

Maximizing Client Engagement

The aim of this chapter is to describe in detail the strategies in RO DBT that are designed to enhance OC client engagement in therapy. The chapter is organized according to three broad classes of elements:

1. Physical and environmental elements

2. Orientation and commitment elements

3. Timing and sequencing elements

Each element is designed to enhance client engagement in therapy by accounting in differing ways for the impact of OC biotemperamental predispositions. The chapter begins by describing how to maximize OC client engagement via adjustments of physical space. Following this, RO DBT orientation and commitment strategies are outlined, including a detailed overview of the first four sessions. The chapter ends with a description of RO DBT timing and sequencing strategies.

Enhancing Client Engagement via the Physical Environment

Though it might seem like a dirty word in RO DBT, "controlling" the physical therapeutic milieu can be a critical factor in enhancing client engagement and achieving a successful outcome. The reason this is given such high priority in RO DBT pertains to the innate biotemperamental predispositions for heightened threat sensitivity that characterize OC clients. OC clients are more likely to respond with low-level defensive arousal to environmental stimuli that might go unnoticed by other people. They are also less likely to admit to anxious defensive arousal when queried. Plus, as discussed in chapter 4, the primary goal of treatment is to help the client learn that social interactions can be intrinsically rewarding and that it is possible to experience feelings of safety when around others, not to overcome, defeat, or control social anxiety by braving it out or going opposite action.

Hence it is important for therapists to proactively control the physical milieu in order to make it less likely for OC biology to interfere with their clients' learning how to have fun, play, express themselves more freely, chill out, and be less serious. This means accounting for a range of often subtle physical and nonverbal factors that can enhance (or diminish) social safety experiences in OC clients. Therapists should not dismiss these factors as unimportant simply because they themselves are not bothered or the client denies discomfort. Thus, before commencing treatment with an OC client, therapists should take into account environmental factors that might potentially influence outcomes.

Chairs in individual therapy settings should ideally be positioned at a 45-degree angle to each other (see figure 5.1). This avoids face-off behaviors or face-to-face body postures linked to highly intimate or aggressive exchanges within our species (Morris, 2002). Furthermore, therapy chairs should ideally have armrests. Armrests allow therapists to easily shift into body postures that nonverbally signal cooperation, safety, and nondominance, postures that are essential when repairing alliance ruptures or when confronting an OC client.

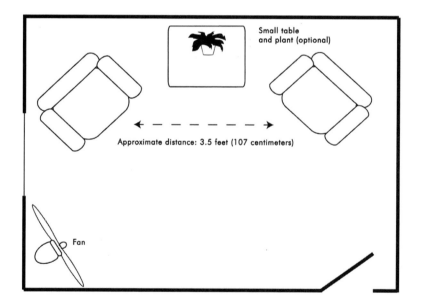

Figure 5.1. Individual Therapy Room Furniture Arrangement

Prior to a session with an OC client, the therapist should arrange the seating in a manner that maximizes physical distance. OC clients generally have a greater need for personal body space relative to others. Close body proximity is a nonverbal signal of intimacy or confrontation (Morris, 2002). The same reasoning applies to the physical layout and seating arrangements used in RO skills training classes. Ideally, the classroom will include a long table with chairs positioned around it in the style of a dining room, and with some type of whiteboard or flipchart at the front of the room for the instructor to write on. Figure 5.2 shows this type of classroom setting. It signals that the purpose of the class is learning skills rather than participating in group therapy, engaging in interpersonal encounters, or processing feelings. The table and room arrangement also provide physical buffers between class members (this functions to reduce their feeling of being exposed) while providing space for note-taking (which allows OC clients time to downregulate without calling attention to themselves). The skills class should also and ideally be conducted in a large and airy room that can accommodate up to nine people. A large room also allows clients greater freedom in how they might adjust their seating or move their chairs farther away from others without calling attention to themselves.

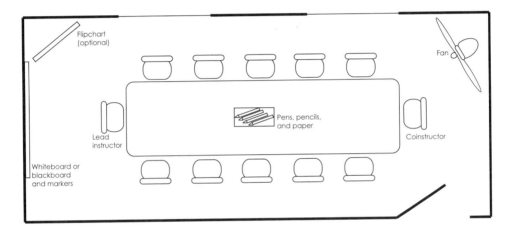

Figure 5.2. RO Skills Classroom Layout

It is also very important that room temperature be considered for both individual therapy sessions and skills training classes. A hot or very warm environment naturally triggers perspiration in most people. For many OC clients, sweating is a conditioned stimulus linked to anxiety and maladaptive avoidance. When working with OC clients, therapists should set room temperatures to be lower than what might be normal; if necessary, clinics should invest in fans or other means to cool rooms, when required. In general, the rule is to keep the room cool unless the OC client requests that the temperature be increased.

Interestingly, most people find it easy to tell others when they are cold, but people are amazingly reluctant to complain when they feel hot, especially in settings that are evaluative or trigger self-consciousness (for example, a job interview). This is because feeling cold is not a symptom of anxious arousal, whereas feeling hot is. Our experience applying this principle in our research trials and clinical work over the years has repeatedly shown this relatively simple factor to oftentimes profoundly influence client behavior and treatment engagement.

For example, one RO DBT therapist during clinical supervision reported that her client had missed several sessions, and that she was concerned about treatment dropout. Review of a videotaped session revealed fidgeting and restless body movements, behaviors that had not been noticed by the therapist. When asked by her supervisor if the cooling fan in the room was being used, the therapist indicated that she had stopped using the cooling fan several weeks earlier and had checked in with her client about it by asking if he still needed the fan on now that autumn had arrived. The client had stated, "No, I'm fine." The supervisor suggested that, despite the client's previous report, the therapist turn the fan back on prior to the start of the next session and begin the session as she normally would, without any mention or reference to the fan unless the client brought it up. To the surprise of the therapist, the behavior of the client seemed more engaged during that session. His body movements appeared less agitated, eye contact improved, and he spoke more freely. The therapist kept the fan on from then on and made sure she had a light sweater available for herself. Weeks later, when the therapist and her client were practicing ways of activating social safety in session, the client revealed that he had been too embarrassed to tell her that he was feeling hot when the fan was not on because he thought his therapist might take it as criticism.

Thus therapists should always assume that seating and proximity factors are important when working with OC clients, regardless of clients' verbal reports to the contrary. So *turn on* the fan and *turn down* the heat when working with OC clients, and bring layers of clothing for yourself if you tend to get cold easily. This simple physical environmental adjustment can make an enormous difference, especially early in therapy, when an OC client is less likely to reveal what he may be truly feeling or thinking inside. Clients in skills class who report the room being too cool can be encouraged to bring a light sweater with them to class, and we always like to have a few sweaters on hand in class to be borrowed if needed. For additional information on managing the environment in skills training classes, see the skills training manual, chapter 1.

Enhancing Client Engagement via Orientation and Commitment

RO DBT individual therapy is designed to be delivered in sequential stages or steps, with each new component building on the previous one. The phase of orientation and commitment is one of these stages, and it occurs during the first four sessions of therapy.

In general, commitment protocols in RO DBT pertain to three issues:

1. Agreement by the client that he is OC and is committed to working on it

2. The client's commitment to return in person and discuss urges to drop out of therapy before actually doing so[35]

3. The client's commitment not to self-injure or attempt suicide without contacting the therapist or another health care professional (assuming this is relevant)

Another major aim of the orientation and commitment stage is to collaboratively identify the client's valued goals, which are used to facilitate treatment targeting. Both the heightened biotemperamental threat sensitivity that characterizes OC and the overall OC tendency to abandon relationships mean that "foot in the door" strategies are more frequently used in RO DBT than "door in the face" strategies when therapists want to deepen commitment.[36]

RO DBT commitment strategies start with a stance of humility and openness on the therapist's part. RO DBT acknowledges that it is the client's right to choose the life she wishes to lead, even if it is a miserable one (or at least to the therapist's eyes appears miserable). RO principles contend that it would be arrogant for a therapist to assume he knows how his OC client should live or what she should consider important. Thus, ultimately, the RO DBT therapist acknowledges to himself (and to his client when needed) that his client is responsible for the choices she makes, including the choice of remaining depressed, anxious, or lonely, and that ultimately the therapist cannot fix his OC client's problems. Similar to the role of a national park ranger helping someone lost in a forest, an RO DBT therapist can walk alongside his OC client and provide a map and compass as a guide (that is, the RO DBT treatment strategies) to help his client find her way home, but he cannot carry her out of the forest—the client must walk out on her own.

Thus the orientation and commitment stage of RO DBT individual therapy sets the stage for the rest of treatment. Since OC clients are highly rule-governed and generally serious about life, it is important for therapists to avoid reinforcing these perspectives by adopting an overly serious, formalistic, or rigid stance suggesting compliance or agreement is essential. RO DBT principles of openness, flexibility, an easy manner (see chapter 6), and self-enquiry guide the therapist's behavior from the moment he first meets a client.[37]

First and Second Sessions

After welcoming and introducing oneself (including one's credentials and therapeutic experience or background), and before actually beginning, it is important in work with OC clients to briefly describe the type of interaction to expect and the overall aims of the first session:

Therapist: Okay, before we start, I thought it might be useful for me to give you a sense of what to expect. The type of therapy I will be using involves a two-way dialogue between the therapist and the client. This means that both of us will be talking during therapy, and sometimes I may need to interrupt you in order to ask a pertinent question. And, by the way, it's okay for you to interrupt me too. *(Smiles.)* Does that make sense? Today's session will involve me learning more about the type of problems that have brought you here, which means that I will be asking some questions about different aspects of your life, which may at times require me to interrupt you or direct us to another topic. Plus, just to let you know, although I already know a little about you from your medical record, I usually find it most useful to hear directly from my clients, in their own words, what their particular struggles might be. So, to begin, can you give me a sense about what brought you here today?

Communicating to an OC client that the treatment will involve a two-way dialogue is essential. This can help prevent problems later, since without it, some more talkative OC clients may believe it unfair or wrong to interrupt them, especially since they were not warned this might occur.

Limiting the Use of Written Material in Individual Therapy

Therapists can enhance clients' engagement when it comes to another aspect of the physical environment: the use of written materials in individual therapy sessions (as opposed to skills training classes).[a] Providing an OC client a copy of a figure, table, or handout during an individual therapy session can sidetrack the intended discussion. The OC client's biotemperamental tendencies to notice details and minor errors may lead her to stop listening to what the therapist is saying and instead intently focus on the written material she was just handed. This can trigger long and convoluted discussions that may have very little to do with the actual content of the material itself, or rejection of the material because of disagreement over word choice or grammar (for example, a grammatical error may be taken to mean that the entire document is useless). As a consequence, the therapist may find himself spending valuable session time justifying, defending, or capitulating in order to keep the peace. Written materials are like plutonium—you only need a little for a major explosion. That said, as with any RO DBT strategy, the key is to be flexible and to take advantage of a client's unexpected reactions as opportunities to lighten up.

For example, in our most recent multicenter trial of RO DBT, during our startup phase, a number of our OC clients at three independent sites were quick to point out a minor error—a misspelling that caused the word "dairy" to be substituted for "diary" in the title of the RO DBT diary card (see "Introducing the RO DBT Diary Card," later in this chapter). To these clients, this minor error seemed major. But instead of immediately rushing out to produce new copies of the handout and correct the misspelling, we played along with the mistake. When a client pointed out that the handout said "dairy card" instead of "diary card," his therapist said, "Yes, isn't that wonderful? I've always wanted to live on a farm." Another therapist said to

It can also be helpful to briefly mention in the first session that the feasibility, acceptability, and efficacy of RO DBT were solidly established and studied for more than twenty years before RO DBT was disseminated more broadly. However, a word of caution here, since OC clients are detail-focused and threat-sensitive: some may wish to discuss further the results of the clinical trials, request to see copies of published studies (immediately), or be dismissive or judgmental if a therapist cannot immediately and precisely answer a question about the research. The issues surrounding the empirical basis of RO DBT are similar to those described in connection with the use of written material during individual therapy (see "Limiting the Use of Written Material in Individual Therapy," below). The best approach to dealing with a client who becomes intent on knowing the data before proceeding further is for the therapist to validate the client's desire for information while continuing to orient the client to the primary aims of the first session:

a client, "Let's take a look at your dairy card and see how productive your cows have been lately." This simple misspelling presented an opportunity to present a major teaching point—namely, that not every mistake in life has to be fixed right now, or ever—and the therapist's playful irreverence provided some minor corrective feedback, without making a big deal of it. (Recall that OC clients are overly serious and need to learn how to play and chill out; see chapter 10 for more details about this strategy.)

These recommendations should be applied flexibly. Most therapists, at least occasionally, bring a handout with them into an individual therapy session, as a reminder of a topic that they wish to discuss or teach on a particular day (for example, the therapist may place a copy of the handout on the clipboard normally used for taking notes during a session, but without giving a copy to the client). Another way to use written material during individual therapy without provoking fruitless discussion or debate is to engage the client's attention in the present by drawing a diagram on a whiteboard, whereas giving a client a copy of a handout and asking her to read it silently before discussing it can lead to the hyperscrutiny just described.[b] If a client requests a copy of a handout, figure, article, or other written material, the therapist can provide it, ideally at the end of the session or via email.

[a] In RO DBT, the aims of individual therapy and RO skills training are different. Individual therapy provides the practice grounds for an OC client to learn how to rejoin the tribe and socially connect with others, whereas skills training classes are didactic in nature and focused on teaching new skills that will facilitate social connection. Therefore, copies of handouts and worksheets are always made available during skills training classes and are considered essential elements of the learning process.

[b] Nevertheless, a therapist teaching a specific RO skill during an individual session should feel free to use handouts and worksheets from the skills training manual, if doing so will enhance the client's learning.

Therapist: I'm really glad to hear that you want to know more about the research. If I were in your shoes, I would probably be asking similar types of questions—the scientific basis behind a treatment really matters. However, since I actually don't have a pile of research article printouts to hand to you right at this very moment, and since it is also our very first session, if it's okay with you I would like to ask your permission to proceed. This will allow us some time to get to know each other—and, hopefully, determine whether RO DBT seems like a good fit for you. *(Smiles.)* Regardless, before we end today, I will give you the name of a website link that you can access yourself, to take a look at what the therapy is all about before our next session. How does that sound to you?

Such comments are rarely needed. Most OC clients arrive at the first session with an open mind and expectation of therapist competence. Thus I would recommend that a clinic not make it a policy to start handing out packets of published empirical research in support of RO DBT prior to the start of treatment. As highlighted earlier in this chapter, written material provided during individual therapy often moves the focus away from the client and onto the written material.[38]

Global Aims and Topics for the First and Second Sessions

▶ Determining the client's reasons for seeking treatment, his past treatment experience, and his family and environmental history

▶ Orienting the client to the type of problems the treatment is designed to help, and confirming the client's agreement with and general commitment to targeting OC as the core issue

▶ Assessing the client's current and past history of suicidal and self-harming behavior

▶ Signaling the therapist's willingness to discuss past trauma, sexual issues, and long-held grudges and resentments

▶ Orienting the client to the overall structure of treatment, including information about the purpose of skills training classes, and giving the client notice that his participation in skills class will begin during the third week of therapy.

Obtaining the Client's Commitment to Target Overcontrol

Maladaptive OC can only be treated if the client recognizes it as a problem. Thus, before commencing treatment, in the very first session, it is essential to obtain agreement from the client that, first, her personality style is best described as overcontrolled and, second, she is committed to target maladaptive OC behaviors as a core part of therapy.[39] This discussion should be time-limited (about ten minutes) and conducted with an easy manner (see chapter 6).

The discussion of this topic (see "Four Steps for Identifying Overcontrol as the Core Problem in the First Session," page 106) is the first of three in the orientation and commitment phase that are fully scripted (see also "Four Steps for Teaching the Biosocial Theory for Overcontrol in the Third Session" and "Four Steps for Teaching That Open Expression = Trust = Social Connectedness in the Fourth Session," later in this chapter). The relatively brief time period allocated for the discussion is purposeful. It helps an OC client obtain a sense of what the core focus in treatment will be while allowing time for other topics. It also avoids reinforcing OC compulsive desires to be fully informed about a topic before making a decision while simultaneously reinforcing OC client self-disclosure by not focusing too much attention on a potentially difficult topic (recall that OC clients dislike the limelight).

This often requires therapists to let go of their own personal needs to fully cover a topic or automatically dig deeper when a potential treatment target emerges during the discussion, and to go opposite to their dislike of or resistance to using protocols or scripts. A script can be likened to a protocol—it reflects accumulated clinical experience and is designed to avoid potential problems. Our clinical experience has repeatedly demonstrated the utility of using scripts as written, across a wide range of settings and differing cultures. Sticking to a script helps keep a discussion short and on topic. Therapists should feel free to photocopy a script and bring it into session on a clipboard (something I still do), as a reminder of the material to be covered.

When describing the differing styles (undercontrol versus overcontrol), it is essential for therapists to act out, using body gestures and facial expressions, the social signals that typify each style rather than simply describing them. Thus, when describing the undercontrolled style, which should be done first in the discussion, therapists should exaggerate facial expressions and body movements, such as gesticulating expansively with their arms as they describe the undercontrolled style. OC clients will immediately recognize that the dramatic, erratic, excitable, and highly expressive nature that characterizes undercontrol disorders does not characterize them. When describing the OC style, therapists should dampen down their affect and adopt a more controlled body posture, thereby making it viscerally easier for clients to identify themselves with an OC style. The importance of this cannot be overstated. Without acting out how each style social signals, OC clients can mistakenly believe that they exhibit some of the core features associated with undercontrol. However, this quickly disappears when the dramatic, erratic facial expressions and body movements associated with undercontrol are shown to an OC client, not just talked about. As one OC client quickly stated after seeing what undercontrolled looked like, "Nope, that's not me." The vast majority of OC clients (who are seeking treatment) quickly recognize themselves as overcontrolled and find the label a useful means for describing a pattern of behavior that they have known about for most of their lives.

Four Steps for Identifying Overcontrol as the Core Problem in the First Session

1. *Say:* As I mentioned earlier, one of the things I wanted to do today is give you a bit of a sense of the treatment approach that I will be using in our work together. Here's what's really interesting—researchers from around the world have reached a type of consensus or agreement that around age four or five it is possible to start to see the beginnings of two differing personality or coping styles that are linked to problems later in life. Have you ever heard about anything like that before?

2. *Say:* One of these styles is known as *undercontrolled*.[a] As children, undercontrolled individuals were often described as highly excitable, overly expressive, conduct-disordered, or impulsive. When they felt something inside, everyone knew about it! Plus, they found it hard to plan ahead or resist temptation. When they saw a cookie, they grabbed it and ate it up, without thinking about the consequences. They also tended to do things according to how they felt in the moment. And now, later in life, if they don't feel like going to work, they just don't go! So when you think about yourself, now or when you were a child, does this type of personality or coping style describe you?

3. *Say:* Perhaps you lean the other way.[b] The other style, known as *overcontrolled* coping, is more cautious and reserved. As children, overcontrolled individuals may have been described as shy or timid. They tend to control or constrain expressions of emotion and are able to delay gratification and tolerate distress for long periods of time in order to achieve long-term goals. They tend to set high personal standards and are likely to work harder than most to prevent future problems, without making a big deal of it. Yet inwardly they often feel lonely, not part of their community or excluded from it, and feeling clueless about how to join with others or form intimate relationships, and they often feel isolated. So when you think of yourself, now or as a child, do you think this style might describe you better?

4. *Say:* Finally, the treatment approach I will be using—RO DBT—was developed for problems of overcontrol but doesn't consider overcontrolled coping as always problematic.[c] On the contrary, not only is high self-control highly valued by most societies, it's what got us to the moon! It takes a lot of planning and persistence to build a spaceship. Thus, rather than attempting to get rid of your overcontrolled coping, I hope to help you learn how to both embrace and relinquish your tendencies toward overcontrol, flexibly and according to the situation. What do you think when I say that?[d] To what extent are you willing to target overcontrolled coping as a core problem in our work together?

During this initial discussion of overcontrolled coping, therapists should choose descriptors that are generally positive or emotionally neutral while noting the types of words clients use to describe their overcontrol, in order to begin the process of understanding how OC uniquely manifests for a client and to improve individualized treatment targeting in later sessions. Using relatively neutral descriptors during initial discussions of OC coping functions as a "foot in the door" technique, making it easier for a client to admit to some habits or possible imperfections without making a big deal of it. Here are a number of descriptors that most OC clients would endorse:

detail-focused

restrained

perfectionistic

cautious

disciplined

structured

conscientious

reserved

planful

dutiful

a   It is essential for the therapist who is describing the undercontrolled coping style to bodily demonstrate what the UC social signaling style looks and sounds like, in order to avoid confusion and misunderstanding. Thus, when describing undercontrolled individuals as overly excitable or overly expressive, the therapist should simultaneously wave his or her arms about in excitement and display an excitable expression and voice tone. This is essential so that the OC client can viscerally experience (in his or her own body) the UC social signaling style instead of having to imagine it.

b   The vast majority of OC clients will quickly reject the undercontrolled (UC) coping style as representative of their own. When they don't, the therapist should consider the following possibilities: (1) the client is actually UC; (2) the therapist's demonstration of UC social signaling was not dramatic enough; or (3) the client is purposefully endorsing the UC style as representative of his own in order to send a message (for example, that he is too complex to understand, is experiencing an alliance rupture, or is hopeless about change).

c   Step 4 assumes that the client has endorsed the OC coping style as most representative of his own.

d   These final questions, known in RO DBT as check-ins, are designed to assess the client's engagement.

It is also important for therapists to avoid adopting a stance that communicates coercion or pressure to agree with an OC label. If a client struggles with recognizing his style as overcontrolled, therapists can take one of the following approaches:

- Consider the possibility that the client is correct, thereby modeling radical openness

- Experiment with different words or phrases (for example, "high self-control" or "hyperperfectionism") to describe the OC style

- Provide homework assignments that might help trigger awareness of overcontrol

To deepen discussions with an ambivalent client, the therapist can also ask the client to complete the instrument called Assessing Styles of Coping: Word-Pair Checklist (see appendix 1), if it has not already been completed as part of a pretreatment assessment interview, or the therapist can assign the checklist as homework to be reviewed at the next session, although this is generally unnecessary. In addition, as seen in the scripted discussion, it is important to note at some point the prosocial nature of overcontrol (refer to table 4.1), without overplaying it—a form of smuggling (see "More About Smuggling," below).

More About Smuggling

In RO DBT, the social signaling strategy known as *smuggling* is used to introduce information to an OC client by planting a seed or a small part of a new idea. This gives the client an opportunity to reflect on the new idea without feeling compelled to immediately accept or reject it. For example, it is not uncommon for an OC client to assume that psychotherapy will focus primarily on exposing his deficits or discussing his problems, and so briefly introducing the prosocial aspects of overcontrol smuggles the idea that the client's personality style has benefits as well as downsides. Nevertheless, a well-meaning therapist's overenthusiastic proclamations or prolonged discussions about the benefits of OC can backfire and trigger an alliance rupture in the very first session. Most OC clients inwardly believe that they are not very nice people, and they harbor harshly negative self-judgments as a function of their past mistakes, incidents of emotional leakage, or hurtful acts directed toward others. Therefore, at this early stage of therapy, the therapist should not only avoid overplaying the prosocial nature of OC but also be alert for possible signs of an alliance rupture.

In summary, the therapist's overarching aim during discussions of self-control tendencies with an OC client is to awaken an appreciation for self-exploration and a recognition that OC coping both solves and creates problems. This involves *asking*, not telling, the client about how OC has prevented her from reaching important

valued goals. Early in therapy, a client's spontaneous disclosures of fallibility and unprompted
curiosity about OC coping are good indicators
of client engagement. Finally, it is important
for therapists to remember that successful
treatment of OC does not mean converting
the client into a dramatic, erratic, undercontrolled person; on the contrary, it involves
helping a client learn how to appreciate her
personality style and yet be able to flexibly
relinquish it when the situation calls for it.

> The therapist's overarching
> aim during discussions of
> self-control tendencies with
> an OC client is to awaken an
> appreciation for self-
> exploration and a recognition
> that OC coping both solves
> and creates problems.

Dealing with Suicidal Behavior and Self-Harm

Despite the fact that OC clients appear composed and self-controlled on the
outside, suicidal and self-injurious behaviors occur at disproportionately high rates in
people with disorders of overcontrol. OC clients tend to feel isolated and alone on the
inside, and social isolation and low social integration are core risk factors for suicide,
over and above demographic and diagnostic covariates (Darke, Williamson, Ross, &
Teesson, 2005). The social signaling deficits and low openness that characterize maladaptive overcontrol are posited to result in repeated experiences of social ostracism,
rejection, and exclusion from an early age, thus exacerbating an OC client's sense of
social isolation, his loneliness, and his sense of himself as outsider—and, as a consequence, making his risk of suicide greater. For example, anorexia nervosa (a prototypical disorder of overcontrol) has the highest mortality rate of any psychiatric
illness. People with anorexia nervosa have a fifty-sevenfold greater risk of death from
suicide than their age-matched peers (Keel et al., 2003). OC traits such as low openness to experience are associated with greater suicide risk (Heisel et al., 2006), and
chronic depression, which is characterized by prototypical OC traits (Riso, et al.,
2003), is also associated with exceptionally high rates of suicidal behavior. For
example, 86 percent of treatment-resistant depressed clients have been shown to
report suicidal thoughts or plans (compared to only 53 percent of nonchronic
depressed clients), and 29 percent attempted suicide during their treatment phase
(compared with only 3 percent of nonchronic clients; see Malhi, Parker, Crawford,
Wilhelm, & Mitchell, 2005).

In addition, nonsuicidal self-injury is also markedly frequent in disorders typifying overcontrol, such as dysthymia, refractory depression, anorexia nervosa, and
Cluster A personality disorders (Claes et al., 2010; Ghaziuddin et al., 1991; Hintikka
et al., 2009; Klonsky et al., 2003; Nock et al., 2006; Selby et al., 2012).[40] For most OC
clients, suicidal behavior and self-harm represent proof that they are fatally flawed
and are a source of deep shame.

Yet, almost paradoxically, OC clients can also appear to relish, romanticize, or
become enveloped in brooding, feeling sad or melancholic, or wallowing in self-pity

or a sense of being a martyr—factors that can heighten suicidal risk. For example, they may write tragic stories and poems, describe despair or melancholy as intellectually pure or noble, delight in nihilistic thinking, enjoy reading obituaries, or write romanticized stories or poems about death or suicide. They may secretly revel in their sense of isolation or estrangement from others because it reinforces their beliefs that no one cares, understands, or appreciates their self-sacrifices or unique talents. Similarly, melancholy, misery, and despair often signal that the OC client experiences herself as the victim, scapegoat, or martyr of an unfair or unjust world (or unjust family). Thus OC clients' suicide may stem from desires for revenge or to punish family members who have failed to recognize their self-sacrifices. OC clients are characterized by high moral certitude (that is, there is a right and wrong way of doing things) and this is often linked to beliefs that good deeds should be rewarded and evil deeds punished. Punishing the transgressor restores a person's faith in a just world. A just world is one where actions and occurrences have predictable and appropriate consequences, and people get what they deserve according to how they behave.[41] This helps explain why many people find it so difficult to forgive—it can feel morally wrong not to punish a transgressor. However, one of the more perplexing behaviors associated with nonsuicidal self-injury is self-reported reasons for engaging in self-injury as a means to punish oneself. Indeed, punishment, by definition, should function to reduce the probability of a particular behavior, but causing oneself pain, at least on the surface, does not seem to be pleasurable. Thus the question becomes, "What is reinforcing about self-punishment?"

RO DBT posits that self-punishment feels "good" because it restores our sense of order. As mentioned earlier, most OC clients inwardly believe that they are not very nice people, and they harbor extremely negative self-evaluations. RO DBT posits that this often stems from intense shame for not ever having been caught or punished for behavior they consider reprehensible, morally wrong, or harmful to others (perceptions that may often have validity). From an OC client's perspective, the inability to admit to prior wrongdoing is proof of a fundamentally flawed character. According to Swann's self-verification theory (Swann, 1983), nonsuicidal self-injury is posited to verify a sense of oneself as bad or evil and deserving of punishment (T. R. Lynch & Cozza, 2009). Indeed, self-verification is so powerful that it is preferred even when it means enduring pain and discomfort (Swann, Rentfrow, & Gosling, 2003). In addition, the OC client's silence makes it impossible for him to be punished by his tribe, and so he may believe that the only way to restore his sense of self is to pay for his sins through self-harm or self-sacrificial suicide. Indeed, in a sample of chronically depressed people, feeling guilty, sinful, or worthless has been shown to be associated with a six times greater chance of having suicidal thoughts (T. R. Lynch et al., 1999). Thus acts of self-harm are reinforcing because they function to verify or confirm an OC client's pathological sense of self and restore a sense of safety (for example, through restored faith in a just world).

Plus, self-harm is often described as negatively reinforced because it appears to provide a momentarily efficient means of reducing arousal and removing negative emotions; self-injurious behavior has been shown to be associated with reduced pain perception (Gardner & Cowdry, 1985). From an RO DBT perspective, the mechanisms behind this may involve activation of two differing neural substrates that function to reinforce self-harming behavior via changes in emotional experience:

1. The first mechanism is posited to reinforce self-harm by triggering positive emotions linked to a sense of accomplishment, pride, and achievement (positive reinforcement). Here, top-down regulatory processes use self-harm as evidence for negative self-beliefs ("My self-harm proves that my belief that I am fatally flawed must be correct") or as a valid means of communication ("By harming myself, I am repairing a wrongdoing") or as evidence of the OC client's superior self-control capacities ("Harming myself proves that I have the courage to do the right thing"), thus triggering SNS positive affectivity.

2. The second mechanism is posited to reinforce self-harm via bottom-up regulatory processes that function to provide relief from overwhelming stress (negative reinforcement). Specifically, self-inflicted tissue damage that is severe or prolonged (and that may include the sight of copious amounts of blood) is posited to be evaluated at the sensory receptor level as an overwhelming threat, thus triggering automatic shutdown responses, such as fainting, immobilization, a lowered heart rate, reduced pain perception, and withdrawal of SNS approach, fight, and flight responses, as described in chapter 2.

Plus, OC clients tend to be rule-governed. A rule-governed behavior specifies a relationship between the behavior (cutting my wrists) and a consequence (self-punishment and restoration of a just world, a less aversive emotion). Since the behavior is based on rules (that is, historical experiences or societal expectations), it can become problematic precisely because the rule-governed behavior is less responsive to current contingencies (what is occurring in the present moment). For example, studies have demonstrated that individuals who are verbally instructed on a task do not change strategies when contingencies change; rather, they persist in a given strategy because it is consistent with a rule that verbally specifies contingencies (Hayes, Brownstein, Haas, & Greenway, 1986). A literal belief in rules may lead to beliefs that thoughts or emotions are dangerous ("If I think x, then a very bad thing will happen") and that certain thoughts are in themselves bad or equivalent to unwanted actions (Rachman, 1997). As a consequence, an individual may come to believe that she must punish herself via self-injury whenever she experiences certain taboo thoughts or emotions, or she may try to suppress emotional thoughts, which research has shown to be a particularly ineffective strategy (T. R. Lynch et al., 2001; T. R. Lynch et al., 2004; T. R. Lynch, Schneider, Rosenthal, & Cheavens, 2007). Unfortunately, this can develop into a vicious self-confirming cycle, leading to further rigid rule-governed behavior: "Since I am hurting myself, it must be true that I am evil; therefore, I must be punished by continuing to injure myself."

OC tendencies to mask inner feelings and minimize distress can sometimes make suicidal risk assessment challenging. For example, unless directly asked about suicidal thoughts and behavior, most OC clients are not likely to independently report them (especially in the first session). Moreover, their natural tendencies to mask inner feelings and minimize distress make their underreporting of suicidal behavior more likely than underreporting of suicidal behavior in other clinical groups. In addition, OC clients are experts at blocking discussion of topics they don't want to discuss, without making it obvious. The good news is that, in general, OC clients are less likely to overtly lie or deceive a therapist when asked directly about suicidal behavior (recall that OC clients value honesty and integrity). However, they will covertly lie in order to avoid imagined disapproval or maintain an appearance of competence by not disclosing important facts or details unless they are specifically asked. Examples of downplaying or avoidance include changing the subject by bringing up a new one that seems equally significant ("Before I answer that question, I think you should know that I haven't been touched by another person for seventeen years"); talking a great deal but never answering the question ("I do occasionally think about death—I was raised Catholic, and as an altar boy I had to attend funerals at a young age"); and implying that prevention concerns are unnecessary ("My previous therapist said suicidal thoughts are normal") or inappropriate, since further discussion would be damaging, too painful, or too revealing, or because the client's "other doctor" is already taking care of the issue. There are many other ways in which covert lying can manifest; most of them involve indirect rather than direct methods of communication, and that makes them plausibly deniable, or difficult to challenge.

However, occasionally the reasons behind this type of avoidance are much more serious. For example, although this is rare, some OC clients arrive at their first session with an already established plan to kill themselves—that is, they have decided on the exact date, time, place, and method of suicide and have also decided not to reveal these plans to the therapist. Most often they have chosen to attend therapy in order to prove to themselves (beforehand) and family (afterward) that they have dutifully strived to solve the problem, thereby rendering suicide justifiable. However, regardless of the underlying motivations, the situation poses a problem for the therapist that is multifold. For one, the client's decision not to reveal his suicide plan not only makes a genuine commitment for change less likely but also negatively impacts the development of the genuine working alliance that is considered an essential part of successful RO DBT therapy. Fortunately, it is possible to get past this apparent impasse via a strategy often referred to in RO DBT as therapeutic induction of guilt. If the stance could speak, it would say, "I trust you to do the right thing. I believe in you. I have faith in your ability to follow through with your commitments." The stance takes advantage of core OC client values for honesty, integrity, and dutifulness, with the therapeutic guilt emerging gradually over time. In this example, the first inkling of therapeutic guilt is likely first experienced by the OC client almost immediately after the therapist obtains a verbal commitment from the client that he will report any urges, thoughts, plans, or actions pertaining to suicide or self-injury over the course of treatment. This commitment is obtained from all OC clients—including those reporting no prior history of suicidal or self-injurious behavior—and is easy to obtain from a client who is attending therapy in order to improve his life. However, for the OC client with other ideas, this commitment creates cognitive dissonance, since it requires the client to overtly lie to the therapist and goes against core values. Thus, rather than adopting a stance of suspicion or distrust (for example, out of fear of a potential suicide), RO DBT therapists are encouraged to adopt a stance that signals trust and belief in the client to do the right thing while simultaneously being prepared to do what is necessary to keep a client alive or safe when new information emerges suggesting imminent threat. The good news is that our experience has shown that almost invariably the OC client himself will be the one who steps forward and reveals the truth, which is welcomed by the therapist and most often serves as a critical change point in therapy. OC clients give a damn; even when hopelessly lost, they retain an ability to be touched by kindhearted actions and reciprocate if possible (in this example, by revealing suicidal plans to the therapist despite prior decisions to avoid doing so).

In conclusion, OC life-threatening behaviors are often qualitatively different from those displayed by other clinical groups. Awareness of these features can facilitate understanding of an OC client and improve treatment targeting. A summary of these features follows:

- OC client suicide and self-harm are usually planned, often hours, days, or even weeks in advance (and sometimes longer).

- OC self-harming behavior is usually a well-kept secret. It may have been occurring for years without anyone knowing, or knowledge about it may be limited to immediate family members (or very close friends and therapists). Thus OC self-harm is rarely attention-seeking. The severity of self-inflicted injuries is carefully controlled in order to avoid medical attention, and scars are carefully hidden. An OC client may acquire first aid or medical training in order to treat self-inflicted wounds on her own and avoid having to go to a hospital. Exceptions to hiding behavior can occur, most often among OC clients with a long history of psychiatric hospitalization, whereby dramatic displays of self-injury are often intermittently reinforced (for example, self-injury gets an OC client placed in a private observation room, which is preferable to the uncertainty of being part of the general inpatient community).

- OC clients may attempt suicide to punish family or close others ("When I'm gone, you'll be sorry") or to get even, make a rival's life difficult (for example, the hope is that the client's death will make it impossible for the rival to achieve an important goal), or expose moral failings.

- OC self-harm or suicidal behavior is more likely to be rule-governed than mood-governed (for example, its purpose may be to restore the client's faith in a just world through self-punishment for perceived wrongs).

- Some OC clients may romanticize suicidal behavior and consider brooding or melancholy to be noble or creative.

Assessing OC Life-Threatening Behaviors

The primary aim of this initial assessment is to ensure client safety and to determine the extent to which suicidal behaviors and deliberate self-harm may need to be targeted during treatment. Imminent life-threatening behaviors are defined as follows:

- Actions, plans, desires, urges, or ideation, the goal of which is to intentionally cause tissue damage or death (for example, nonsuicidal self-injury, suicidal ideation or urges, suicide attempts)

- Behaviors that are not intentionally aimed at dying or causing tissue damage but are an imminent threat to life (imminent life-threatening behaviors take precedence over other targets or treatment goals; see chapter 4)

Thus, the therapist should be prepared to adjust her planned agenda for the session or may need to extend the orientation phase of treatment when imminent life-threatening behaviors are revealed, in order ensure client safety. In general, it is recommended that the therapist introduce the topic and begin the assessment approximately thirty minutes into the session (or midpoint). This allows some time to get to know the client and orient him to some aspects of the treatment (for example, the focus on overcontrol) yet allows sufficient time for a risk assessment and a suicide-prevention plan or self-injury-prevention plan, if needed.

The single most important risk factor for a completed suicide is a previous attempt. Essentially, the more recent the attempt, and the more lethal the means used, the higher the risk. An important outcome of this assessment is to obtain a commitment from a client who reports urges, thoughts, or plans to kill or harm himself in the near future that he will not engage in self-harm or attempt suicide before the next session and, ideally, will commit to working on eliminating self-harm and suicidal behaviors as a core aim of treatment. The therapist can use the following script to introduce a discussion of life-threatening behavior with an OC client:

Therapist: It turns out that research shows that many people struggling with the kinds of problems you are experiencing can get so depressed or hopeless that they start thinking about killing themselves or hurting themselves, and this can start at a young age. So what I would like to do next is spend some time talking about these types of issues with you in order to understand whether these types of issues have been a problem for you, and the extent to which we may need to focus on them during our work together. So my first question is…

At this point, to guide the discussion with a set of questions derived from clinical experience, the therapist can turn to the RO DBT Semistructured Suicidality Interview (appendix 4); the greater the number and the severity of the client's past or current problems involving self-harm or suicidal behavior, the more questions the therapist should expect to ask, and the more time the therapist should expect to spend on this topic.[42] The therapist should also feel free to augment this approach with structured interviews, such as suicide and self-injury assessment protocols (Linehan, 1993a, pp. 468–495), or self-report questionnaires, such as the Scale for Suicide Ideation (A. T. Beck, Kovacs, & Weissman, 1979) and the Adult Suicidal Ideation Questionnaire (W. M. Reynolds, 1991; Osman et al., 1999).

The RO DBT Crisis-Management Protocol

This protocol is only needed when an OC client reports urges to harm himself or kill himself in the near future (that is, the same day or before the week is out) or when there is a similar serious and imminent life-threatening event. The good news is that when working with OC clients, crisis management is rarely needed. OC clients are conscientious and cautious; they prefer stability and dislike chaos. Thus, for an OC client who has voluntarily chosen to participate in therapy, his sense of dutifulness is likely to make a crisis during the first session an unlikely event. From the OC client's perspective, since he was the person who decided to seek treatment, it seems unfair to tell a therapist he has just met that he plans on killing himself or engaging in self-harm the very next day or within days (that is, he hasn't given the therapy or therapist much of a chance). Yet therapists should not take this to mean they can relax. OC clients have high standards and are likely to expect quick results. Plus, if an OC client has a recent history of suicidal or self-injurious behavior, therapists can anticipate it to reemerge at some point during therapy; that is, old habits are hard to change.

The crisis intervention principles and strategies discussed in this section focus on management of imminent life-threatening behaviors with a client in the very first session but can also be applied to similar high-risk situations if they occur later in therapy. The protocol is activated whenever a client reports imminent life-threatening behavior but is unwilling to provide a commitment to the therapist not to kill himself prior to the next scheduled session. Although in general the steps outlined here are intended to be sequential, not every step has to be included. The goal is to end the session with the client's commitment not to kill himself (or cause himself serious harm) prior to the next session. Once this commitment has been obtained, the therapist can end the protocol and either move to another topic (if time remains in the session) or end the session altogether. It is important to engage in frequent check-ins about suicide risk level at each step. It is also important for either the therapist or a designee to remain with the suicidal or distressed client until risk is lowered.

RO DBT Crisis-Management Protocol

1. Thank the client for the gift of truth. Express your appreciation that he has been honest about his feelings (instead of hiding them), and link this to his therapeutic progress. Tell the client, for example, "Okay…I suppose the first thing I would like to say is thanks for being honest with me about what's going on inside."

2. Ask the client, "What set this off?" Say, for example, "Do you have a sense of what might have triggered your reaction?"

3. Ask the client to help you understand. Say, for example, "I am aware of imagining that at least part of your disclosure is also a social signal. What is it that you are trying to say to me or other people when you engage in self-harm or think about dying?"

4. Encourage criticism. Say, for example, "I am also thinking that perhaps the reason this might be happening is because I missed something, did something, or said something that triggered your reaction. Assuming this might be the case, can you tell me what I may have done to contribute to the problem?"

5. Validate feelings. Say, for example, "Based on your history, it's understandable that you are feeling despair."

6. Signal concern. For example, rather than trying to appear calm, signal caring by viscerally showing your distress.

7. Signal openness. Balance signals of concern with signals communicating openness. For example, while listening to the client, use an eyebrow wag. Lean back in your chair. Slow the pace of the conversation by taking a deep breath. Allow the client time to respond to questions or complete observations before you speak. Use openhanded gestures. Signal nondominance by shrugging your shoulders when uncertain. Maintain a musical tone of voice.

8. Take the heat off by taking a break. For example, suggest taking a brief walk together or getting some food or coffee before continuing the discussion. If the client is reluctant to take a break, acknowledge his wishes—"Okay, no problem"—but then ask, "But would you mind joining me as I make myself a cup of coffee?" The aim of this is not to get the client to have a cup of coffee but to change the emotional intensity of the discussion by altering the social or physical environment (that is, coffeemaking behavior is something done with family or friends). Essentially, the goal of a short break and shift in physical context is to provide the OC client the time and space to down-regulate and reconsider how he is behaving, without making a big deal of it. Thus, it's important for therapists to purposefully drop the discussion of the life-threatening behavior during the break unless the client independently brings it back up.

9. Focus on removing available lethal means. The aim is to work with the client on finding practical ways of removing objects in his environment (such as razor blades, pills, or guns) that can be used to cause self-harm or death. For example, obtain the client's commitment that he will flush down the toilet any pills that were to be used for a planned overdose and that he will text you afterward to confirm that the pills are no longer available.

10. Practice radical openness and self-enquiry by silently asking yourself, *To what extent am I willing to examine my personal responses to the client's behavior? What is it that I might need to learn?*

11. Explore the client's crisis behavior from the perspective of social signaling. Ask yourself, *What might the client be trying to tell me by behaving this way?*

12. Use a strong emotional appeal—for example, "Please stay"—to encourage the client to join you in finding an alternative solution to his dilemma, one that does not involve him taking his life, and let the client know that you care. Essentially, this message says, "Please stay with me. I care about you. Don't go away. Hang in there. We can sort this out. Give me a chance to help you."

13. Say to the client, "I believe in you." Signal that you believe he can get past this, despite his current suffering and despair. Ask him to give you a chance to sort things out. Remind him that he is early in treatment.

14. Say to the client, "You can't do this." Emphatically tell him that you don't want him to kill himself.

15. Say to the client, "Use your self-control." To stop self-harm or suicidal behavior, at least for the time being, encourage the client to take advantage of his superior capacity for self-control.

16. Encourage self-enquiry. Ask, "What is it that you might need to learn from this experience today? Is it possible that you are stronger than you think you are?"

17. Remind the client of his prior commitments. If the client has previously committed not to engage in self-harm or commit suicide, remind him of this commitment and of his core values linked to doing the right thing, honoring commitments, and having integrity.

18. Arrange for emergency backup. Make sure the client has emergency contact numbers.

19. Contract with the client not to engage in suicidal acts. Ask the client to call someone to pick him up or be with him as he travels home, if the client remains at high risk at the end of the session. If the client appears unwilling to make the call, offer to call for him.

20. Obtain contact information. Get phone numbers and email addresses of people who are in the client's support network.

21. Accompany the client to the emergency room, or call emergency services or the police if suicidality cannot be reduced, risk is high, no other support can be found, and the client refuses help.

Finally, the high social comparisons that characterize overcontrolled coping can result in frequent experiences of unhelpful envy and desires for revenge. OC individuals are more likely to hold grudges and believe that it is morally acceptable to punish a wrongdoer. Thus it is important to also assess desires for revenge and urges to harm others—at least briefly—during an initial OC client risk assessment. Contrary to common assumptions that all (or most) violent acts stem from poor impulse control, emotion dysregulation, and low distress tolerance (that is, undercontrolled coping), our work in forensic settings with violent criminal offenders and prior research have identified two subtypes of overcontrolled violent offenders (Hershorn & Rosenbaum, 1991; P. J. Lane & Kling, 1979; P. J. Lane & Spruill, 1980; Quinsey, Maguire, & Varney, 1983). Overcontrolled violent offenders are characterized as introverted, shy, timid, and apprehensive and have significantly lower criminal histories and less institutional misconduct, compared to other violent offenders. However, their acts of violence, though often occurring only on one occasion, are disproportionately more violent and more likely to be revenge-focused and planned, compared to the violence of nonovercontrolled offenders. An OC client's superior inhibitory control allows him to plan his revenge carefully, and his moral certitude can make physical harm directed toward others seem like the right thing to do (recall the Columbine massacre). Thus, when signaling a willingness to discuss past traumas and sexual issues (see the following section), it is also important to signal a willingness to discuss past grudges, revengeful desires or acts, and past violence.

Signaling Willingness to Discuss Past Traumas, Sexual Issues, and Grudges

Many OC clients have engaged in hurtful, vengeful, socially inappropriate, or passive-aggressive behaviors; have a history of abuse; or have sexual difficulties, fears, or problems that if not brought up first by the therapist are unlikely to be brought up by the client. For example, in one of the treatment development trials for RO DBT, we anecdotally noted that approximately 45 percent of clients were holding on to a past transgression, perceived mistake, or grudge (often for thirty years or longer; see T. R. Lynch & Cheavens, 2007). A client may have stolen mail from a neighbor who angered her, covertly sabotaged an envied colleague's career, punctured a transgressor's automobile tires, or intentionally spread false gossip. In addition, since most OC clients have struggled to form intimate relationships, it is not uncommon for them to have developed unusual, deviant, or peculiar sexual habits or behaviors (such as sex with animals, cross-dressing, anonymous sex with strangers or prostitutes, addiction to internet pornography, sexual fetishes, stalking behaviors, and fantasies or misinterpretations regarding the sexual intentions of others). These atypical sexual behaviors are rarely predatory in nature (as in forcible rape). Nonetheless, they are often a source of great shame and self-hatred or affirm a self-construct of being a fatally flawed outsider. Clients may never have discussed any of these issues with anyone in the past (a therapist or someone else), and strong desires to be seen as socially acceptable may make it difficult for them to bring such issues up on their own. Crucially, if these issues are not addressed at some point during treatment, it may be less likely for the client to genuinely rejoin the tribe because the secret shame associated with these behaviors helps maintain "outsider" convictions. Consequently, when treating OC, therapists should matter-of-factly orient the client to the possibility of long-standing grievances, shameful revengeful acts, and the presence of sexual issues early in treatment. The presence of these issues is usually assessed as an addendum to the suicide risk assessment:

Therapist: One of the things we know, based on research, is that a number of people have had painful experiences in their past or may have done things they feel ashamed about, such as holding a grudge for thirty years or harming someone. In addition, many people have had problems related to sex or sexual relations. So, although this is our first session, I thought it might be important for me to let you know that our therapy together can include discussion of any topic or issue you think is relevant or important, including past traumas, behaviors you may not be proud of, or sexual problems. We don't need to go into any detail today about these, but I thought it important to let you know that if you have anything related to these that you might at some point like to discuss, I am more than willing to do so. In fact, doing so might prove important. Does that make sense? Do you have any questions, or is there anything you might want to say, right now, about this?

If an OC client does reveal concerns related to such issues when queried, the therapist should adopt a nonjudgmental stance and, if possible, normalize or validate the behavior. For instance, the therapist can provide reassurance that differing sexual behaviors or expressions are common and normal and that it is understandable that the client developed this type of sexual behavior, considering how isolated and alone she has felt, or considering the struggles she has had locating romantic partners who share her values.

The general rule when working with OC clients is to delay detailed assessment of potentially embarrassing, shameful, or traumatizing experiences until a solid working relationship has been established (recall that this is not expected until the fourteenth session; see "Repairing Alliance Ruptures," chapter 4). Instead, therapists should thank clients for revealing the issue, highlight the importance of the issue, signal they are comfortable discussing the issue, and then assure clients that they intend to discuss the issue with them in the future. Well-intentioned attempts to explore these issues prior to the establishment of a solid working alliance can at the time they are discussed appear to go well but lead to treatment dropout. The most typical response by an OC client might look something like this: The client reveals, when asked about sexual issues, a previously undisclosed atypical sexual behavior (for example, cross-dressing). The therapist, recognizing the potential significance of this, asks the client for more details. The client, believing it important to comply with the therapist, or desiring to be a good client, complies by revealing more details, which triggers intense emotion that the client is unable to fully control (for example, he may become tearful or cry). The session ends with the client reporting that he found the session very helpful, that he is feeling fine, that he appreciates the efforts of the therapist, and that he is looking forward to the next session. Three days later, the therapist receives an email from the client stating that he is dropping out of treatment because he has decided that this type of therapy is not for him, with a request that the therapist not attempt to contact him about this issue, because his decision is final.

The preceding scenario has many different versions, most of which don't have a happy outcome. The problem is not the targeting by the therapist—learning how to make contact with and disclose emotionally charged experiences and vulnerability is a core target in treatment of OC. The problem is timing—the therapist assumed her relationship with the client was stronger than it actually was and that the client's self-reports of feeling fine and appreciating her efforts were accurate indicators of his inner experience. Instead, however, the client's outward calm actually reflected inward numbness or shutdown responses secondary to overwhelming threat and partial activation of the PNS-DVC (see chapter 2). The preceding example represents the powerful influence biotemperament can have when working with OC clients (the client's innate self-control had been successfully regulating attention away from the emotionally charged event) and also highlights the importance of sequencing treatment strategies when working with hyper-threat-sensitive clients. For example, discussing the same problem at a later stage in therapy is likely (in our experience) to be much more helpful for the client. Exceptions to this include times when an OC client hints at the existence of urges to exact revenge or punish others. When this occurs, therapists should assess the behavior more thoroughly at the time it is reported (regardless of the stage of treatment) in order to determine the extent to which the behavior should be targeted as representing high risk.

When the Client Wants to Drop Out of Therapy

Our quest to understand the inner experience of an OC client has repeatedly revealed that things aren't always as they seem. Over the years, as a consequence, our clinical research team has recognized the importance of building into the treatment a means of blocking OC clients' automatic tendencies to walk away or abandon relationships when conflict emerges. It involves obtaining a commitment from the client in the first RO DBT session (most often just before the session ends) to return in person and discuss any desire to drop out of treatment before actually doing so. It works by taking advantage of the OC tendency to value the importance of keeping a promise and the high OC sense of moral duty and obligation. Our clinical and research experience has demonstrated that obtaining this commitment (and reobtaining it frequently throughout the course of therapy) functions to substantially reduce the possibility of premature termination of therapy (see chapter 8 for details). Here is a script that touches on the essential points of asking for this commitment:

> Research shows that it is likely that at some point during our work together you may not feel like coming to therapy, or you may want to drop out of treatment. What I would like to ask is if you would be willing to commit to coming back in person to discuss your concerns before you actually make the decision to drop out. Would you be willing to give me this commitment?

Eliciting the Client's Commitment to Attend RO Skills Training Classes

During the second session, the therapist should briefly outline the rationale and structure of the RO skills training classes. The client's commitment should then be obtained to attend the very next scheduled class. The therapist should discuss skills training in a matter-of-fact way that signals class attendance as important, expected, and something that the client will enjoy. The skills training component is referred to as a "class" rather than "group therapy" because this accurately reflects its primary purpose of learning new skills, not processing feelings or providing feedback to other class members.

Therapists should not assume that OC clients will automatically resist participating in skills classes or find the idea of a group skills class frightening. Well-intentioned attempts by a therapist to prepare a socially anxious OC client prior to attending the first class can signal that fear is justified and also unnecessarily lengthen the commitment process, sometimes for months. It is like telling someone that horses are not dangerous while placing full body armor on the person prior to the first ride. Therapists can also be influenced by the opinions of other professionals, or by warnings from family members about how a client might be expected to respond, and as a consequence may unintentionally reinforce avoidance. Thus it is important for therapists to examine their own personal reactions whenever they observe strong desires to prepare, soothe, or behave cautiously when introducing the necessity of attending skills classes. The following questions can help: *What do I fear might happen if I do not behave cautiously? Is it possible that I am treating the client as fragile? Why do I believe it is so important to prepare the client for class participation? Is it possible that I have been subtly shaped by my prior experiences, or by this client, to assume that skills classes will prove extremely difficult for her?*

The best approach is to behave in a manner that communicates confidence in the client's ability to attend the class and in a manner that is not defensive, coercive, or apologetic. If needed, clients can be reminded that they already have a great deal of experience in similar situations (that is, most OC clients have been highly successful in school and similar classroom settings; attending an RO skills training class is like going back to school; the focus is on the material being taught, not the individual being taught). Therapists can also matter-of-factly emphasize the importance of receiving a full dose of treatment—for example, not attending skills classes is like deciding to take only half a dose of antibiotics to cure a severe infection. The attitude needed is similar to one adopted by a nurse in a hospital who requests a client to undress and put on a hospital gown before surgery; despite the fact that most people experience anxiety or mild embarrassment when asked to do this, the nurse, via a relaxed and matter-of-fact tone, communicates that the request is a routine part of treatment, not a problem.

Third and Fourth Sessions

The third and fourth sessions of the orientation and commitment phase are designed to introduce some of the core features of RO DBT that set it apart from other approaches (such as its emphasis on social signaling) and begin the process of establishing individualized treatment targets. Two core teaching scripts are used to facilitate the introduction of the RO DBT biosocial theory for overcontrol and the core RO DBT hypothesized mechanism of change linking the communicative functions of emotion to the formation of close social bonds essential for individual and species well-being. A key task during these sessions is for therapists to identify important valued goals that will be used to guide the development of treatment targets over the course of treatment.

Global Aims and Topics for the Third and Fourth Sessions

- Identifying four to five valued goals that are important for the client, with at least one pertaining to social connectedness

- Teaching the biosocial theory for overcontrol (typically in the third session)

- Teaching the key mechanism of change, linking open expression of emotion to increased trust and social connectedness and to the importance of social signaling in human relationships (typically in the fourth session)

- Introducing the RO DBT diary card (typically in the fourth session)

Identifying Values and Goals Linked to Social Connectedness

Values are the principles or standards that a person considers important in life and that ideally function to guide how a person lives his life. They help us determine our priorities in life and help us assess the degree to which our life is turning out the way we envisioned it. When our way of living matches our values, we experience a sense of contentment or satisfaction, whereas when we fail to live by our values, we often feel an underlying dissatisfaction or discomfort. Goals are the means by which a personal value is achieved—they are how we express our values. Valued goals represent a combination of both constructs. Thus, if a person values family, her valued goal might be to find a romantic partner. Valued goals change over time, depending on our stage in life or life circumstances. Plus, how they are expressed and the importance assigned to them will vary as a function both of culture and of individual experience.

Perhaps not surprisingly, OC clients tend to underreport values and goals that have obvious links to interpersonal relationships (such as a goal of being intimate with another person) and overreport valued goals associated with self-improvement (to work harder), autonomy (to live independently), achievement (to be productive), and self-control (to think before they act). Examples of common OC values linked to self-control include competency, achievement, restraint, temperance, fairness, politeness, self-sacrifice, accuracy, integrity, service, responsibility, dedication, self-improvement, honesty, accountability, and discipline.

Yet all of these values depend upon a social context for meaning; that is, they are virtuous not just because they are difficult to live by but also because they function to contribute to the well-being of one's tribe. For example, values for service, fairness, and honesty are cherished because they place the needs of others over the needs of the individual. RO DBT posits that our core values as a species are considered "good" because they function to contribute to the well-being of our tribe. This is why most people dislike being labeled selfish or self-centered. Our unique capacity to form strong social bonds, work together, and share valuable resources with genetically dissimilar others is unprecedented in the animal world. Even values for independence contribute to the welfare of others by lessening the need for assistance. Thus our cooperative nature represents a core part of who we are as a species, and our values reflect this.

Consequently, when identifying valued goals with an OC client, it is important not to rely solely on clients' self-reports, particularly when a client reports no valued goals directly linked to social connectedness. Since OC is fundamentally a problem of emotional loneliness, it is essential for therapists to help OC clients find at least one valued goal linked to intimate relationships. To facilitate this, it can help to reframe an OC client's valued goals as fundamentally prosocial, thereby circumventing protests or contentions from the client that he doesn't care about people or need others. For example, valuing correctness, accuracy, and high performance is essential for tribal success. Valuing rules and fairness is needed in order to resist powerful individuals who intentionally harm or exploit others for personal gain, whereas valuing prudence and restraint helps save valuable resources for less abundant times. Linking OC valued goals to the benefits they provide for society helps smuggle the idea to despairing, isolated, and highly self-critical OC clients that not all of their behavior is negative (which is what many inwardly believe) and can help them take the first step toward rejoining their tribe.

Thus, according to RO DBT, valued goals function both to guide our actions and to socially signal our intentions to others. The good news is that we can adjust our social signaling to support living by our values. For example, if you value being fair-minded, then signal openness by allowing time for the other person to respond to questions or complete observations before jumping in with your opinion, whereas if your valued goal is to be taken seriously, then signal gravity and confidence by looking the other person in the eye, speaking calmly but firmly, and keeping your shoulders back and chin up. And if you value being forthright and honest, then—when the situation calls for it—express what you are feeling inside on the outside. Therapists can begin to introduce these core RO DBT principles early in therapy. Most OC clients immediately grasp their significance and are eager to learn more. However, to match social signaling to valued goals, one must first know what one values.

Yet identifying valued goals can be difficult—many people struggle with knowing what they want or desire out of life because they have spent a lifetime focusing on what they *don't* want. Therapists can facilitate values clarification by asking questions such as these:

- When it comes to family, friends, and work, what are the things you consider most important?

- What attributes do you admire in others?

- What ideals would you consider important to teach a child?

- How would you like others to describe you? How would you like others to describe you at your funeral?

Plus, for some clients, to further facilitate values clarification, it can be useful to assign as homework worksheet 10.A ("Flexible Mind Is DEEP: Identifying Valued Goals"), found in the skills training manual.

However, valued goals can also be obtained less formally, which can often prove therapeutic for rule-governed OC clients (formal assessments using written materials may inadvertently reinforce compulsive desires for structure and order). Informal values clarification begins by noticing what appears to be important for a client— that is, our values are often reflected in the words we use to describe ourselves and the things we like or dislike about other people or the world. For example, a client reporting that she is not easily impressed may be signaling a value for precision and thoughtfulness, whereas a client reporting anger at a neighbor for telling him how to improve his internet connection might value independence or self-sufficiency. Therapists can help clients identify their values in these moments by asking about the value behind a reaction or statement: "It sounds like you value independence and solving problems on your own. Do you think this might have been linked to the way you responded to your neighbor?" The advantage of this type of interactive dialogue is that it smuggles the idea of self-exploration, and therapists can model radical openness when guesses are rejected by a client by not holding on to their guesses as truth. Sometimes simply asking a relevant question is all that is needed to pull out a valued goal. For instance, a client was discussing that she no longer had relationships with her grown son and daughter, and her daughter had recently had her first grandchild. The therapist might simply ask, "Would you like an improved relationship with your children?" If the client says yes, this can be highlighted as a treatment goal linked to values for close social bonds. The therapist can delve deeper by assessing the degree to which the client's family problems might function to exacerbate her distress.

Discovering valued goals and linking them to problem behaviors and emotional reactions can help OC clients begin to recognize that most of their difficulties, although often self-created, arise from heartfelt desires to live according to prosocial values. For example, the OC client who is horrified by her emotional leakage on a bus after yelling at a passenger for not giving up his seat for an elderly person can be encouraged to recognize that her leakage represents a social signaling error rather than a fundamental flaw in her character and the source of her emotional outburst stems from a prosocial value (that is, a value to care for those in need). Ideally, by the end of the commitment and orientation phase (that is, the first four sessions), the therapist and client have mutually identified four to five valued goals, with at least one pertaining to social connectedness.

> Discovering valued goals and linking them to problem behaviors and emotional reactions can help OC clients begin to recognize that most of their difficulties, although often self-created, arise from heartfelt desires to live according to prosocial values.

The importance of values clarification when treating problems of overcontrol cannot be overstated. OC clients are perfectionists who tend to see mistakes everywhere (including in themselves) and work harder than most others to prevent future problems. Thus, rather than focusing on what's wrong, values clarification focuses on what's right by identifying what a client wants or desires out of life (that is, his valued goals), which facilitates engagement in therapy; committing to change is easier when a person is able to recognize that it is his own behavior that appears to be blocking him from achieving his valued goals.

Here are some examples of values and goals:

To raise a family

To be a warm and helpful parent to one's children

To be gainfully and happily employed

To be more spiritual or self-aware

To find more time to contribute to others

To find more time to relax and fully appreciate one's life

To develop or improve close relationships

To form a romantic partnership

To develop a wider network of friends

To behave more altruistically toward others or be more nonjudgmental

To get married

To be better educated (go to college or university)

To participate more freely in community activities or events

To be able to dance, sing, or socialize without self-consciousness

To learn compassion for self and others

To learn how to forgive oneself or others

To be more open to feedback and others

To laugh easily

To play more often

To find time for oneself

To accept those things that cannot be changed, without hopeless resignation or despair

Teaching the Biosocial Theory for Overcontrol

An important goal of the orientation and commitment stage is to help OC clients learn more about overcontrolled coping. Providing a brief overview of the RO DBT biosocial theory for overcontrol is an important part of this. As outlined in detail in chapter 2, the theory contends that an OC style of coping develops from transactions between biotemperamental predispositions for heightened threat sensitivity, diminished reward sensitivity, high inhibitory control, and preoccupation with details, and these biotemperamental dispositions are posited to transact with early family, environmental, or cultural experiences emphasizing mistakes as intolerable, achievement as essential, and self-control as imperative. The individual learns that if she avoids unplanned risk, masks inner feelings, and adopts an aloof interpersonal style, she can avoid making mistakes or appearing out of control. Unfortunately, overcontrolled coping has hidden costs. Avoidance of unplanned risks makes new learning less likely, masking inner feelings makes it harder for others to know you, and behaving in an aloof and distant manner makes it more likely for people to avoid you. Plus, excessive self-control is exhausting.

Teaching the OC biosocial theory should be planned for the third session (see "Four Steps for Teaching the Biosocial Theory for Overcontrol in the Third Session," page 129). It represents the second of three discussions occurring during the orientation and commitment phase of RO DBT that are fully scripted. As in the first scripted discussion (see "Four Steps for Identifying Overcontrol as the Core Problem in the First Session," earlier in this chapter), the overview of the OC biosocial theory should be limited to approximately ten minutes, and therapists are strongly encouraged to stick to the script. Teaching the OC biosocial theory should only occur if a client has agreed that OC represents his style of coping and has committed to target maladaptive overcontrol as a core part of treatment (see the commitment protocols for the first and second sessions). Therapists should feel free not to cover every single aspect of the theory, since it will reappear multiple times throughout treatment. What follows is a transcript of a therapist teaching the biosocial theory for OC:

Therapist: As I mentioned during our agenda setting today, one of the things I want to do today is tell you about the RO DBT biosocial theory for overcontrol. Are you okay with us doing this now?

Client: Sure. I definitely want to know more.

Therapist: Okay. The biosocial theory posits that overcontrolled coping is the result of three transacting elements. The first pertains to biological and genetic influences—or nature. The second pertains to family history, learning, and culture—or nurture. And the third pertains to OC coping itself—or coping. The nature component of the model posits that, just like we are all born with different eye colors, we are all born with different brains, and our brain influences how we perceive the world. Now, imagine a person born with a brain that is highly detail-focused. They can see the trees, but they often miss the forest. Thus their brain is hardwired to automatically notice minor errors, like a misplaced comma. Plus, their brain is also hardwired to notice the potential for harm over the potential for reward in any given situation. So when they walk into a rose garden, their brain automatically notices the thorns more than the flowers, or going to a party seems potentially dangerous, not fun. They also possess a biological predisposition for being able to inhibit impulses or emotional expression, so they might feel anxious on the inside but are able not to show it on the outside. When you think of yourself, now or as a child, to what extent do you think this might describe how you cope or perceive the world?

Client: Well, not only do I obsess about details, I definitely notice the thorns. When I walk into a room, I immediately start scanning for signs of disapproval. Very few people know about this, because I am expert at not showing it. I guess I'm one of those downers—one of those people who always see the cup half empty.

Therapist: Okay, that makes sense to me. Now imagine this very same person growing up in a family, a culture, or social environment that highly values self-control, performance, and not making mistakes. Do you think you were ever given the message that mistakes were intolerable, that you could always do better, or that it was important to never show emotion?

Client: Of course. I've known that for some time. My family—in particular, my mother—has a long history of insisting that things be done right. We were expected not to complain or cry. Whining was for losers. I learned early on not to make waves. I was always told that I should be better than other people—and that I could do better. I suppose the message was that I was never good enough.

Therapist: I really appreciate your sharing this. What you said fits with the kind of messages that a lot of people with OC have said about their past.

Client: Yeah, that makes sense.

Therapist: Great. So—back to our imagined person. The third component of the theory pertains to OC coping that emerges from the first two elements, which are nature and nurture. Perhaps the question now becomes, what might this highly threat-sensitive yet controlled person learn to do? How might they cope?

Client: Yeah, that is a good question. I suppose I just started to become quieter and quieter, and more aloof from people every day. I felt like an outsider.

Therapist: That makes sense, based on what you've told me. When we go back to our imagined overcontrolled person, one aspect of the theory posits that a child may avoid taking risks so as not to ever make a mistake. Unfortunately, the only way to learn is to take a risk. Also, they might learn to avoid showing any vulnerability, even when distressed, in order to avoid appearing out of control. And, as a result of this, they may tend to mask their inner feelings—which, as research shows, makes it harder to make friends. Plus, they may acquire an aloof and distant relationship style, making them slow to warm up in new relationships. What are the pros and cons of behaving this way? How do you think this way of coping might be linked to depression or interpersonal relationships?

From here, the therapist and the client continued to explore how the client's temperamental threat sensitivity and family, cultural, and environmental influences may have functioned to lead to an OC coping style. Additional discussions of the biosocial theory in later sessions helped refine treatment targets pertaining to difficulties in revealing inner feelings, showing vulnerability, and pretending not to care about relationships.

Four Steps for Teaching the Biosocial Theory for Overcontrol in the Third Session

1. *Say:* Just as we are all born with different eye colors, we are all born with different brains. Our brain influences how we perceive the world. Now, imagine a person born with a brain that is more sensitive to negative things and less sensitive to positive things. When this person walks into a rose garden, his or her brain is more likely to notice the thorns than the flowers. When you think about yourself, now or as a child, do you think you've tended to notice the flowers or the thorns more?

2. *Say:* Imagine this same person growing up in a family, a culture, or a social environment that highly values self-control, performance, and not making mistakes. Do you think in any way your family or early environment could have given you the message that mistakes are intolerable, or that you should strongly avoid ever showing weakness or vulnerability?

3. *Say:* What might this person learn to do? What ways of coping do you think you learned from these expectations or family rules, so to speak?

4. *Say:* First, this person might avoid taking risks, so as not to ever make a mistake. Second, this person might learn to avoid showing any vulnerability, even when distressed, in order to avoid appearing out of control, by masking inner feelings or keeping a poker face. Third, this person might learn to be cautious when getting to know new people, which might lead others to believe that this person is aloof and distant. What are the pros and cons of behaving in this way? How do you think overcontrolled coping might be linked to some of the problems you are seeking treatment for today? How might it impact other areas of your life, such as your relationships or your success in living according to your valued goals?

Linking Social Signaling to Social Connectedness

Typically by the fourth session, the therapist is ready to discuss the key mechanism hypothesized to lead to an OC client's sense of isolation, ostracism, and loneliness. The discussion of this topic (see "Four Steps for Teaching That Open Expression = Trust = Social Connectedness in the Fourth Session," page 131–132) represents the last of the three that are fully scripted and that occur during the orientation and commitment phase of RO DBT. It is also the most challenging of the three because it is the first to provide direct corrective feedback. The good news is that OC clients are stronger than you think (or even *they* think). The therapist should adopt a stance that communicates confidence in the client's capacity for self-examination while simultaneously signaling a willingness to be open to feedback. Plus, it should be explained that this topic will be revisited multiple times throughout course of treatment.

Like the two scripted discussions presented earlier in this chapter, this one should be collaborative and time-limited (ten minutes) and should allow time for questions. In the first step, the therapist asks the client if he is familiar with research examining the negative effects associated with inhibiting emotional expression, and the therapist corrects any misinformation before proceeding. What follows is a session transcript of a therapist introducing the topic:

Therapist:	One of the things I wanted to talk about today was the key mechanism of change in RO DBT, or the factor that is believed to be the primary underlying factor for treatment success. Last week you mentioned that you have learned not to show your feelings to others—that way, you couldn't be hurt.
Client:	I always was a wallflower—don't think it, don't show it, stay out of trouble. But I also felt different from the other kids.
Therapist:	Well, there is growing research showing that hiding feelings and not expressing our emotions can actually lead to being socially ostracized. Have you ever heard about anything like that?
Client:	Nope. I eventually came to the conclusion that everyone was fake and phony. But this sounds different.
Therapist:	I'm imagining that you are starting to consider how some of the ways you learned to cope with your anxiety and other emotions—not only when you were young but also now as an adult—kept you safe but also had some downsides, too. Am I sensing things correctly?
Client:	I think I am beginning to understand this more. I was an outsider, always looking in, and angry that others seemed to find it easy. It was a…oh, wait, it *is* a lonely existence. *(Pauses.)* Eventually, I just assumed I was better off without relationships. *(Smiles.)*
Therapist:	Being or feeling on the outside of one's tribe is not a lot of fun.

The second step in this scripted discussion is perhaps the most important. It begins with the therapist telling a story that is related to the topic of social signaling but unrelated to the specific social signaling style most often exhibited by the client. This takes the heat off the client without losing the point of the discussion. While telling the story, it is essential for the therapist to act out or model the social signaling deficits of the protagonist in the story rather than intellectually describing or talking about what the social signals might look like. This allows the OC client to viscerally experience what it might feel like to be on the receiving end of her own social signaling deficits, but without having her nose rubbed in it. The two recommended stories presented later in this chapter playfully demonstrate how constrained and disingenuous expressions can negatively impact the social environment. The first story, "'Twas a Lovely Affair," is about a coworker with a fake smile; the second story, "I Have Some Really Exciting News," is about a coworker with a flat, frozen affect. Only one story should be used, and the therapist should pick the story that is least likely to reflect the social signaling style of the client. Thus, if the client tends to be more flat-faced during interactions, the therapist should choose to tell the first story (about the coworker with the fake smile), whereas the second story (about the flat-faced coworker) should be used when working with an OC client who tends to socially signal in an overly agreeable or phony manner. Choosing the style opposite to that of the OC client is working with functions to take the heat off the client by not making the story about her, while playfully keeping the heat on by providing an opportunity for the client to be on the receiving end of a social signaling deficit.

Four Steps for Teaching That Open Expression = Trust = Social Connectedness in the Fourth Session

1. *Say:* As I mentioned at the start of our session, one of the things I want to talk about today is the key hypothesized mechanism of change in RO DBT. It is based on the assumption that our species' survival depended on our ability to form long-lasting bonds and work together in tribes or groups. This evolutionary advantage required the development of complex social signaling capabilities that allowed for a quick and safe means to evaluate and/or resolve conflict and manage potential collaborations. Thus, when it comes to being part of a tribe, social signaling matters! Plus, in support of this, research shows that what may matter most in intimate relationships is not what is said but how it is said. What comes to mind when I say this? Have you ever heard about anything like that before?

2. *Say:* Okay, but before we proceed, rather than just talking about social signaling, I would like to conduct a little demonstration that I hope you will find both entertaining and educational. (Use one of the recommended stories to ensure a pithy delivery[a] and maximize client learning and engagement; see "'Twas a Lovely Affair" or "I Have Some Really Exciting News,"[b] later in this chapter.) After the demonstration, ask: What was it like to interact with the person I was role-playing? Would you like to spend more or less time with this person after this interaction? What might this tell us about the importance of social signaling?[c]

3. *Say:* The way you responded to my extremely odd social signaling behavior is exactly how most people would respond.[d] Plus, there has been a wide range of research reporting similar conclusions. For example, experimental research has shown that suppressing emotional expression interferes with communication, impedes relationship development, and increases anxious arousal in both the suppressor and those with whom they interact. Interestingly, a wide range of studies have also shown that people like people who openly and freely express their emotions, even when they are negative—they are perceived as more genuine and trustworthy, compared to those who suppress or mask their emotions. To what extent do you think

your social signaling style impacts your social relationships? How frequently do you openly reveal inner experience or vulnerable emotions to another person?

4. *Say:* Okay, it seems that we both agree that how a person social signals really matters, especially when it comes to long-term intimate relationships.[e] However, it is perhaps equally important to recognize that open expression does not mean expressing emotions without awareness or consideration. On the contrary, effective emotional expression is always context-dependent. Lastly, it is important that we take our time to learn more about your social signaling style before deciding to target it for change. What do you think or feel when I say this? How willing are you, in this moment, to target social signaling in our work together?

[a]   It is essential for the therapist to mimic or playact the facial expression and voice tone of the central character. This enables the OC client to viscerally understand (in his or her body) the impact that social signaling has on others.

[b]   Key point: Always pick the story that is least likely to reflect the social signaling style of the client.

[c]   The therapist should be prepared to discuss supporting research (for details, see especially chapter 2). For example, a number of studies have shown that people become anxiously aroused when interacting with a nonexpressive person and prefer not to spend time with that person, and emotionally constricted children have been shown not only to experience more peer rejection during childhood but also to be more likely to become increasingly depressed, anxious, and socially isolated over time.

[d]   This statement assumes that the client has reported finding the social signaling style portrayed by the therapist to be off-putting.

[e]   It is important for the therapist be prepared for and to address self-deprecating statements and Fatalistic Mind thinking from some clients—for example, "This just proves that I'm no good, because if what you say is true, then I could have fixed myself years ago." (For an explanation of the concept of Fatalistic Mind, see the skills training manual, chapter 5, lesson 11.) The therapist should help a client who responds in this manner to recognize that getting down on himself for not recognizing a problem earlier is not only a good way to stay miserable but also to avoid the necessity of having to change. The therapist should encourage the client to practice seeing problems as opportunities (for new learning and growth). From an RO DBT perspective, if you hate the color purple but live in a purple house, you can't do anything about it until you notice that your house is purple.

"'Twas a Lovely Affair"

For this story, it is essential that the therapist put on an overly polite or pro-social voice and a phony smile that remains frozen whenever he or she is speaking the words attributed to the coworker. Seeing a phony smile enables the client to viscerally experience what it would be like to interact with that person; without the phony smile, the learning that is possible from this story would remain intellectual rather than experiential. A phony smile involves moving only the lips, with the eyes flat, and with the eyebrows kept still. The therapist should also exaggerate the phoniness of the smile, displaying his or her teeth while making sure the smile remains static. This drives home the point of the story, and it smuggles humor as well as the notion of not taking oneself too seriously:

Therapist: Imagine that you're out to lunch with a new coworker, and during the meal she reveals some very personal information. *(Begins smiling.)* While smiling and nodding, she says, "Last night I discovered that my husband is having an affair." *(Keeps smiling.)* "Plus, I found out we are now bankrupt because he has spent all of our money on the other woman." *(Keeps smiling.)* "So I decided to set fire to the house." *(Keeps smiling.)* "How was your evening?"

After reading the story aloud, the therapist asks the client to respond to the following questions:

- What would you think or feel if you interacted with someone who behaved like this?

- Did the coworker's description of her evening warrant smiling?

- Would you like to spend more or less time with this coworker after this interaction?

- What emotion was the coworker likely feeling but not showing? (Answer: Most likely bitter anger.)

- How might this impact a relationship?

"I Have Some Really Exciting News"

For this story, it is essential that the therapist put on a completely unemotional, flat facial expression and use a flat tone of voice whenever he or she is speaking the words attributed to the coworker. Seeing a flat face enables the client to viscerally experience what it would be like to interact with the person described in the story; without the flat face, the learning that is possible from this story would remain intellectual rather than experiential. In order to read the story effectively, the therapist will have to behave like a zombie. This drives home the point of the story and smuggles in the idea that it's okay to be silly, and that learning can still happen even—and perhaps especially—when one is having fun:

Therapist: *(Using normal tone of voice)* Imagine that you're out to lunch with a different coworker. During the meal, he reveals some very exciting news. *(Begins using a flat face and a monotone.)* He says, "Last night I discovered that I won ten million dollars in the lottery. I was thrilled." (*Continues flat face and monotone.*) "Plus it was Steven Spielberg, the movie director, calling from Hollywood. He had just read the script that I'd sent him on a whim, and said he loved it so much that he was sending first-class tickets to fly me to Los Angeles to discuss making my script into a movie. I was so happy." (*Continues flat face and monotone.*) "Can you pass me the salt?"

After reading the story aloud, the therapist asks the client to respond to the following questions:

- What would you think or feel if you interacted with someone who behaved like this?

- Did the coworker's description of his evening warrant a flat face?

- When we are flat-faced, what are we signaling?

- How might this impact a relationship?

After telling the story, the therapist should discuss with the client what the client observed and learned from the story and then use this to move back to the script and assess willingness on the client's part to target social signaling as a core part of treatment. The transcript that follows shows how a therapist transitioned from the story back to the client and obtained commitment to target social signaling as a core part of therapy:

Therapist: Now that we have had fun with our story, I am curious. Do you think it's possible that your habit of not expressing vulnerable feelings to others may have inadvertently affected your relationships?

Client: Yeah. I hate to admit it—my blank face is my suit of armor.

Therapist: Sometimes, though, it might be nice to take off the armor. (*Chuckles slightly.*) After all, it must get hot in there sometimes. (*Pauses.*) What is really strange, though, is that research shows that open expression and self-disclosure, instead of making people run away, are actually perceived by others as a safety signal. We tend to trust those who freely express their emotions, particularly when the situation calls for it. It seems that when we take our armor off, others feel that it is safe to take theirs off, too, and then we can all have a picnic! (*Laughs.*)

Client: (*Smiles*) Yeah, I see your point. I guess it would be hard to eat a sandwich with a helmet on. (*Chuckles.*)

Therapist: I am glad we are discussing this, because this is one of the things we believe may be keeping you stuck in some way, with both your depression and your anxiety, but also making you feel like an outsider. Would you be willing to consider working on changing this in some way?

Client: What? You want me to just start expressing myself willy-nilly?

Therapist: *(Senses a potential alliance rupture)* No, certainly not! And don't you dare start! *(Smiles.)* Actually, though, perhaps just a little bit, with the understanding that open expression will not involve simply having you go out and express emotions without awareness or consideration. On the contrary, effective emotional expression is always context-dependent. What I would like to start working on with you is the idea of learning how to take off your armor when the situation might call for it. I think in some ways you've been doing this already in our relationship. How does this feel to you?

Client: A bit scary.

Therapist: *(Uses soft tone of voice)* Yeah, makes sense. It's hard to change habits. What is most important is that we work at a pace that makes sense to you. We will not lose the essence of who you are. You have a style of your own, and we don't want to change everything—that just doesn't make sense. How are you feeling now, right in this moment?

Therapists should be alert for and block harsh self-judgments, and clients can be reminded that social signaling styles are influenced by a wide range of biotemperamental and sociobiographical factors. Thus, although each of us is responsible for how we socially signal, our social signaling can be highly influenced by factors outside our control. The good news for the client is that she is now more aware of how her social signaling may impact others, making change more likely. Plus, RO DBT is designed specifically to target social signaling deficits, particularly those that negatively impact social connectedness.

Therapists should also emphasize that effective emotional expression is always context-dependent; sometimes constraint or controlled expression is what is needed to be effective, avoid unnecessary damage, or live by one's values (consider a police officer arresting a suspect, or a game of poker, or a charged discussion with one's adolescent child). Plus, therapists should explain that the goal of treatment is not to completely change how clients express themselves, because everyone has a unique style. There is no right or optimal way to socially signal; each of us has our own unique style of expression. What is important is that our style actually functions to communicate our intentions and inner experiences to other people, especially those we desire a close relationship with.

Finally, during the orientation and commitment stage of RO DBT, therapists should not feel compelled to go into greater detail than what has been described so far in this chapter. The aim is to smuggle a few new ideas to spur new ways of thinking and behaving over time, with the understanding that the topic will reappear multiple times over the course of therapy.

Introducing the RO DBT Diary Card

Diary cards are designed as a means for the client to record the presence, frequency, or intensity of targeted behaviors on a daily basis, with an emphasis on social signaling targets. The therapeutic rationale for a daily diary card should be explained to the client, usually during the fourth session. The rationale includes the following considerations:

- Diary cards enhance memory about problematic events that will be analyzed during individual therapy.

- Diary cards reduce the amount of time spent determining the session's agenda by providing a quick overview of the client's prior week.

- Monitoring the frequency of a behavior can often change the behavior.

- Diary cards can be used to monitor treatment progress and remind clients to practice skills.

Diary cards are reviewed each week at the beginning of the individual therapy session (including use of skills), and a blank card is provided each week to the client at the end of the session. Diary cards should not be reviewed during group skills training classes because this limits time for teaching. In RO DBT, diary cards are intended solely to be used in individual therapy.

Therapists should obtain their clients' commitment to discuss any desires not to complete the diary cards before the clients stop filling them out. The following transcript provides an example of obtaining this agreement:

Therapist: As I mentioned, the diary card is a really important part of treatment. It will not only speed things up for us but also be a way for us to assess your commitment to change and to treatment. Since we both know that you are here to change *(Smiles)*—that is, here for treatment—we can assume this means you want to feel or get better. Is that true?

(Client nods in ageement.)

Therapist: So I think it is important for you to know that if for some reason you don't complete a diary card, regardless of the reason, I will consider this a nonengagement signal that suggests the presence of an alliance rupture. This means either that you are not finding the treatment relevant to your unique problems or that you feel misunderstood. Most often it means that my treatment targeting is poor—that is, it usually means that you don't find the targets I have identified interesting or personally relevant. So I would like to ask for a commitment that you talk to me in person about your problems with completing the diary cards before you stop using them. Would you be willing to do this?

This commitment strategy works to enhance diary card completion by taking advantage of the OC client's natural tendencies for dutifulness and dislike of the limelight. The efficacy of commitment involves the highlighting of a noncompleted diary card as a social signal (that is, a signal that an alliance rupture has occurred). When presenting the concept of the diary card for the first time, the therapist should not rush to cover every possible target or explain every detail on the diary card. In fact, not covering every detail on the card provides the perfect (pun intended) opportunity for clients to practice letting go of rigid needs for structure and perfect understanding. This opportunity should ideally be revealed in a slightly tongue-in-cheek or playfully irreverent manner by therapists. Finally, it should be explained to clients that the primary targets on the diary card will be social signaling behaviors (for more about diary cards, see chapter 9).

Commitment Problems Unique to Overcontrol

OC threat hypersensitivity combined with tendencies to mask inner feelings can make the task of gaining genuine commitment a daunting enterprise. Therapists may find OC clients readily agreeing and committing to treatment principles and expectations early on, only to later discover extreme ambivalence, strong aversion, or anger directed toward the treatment or the therapist. It can appear suddenly and without apparent warning. Additionally, OC self-disclosures, particularly early in treatment, may not necessarily reflect inner experience, and OC declarations of commitment may be based on misinformation or differing expectations about what therapy should be. Many OC clients, for instance, fail to comprehend the radical nature of the changes that may be needed or may fail to grasp that practicing new skills, self-enquiry, and openness can sometimes be humbling, disconcerting, and embarrassing. Furthermore, most OC individuals consider it important to be respectful, dutiful, and polite when in public or when they first meet someone. Early in therapy, they may agree, comply, or commit out of a sense of obligation or duty rather than actual agreement or understanding. At the same time, they may consider it improper to disagree with a person in a position of authority (that is, the therapist). Client politeness, commitment, agreement, and positive reports by OC clients should be viewed as possibilities rather than truths.

It is not uncommon for an OC client to report that she has found prior experiences of psychotherapy humiliating, embarrassing, exposing, or fear-evoking, and as a consequence she may have a history of premature dropout. Experiences of humiliation may have followed emotional leakage, those times when the OC individual's self-control failed and her inner feelings were revealed or expressed more intensely than she would have preferred. This control failure is considered a sign of weakness or a source of embarrassment or shame. Unjustified fears of emotional leakage may underlie OC tendencies to avoid interpersonal experiences that involve direct conflict. During the commitment phase of treatment, it is important for therapists to discuss emotional leakage and orient clients to the fact that emotional expression will not be seen as a problem during therapy; on the contrary, expression is considered a sign of therapeutic progress. At the same time, it is explained that the treatment will involve slowly learning how to express more emotion in a manner that works for the client and does not consider flooding or extreme exposure to emotional expression useful. The emphasis on the pace of therapy is important and is similar to learning how to swim in that the therapist explains that the process first involves teaching the principles of swimming, then practicing the movements on dry land and dipping one's toes in the water before immersing oneself in the shallow end to practice the newly learned strokes, skills that are all mastered prior to moving to deeper waters.

Since OC clients are highly rule-governed, they often have developed rules not only about what should happen during a therapy session but also about how the therapist should behave when delivering therapy. For example, an OC client may believe that therapists should always be in control and never exhibit personal weakness or disclose personal information. Therapists should assess potential rules that clients may have about therapy by asking them about their expectations while providing various examples of common rules that many OC clients have been shown to privately have about therapy. Ideally, this can begin the process of ensuring the basis for a common ground of expectations for both the client and therapist, making it easier for a collaborative relationship to develop. Throughout therapy, the therapist should be alert to signs that might suggest a client's expectations or rules have been broken and ask about them as a means for discussion.

As outlined elsewhere in this chapter, the first four sessions primarily focus on orienting the client to the theory and structure of the treatment, assessing willingness to change, and taking the first steps needed in order to develop a strong therapeutic relationship. Nonetheless, perfect agreement, compliance, or commitment is not expected at any time during these early stages or throughout the entire course of treatment. Indeed, alliance ruptures, disagreements, and misunderstandings are expected and considered a core part of client growth. The therapist should explain to clients that she practices radical openness skills herself and that part of this means practicing openness to criticism and disconfirming feedback. The therapist should encourage clients to feel free to criticize, voice disagreement, or express concern either about how she is delivering the treatment or about the treatment itself.

In summary, RO DBT considers alliance ruptures as opportunities for growth, disagreement as representing therapeutic progress, and ambivalence as a sign of engagement because the client is trying to understand fully the relevance of the treatment. To avoid commitment problems, therapists should shape rather than demand commitment when working with OC clients by smuggling new ideas under the OC barbed wire.

Tips for Maintaining the OC Client's Engagement

- Handouts don't matter—relationships matter.

- When you sense the client's nonengagement, explore what is happening in the moment.

- Be open to being incorrect or mistaken. Model radical openness.

- Avoid behaving impersonally, and be willing to deviate from the RO DBT protocol.

- Instead of being directive or authoritative, adopt an inquisitive, collaborative manner that allows the client to save face.

- Ask, don't tell. Inspire the client to be the discoverer of his maladaptive behaviors.

- Take responsibility for your observations by saying, "I am aware of imagining..." Avoid statements implying that you possess ultimate knowledge.

- Provide the gift of truth by honestly revealing your perceptions, and encourage the client to return the favor.

- Functionally validate the client's desire to change by solving one problem at a time, to build mastery. Avoid being distracted by apparently relevant topics.

- Focus on the quality rather than the quantity of potential solutions.

- Check in frequently regarding the client's experience of therapy, especially after you have provided didactic instructions or confronted problematic behaviors.

- Don't assume that the client's lack of disagreement means engagement.

- Expect the client's commitment to vary over time, and assess it frequently.

- Encourage disagreement and dissent. Remind the client that alliance ruptures are opportunities for growth, not problems.

- Adopt a light and easy manner (see chapter 6). Model nonuptight problem solving, and playfulness balanced by compassionate gravity.

Enhancing Engagement Through Sequencing

The timing or sequencing of interventions is crucial when treating OC clients. OC biotemperamental predispositions for heightened threat sensitivity and detail-focused processing make it more likely for them to respond to therapist interventions that most others might find helpful as threatening, critical, or imprecise. Yet their superior inhibitory control and tendencies for masking inner feelings make it less likely for them to reveal their concerns to their therapists, particularly early in therapy. This can sometimes lead to premature dropout. In addition, in order to maximize learning and engagement in therapy, it is essential to introduce particular skills at particular times during individual therapy and not wait for them to be taught in skills class. Thus individual therapists are expected to incorporate a select number of skills into individual therapy, regardless of when they may be taught in the skills training class. The advantage for the client is that he is often able to have exposure to the same skill twice during treatment, once informally in individual therapy and once formally within skills class.

Sequencing strategies are also used in RO DBT to enhance engagement in therapy and shape new behaviors incrementally by starting with low-level and less intense practices before having the client attempt more difficult behaviors. A therapist who is targeting increased opinion giving in the client may, for example, have the client begin by stating opinions about the weather and achieve success with this prior to increasing the difficulty level. This does not mean that an RO DBT therapist does not confront maladaptive behavior; on the contrary, confrontation is essential when working with OC. However, rather than telling clients about their problems, providing feedback, or revealing interpretations, RO DBT encourages the client to learn how to challenge his own behavior. This is facilitated by the therapist modeling radical openness principles and adopting an openhearted yet inquisitive stance that ideally serves as a catalyst for client self-enquiry.

The following list outlines the recommended sequence for delivering the major treatment components of individual therapy and the suggested week(s) for their introduction, assuming one individual therapy session per week. The first ten steps are considered essential and ideally should be delivered in the order and time frames specified. The eleventh through twentieth steps should be considered as general guidelines and reminders for individual therapists, thereby allowing more flexibility.

1. The therapist orients the client to the two-way dialogue and collaborative stance between client and therapist (week one).

2. The client self-identifies (with help from the therapist) his or her OC coping style as the core focus in treatment (week one).

3. The therapist assesses current and past history of suicidal and self-harming behavior and signals a willingness to discuss past trauma, sexual issues, and long-held grudges or resentments of the client (week one).

4. The client commits to discussing in person (that is, not via email, text message, or telephone) urges to quit therapy before making the decision to drop out of treatment (week one).

5. The purpose of skills training class is briefly explained and plans are made for attendance during the third week (week two).

6. Four to five valued goals are identified, with at least one pertaining to social connectednesss (weeks one to four).

7. The therapist orients the client to the biosocial theory for overcontrol (week three).

8. The client begins skills training class (week three).

9. The therapist briefly introduces the key hypothesized mechanism of change, which links social signaling to social connectedness (week four).

10. A blank diary card is introduced and one or two behaviors are assigned to be monitored as practice (week four).

11. Individualized treatment targets linked to OC themes are identified and monitored on RO DBT diary cards (weeks four to twenty-nine).

12. Weekly chain and solution analyses targeting social signaling deficits are conducted, each lasting about twenty to twenty-five minutes per session (weeks six to twenty-nine).

13. Radical openness and self-enquiry skills are introduced, and the client is encouraged to begin a practice of self-enquiry and purchase a journal to record her practice (weeks five to thirty).

14. The importance of the social safety system is introduced, and RO skills designed to activate the social safety system are taught (weeks five to six).

15. Loving kindness meditation (LKM) is practiced in individual therapy. The LKM practice is recorded in session and provided to the client to help facilitate the development of a daily practice. Individual issues and difficulties regarding LKM are dealt with (weeks seven to eight).

16. Therapists should anticipate the first alliance rupture around the sixth session (weeks four to seven).

17. The therapist teaches twelve questions from Flexible Mind ADOPTS that are used to assess whether to accept or decline critical feedback and encourages the client to practice using them when feeling criticized (weeks ten to twelve).

18. The therapist informally teaches Flexible Mind REVEALs skills, with a particular emphasis on "pushback" and "don't hurt me" responses, and uses this

to facilitate targeting indirect social signaling on the diary card (weeks thirteen to seventeen).

19. The therapist discusses the importance of personal self-disclosure in developing relationships, practices Match + 1 skills from Flexible Mind ALLOWS in session, and assigns related homework (weeks eleven to eighteen).

20. The therapist introduces the concept of forgiveness and informally teaches how to grieve a loss using Flexible Mind HEART skills (weeks thirteen to twenty-four).

21. Ideally, by the fourteenth session the client and the therapist have had multiple opportunities to practice repairing alliance ruptures, which in RO DBT is considered proof of a good working relationship. Each repair (even if minor) has ideally been linked to important treatment goals (revealing rather than masking inner feelings, practicing openness to feedback, recognizing that conflict resolution can be intimacy-enhancing). If there has not been an alliance rupture by the fourteenth session, the therapist should consider the possibility that his relationship with the OC client is superficial.

22. Once a successful working alliance has been established—evidenced by success at repairing alliance ruptures—the therapist can be more confident that the OC client will be willing to genuinely reveal her inner experience over the course of treatment. Consequently, the therapist can purposefully move from an inquisitive (asking) stance to a more directive or prescribing stance, since he can trust his OC client to tell him directly when she disagrees or feels misunderstood (rather than bottling it up inside). This therapeutic process of giving and receiving feedback (between client and therapist) enhances opportunities for new learning and hastens growth (weeks fourteen to twenty-nine).

23. At the twentieth week, the therapist reminds the client that therapy will be ending in approximately ten weeks and then continues to briefly touch upon it each week and to practice skills linked to grieving relationships (weeks twenty-one to thirty).

24. Troubleshooting regarding potential problems and relapse-prevention strategies is outlined (weeks twenty-five to twenty-eight).

25. The final session is celebrated with a ritual of breaking of bread. Food and tea or coffee are shared to symbolize the transition. Mutual reminiscence is encouraged, highlighting notable moments and lessons learned; plans for preventing relapse are reviewed. To close, the therapist encourages the client to keep in contact and expresses a desire to know how the person progresses over time.

Now You Know...

▶ RO DBT posits that OC biotemperamental predispositions are powerful because they can impact perception and regulation at the sensory receptor (preconscious) level of emotional responding.

▶ They make behavioral responding more rigid and less adaptive to changing environmental contingencies—and, as a consequence, can negatively impact an OC client's engagement in therapy.

▶ The engagement strategies outlined in this chapter are designed to account for the unique biotemperamental perceptual and regulatory predispositions that characterize overcontrolled clients in order to enhance engagement in therapy.

CHAPTER 6

Social Signaling Matters: Micromimicry, Mirror Neurons, and Social Connectedness

Evolutionary scientists hypothesize that approximately 160,000 years ago, modern humans developed genetically unique traits enabling unprecedented collaboration among unrelated individuals, a unique human feature that to this day is unparalleled in the animal world (Marean, 2015). Our hypercooperative nature, combined with superior weapon technology (such as projectile weapons; see Marean, 2015), allowed us to form large networked units that could coordinate actions and work together to achieve long-term goals, making it possible for us to decimate previously feared predators, defeat rival humanoids (for example, Neanderthals in Western Europe and the Denisovan lineage in Asia), and thrive in harsh environmental conditions in a manner that less cooperative species found impossible.

A core component of this evolutionary advantage involved the development of complex social signaling capabilities that allowed for a quick and safe means to evaluate and resolve conflict and manage potential collaborations. Yet these advantages came with hidden costs. The sheer number of possible social signals available to our species (both verbal and nonverbal) makes misinterpretation likely, especially when the meaning of the signal is ambiguous. Plus, social signals can be used to deceive others in order to gain unfair advantage, making members of our own species the most dangerous enemy of all. Despite the high costs of betrayal, we are poor detectors of deception. For example, research shows that most people do little better than chance when it comes to determining whether a person is lying or telling the truth (for a review, see C. F. Bond & DePaulo, 2006). In contrast, we are excellent social safety detectors. We are adept at knowing whether a smile is genuine or phony and can accurately detect tension in the voice of a person, even over the telephone

(Pittam & Scherer, 1993; Ekman, 1992). Exposure to a few minutes of nonverbal behavior, or even just a picture of the face, leads observers to form reliable impressions of a stranger's personality traits, socioeconomic status, and moral attributes like trustworthiness and altruism (Ambady & Rosenthal, 1992; W. M. Brown, Palameta, & Moore, 2003; Kraus & Keltner, 2009). RO DBT extends these observations by linking current brain-behavioral science and the communicative functions of emotional expression (Darwin, 1872/1998) to the formation of close social bonds essential for individual and species well-being (via micromimicry and mirror neurons) and uses this to develop unique social signaling interventions, described next.

Social Bonds, Mimicry, and Mirror Neurons

Robust research shows that humans reciprocally mimic the facial expressions exhibited by an interacting partner, and facial micromimicry functions to trigger similar emotional experiences in the receiver (Hess & Blairy, 2001; Moody, McIntosh, Mann, & Weisser, 2007; Vrana & Gross, 2004). We unconsciously adopt the postures, gestures, and mannerisms of our close companions and we desire to affiliate with those who mimic us (Lakin & Chartrand, 2003; Lakin, Jefferis, Cheng, & Chartrand, 2003). Slow-motion film analysis has robustly revealed that we react to changes in body movement, posture, and facial expressions of others during interactions without ever knowing it (see chapter 2). For example, we need at least seventeen to twenty milliseconds (recall that one second is equal to one thousand milliseconds) to be consciously aware of an emotional face, yet our brain-body is already physiologically reacting at durations as low as four milliseconds (L. M. Williams et al., 2004, 2006).

The neuroregulatory theory underlying RO DBT (T. R. Lynch et al., 2015) contends that human survival depended on our species developing a supercooperative gene that enabled us to form strong social bonds and work together with others who were not genetically related to us. The biological basis underlying this advantage is posited to involve transactions between social signaling, micromimicry, and the mirror neuron (Schneider, Hempel, & Lynch, 2013). A mirror neuron fires when a person acts or when a person observes another person performing an action. Neuroimaging studies examining the mirror neuron system have shown that viewing facial expressions automatically activates brain regions that are involved in the production of similar expressions (Montgomery & Haxby, 2008; Van der Gaag, Minderaa, & Keysers, 2007). For example, when interacting with a person who suddenly grimaces in pain, we automatically microgrimace (that is, mimic the person's facial expression in milliseconds), thereby triggering or mirroring the same brain regions and physiological arousal inside ourselves that are being activated within the other person (albeit at lower intensity). Our mirror neuron system makes it possible for us to literally experience the pains and joys of nearby others, making empathy and altruism a reality. The stranger suddenly becomes part of our family, self-sacrifice feels easy, and we are more likely to behave toward others as we would like them to behave toward us. This helps explain why we are willing to risk our lives to save a stranger from drowning or die fighting for our nation.

Yet imagine this scenario: Two people meet, one demonstrative and emotionally expressive and the other undemonstrative, flat-faced, and nonexpressive. If people mimic an interacting partner, in this situation which style (expressive or flat) is more likely to dominate? The answer is that the flat face predominantly trumps an expressive face. Indeed, the flat face is such a powerful social signal that it is the most frequently used facial expression of villains in Hollywood movies and, unfortunately, often the status quo facial expression among health care providers (see figure 6.1: Dr. Neutral).

To understand why, it is important to take into account three factors our brain uses to evaluate social interactions:

1. Signal detection

2. Context

3. Variability or responsivity

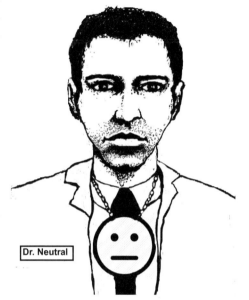

Figure 6.1. The Flat Face Is a Powerful Social Signal

First, for our very early ancestors living in harsh environments, exclusion or isolation from a tribe meant almost certain death from starvation or predation. Similarly, nonhuman primates who are socially isolated from their community die of exposure, lack of nourishment, or predation in a matter of days to weeks (Steklis & Kling, 1985). Thus the cost of not detecting a true disapproval signal implicating tribal banishment was too high to ignore for our very early ancestors, resulting in a signal-detection error bias whereby our modern brains are hardwired to interpret low-intensity, neutral, or ambiguous social signals as disapproving. For example, simply reducing or limiting the amount of eye contact during interactions has been shown to trigger negative feelings associated with being ignored or ostracized (Wirth, Sacco, Hugenberg, & Williams, 2010), and research shows that neutral expressionless faces are frequently interpreted as hostile or disapproving and that they trigger automatic defensive arousal in the recipient (Butler et al., 2003).

Second, the extent to which a flat facial expression emotionally impacts another person depends a great deal on context. Flat or bland facial expressions

> The flat face is such a powerful social signal that it is the most frequently used facial expression of villains in Hollywood movies.

are less likely to be emotionally and socially impactful in situations where dampened expressions of emotion are the norm (such as during a poker game, a business negotiation, or a funeral).

Third, variability and responsivity are relevant in situations where emotional expression is the norm or expected (a party, a therapy session, a romantic date, or an argument with one's spouse); sustained flat or insincere facial expressions are much more likely to trigger negative evaluations from recipients (for example, even seasoned speakers find blank stares and expressionless faces disconcerting). The socioemotional consequences of flat facial expressions appear similar to those arising from stares. Research suggests that the powerful social impact of a stare is not solely due to the amount of time spent staring; instead, the power of a stare most often stems from the starer's lack of responsivity to the prosocial signals or submissive glances arising from recipients of a stare (Ellsworth, Carlsmith, & Henson, 1972). Interestingly, the negative impact of a stare can be mitigated by a simple smile.

Similarly, the powerful impact flat facial expressions exert on others is not solely a function of the absence of expression. Instead, its power is derived from the conspicuous absence or low frequency of expected or customary prosocial signals (such as smiling or affirmative head nods) in contexts that call for free expression of emotion. An individual therapy session represents an example of a context that encourages free expression of emotion. Since our brains are hardwired to interpret neutral expressionless faces as hostile or disapproving (Butler et al., 2003), therapists should expect to experience discomfort (at least occasionally) when treating flat-faced OC clients. Plus, defensive arousal dampens social safety responses, making mutual flattened expressions by both the therapist and the client a likely consequence. Unfortunately, when a therapist unconsciously mimics the deadpan expression of an OC client, the therapist increases the possibility that his flat facial expression will be interpreted as a sign of disapproval or dislike by the threat-sensitive OC client, thereby reinforcing client self-constructs linked to being an outsider or unlovable.

RO DBT incorporates the preceding observations into treatment interventions in the following ways:

- By teaching clients social signaling skills shown to enhance social connectedness

- By teaching clients how to activate the ventral vagal–mediated social safety system and change physiological arousal prior to social interactions

- By teaching therapists how to use nonverbal behavior in session in order to activate social safety experiences in both clients and themselves

Skills linked to the first two components are outlined in the skills training manual. The sections that follow describe how to target the unique social signaling deficits characterizing OC problems and the social signaling strategies employed by RO DBT therapists to facilitate client engagement in therapy and enhance treatment outcomes.

One Size Does Not Fit All

There is no right or optimal way to socially signal; each of us has our own unique style of expression. Yet when it comes to treating socially ostracized and emotionally constricted OC clients, successful outcomes may often require a therapist to socially signal in a manner that goes opposite to his or her prior professional training or ideas about how therapists should behave during therapeutic encounters. For example, OC clients will not believe it is socially acceptable for an adult to play, relax, tease, disinhibit, or openly express emotions unless they see their therapists model such behavior first.

Indeed, most health care provider training programs emphasize the importance of appearing attentive and concerned rather than playful or laid back during therapeutic encounters. Therapists are taught to adopt a neutral or concerned facial expression whenever a client is disclosing something important or distressing and encouraged to sit upright, lean forward, and maintain direct eye contact (without staring). Yet research suggests that one size does not fit all when it comes to therapeutic social signals (Pinto et al., 2012). For example, highly socially anxious individuals experience direct eye gaze as threatening, triggering increased defensive arousal (Wieser, Pauli, Alpers, & Mühlberger, 2009).

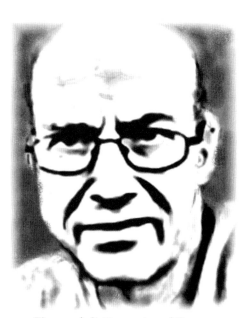

Similarly, OC clients are likely to interpret direct eye contact and an expression of concern (see figure 6.2) as criticism, not compassionate caring. As one OC client explained, "If I wasn't doing anything wrong, then why are you looking so concerned?" Plus, research shows that after a painful experience of social ostracism, people search for signs of social acceptance (for example, a smile; see L. M. Williams et al., 2006), suggesting the importance of prosocial signaling when working with socially ostracized clients (that is, OC clients). This observation underlies the majority of social signaling strategies used by therapists in RO DBT to welcome OC clients back to the tribe.

Figure 6.2. Expression of Concern

Eye Contact

Most people spend approximately 40 percent of their facial gazing time during interactions on the eyes of the other person (J. M. Henderson, Williams, & Falk, 2005). Direct eye contact is most relevant when signaling approach motivations (such as desires to affiliate or intentions to attack). For example, research shows people look more often and longer into the eyes of a dating partner or a person they feel close to as opposed to a stranger (Iizuka, 1992), and faces are perceived to express more anger with direct as opposed to an averted eye gaze from the sender (Adams & Kleck, 2003; Sander, Grandjean, Kaiser, Wehrle, & Scherer, 2007). Direct eye gaze, when combined with specific facial expressions (for example, pursed lips or a furrowed brow), helps facilitate accurate identification of the sender's intentions (see figure 6.3).

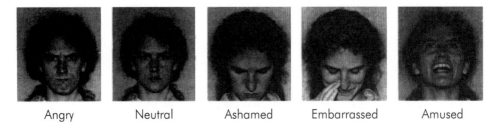

| Angry | Neutral | Ashamed | Embarrassed | Amused |

Figure 6.3. Prototypical Emotional Expressions
Adapted from Keltner, Young, & Buswell, 1997, p. 363.

Interestingly, a blank stare lasting no more than five seconds is all that is needed to trigger defensive emotional arousal and gaze avoidance in all humans (Ellsworth et al., 1972). Furthermore, gaze aversion is essential when appeasement or nondominance motivations are important (such as shame, guilt, or embarrassment). Figure 6.3 also shows the averted eyes that characterize prototypical expressions of shame and embarrassment. Eye contact may be irrelevant, immaterial, or superfluous when it comes to the expression of certain mood states (see figure 6.3).

Therapists treating OC clients should expect to encounter atypical reactions to eye contact gaze behaviors. Heightened biotemperamental threat sensitivity is posited to make it more likely for OC clients to interpret therapist expressions of concern (for example, direct eye contact or a slight furrowing of the brow) as disapproval. Research shows that anxiety-prone individuals with OC features tend to pervasively avoid eye contact, independent of culture, relationship, or context (Yardley, McDermott, Pisarski, Duchaine, & Nakayama, 2008). What is less known is the extent to which gaze aversion or direct stares may be used by OC clients to influence the behavior of others (see the material on disguised demands in the skills training manual, chapter 5, lesson 15) or instead represent a fundamental social signaling deficit.

Regardless, many OC clients have been intermittently reinforced to use signals of appeasement and gaze aversion in order to block unwanted feedback or disapproval from others (see the material on "don't hurt me" responses in chapter 10). For example, it is common for an OC client to look away when someone compliments her or expresses happiness—a response that, if repeated frequently, can function to subtly punish expressions of positive emotion by others when they are around the client— whereas other OC clients may fail to avert eye gaze when it is called for (as when expressing guilt or embarrassment), or they may overuse hostile or blank stares (the "look") to purposefully stop feedback or criticism they do not want to hear but may need to learn from (see the material on "pushback" responses in chapter 10). Finally, OC biotemperamental threat sensitivity is posited to make atypical responses more likely when eye gaze is directed toward the OC client, especially within the context of therapy. Direct eye contact from a therapist that triggers OC client shutdown is referred to in RO DBT as the "deer in the headlights" response. Recognition and treatment of this unique pattern of behavior is described next.

> Therapists treating OC clients should expect to encounter atypical gaze behaviors.

The "Deer in the Headlights" Response

Most therapists, when confronted by an unresponsive or expressionless client, tend to increase the intensity of their social signaling rather than decrease it—for example, by moving closer or leaning forward, attempting to gain eye contact or prolonging eye contact, speaking faster or more adamantly, or repeating themselves. This is done for the following reasons:

- To ensure that the therapist has the client's attention (by gaining direct eye contact)

- To ensure that the client understands the importance of what is being discussed or that the therapist cares about the client (by leaning in or using an adamant tone of voice)

- To ensure that the client understands what the therapist is saying (by repeating what is said)

However, OC clients tend to experience this kind of intense engagement as overwhelming, intrusive, or threatening. For many OC clients, this type of enhanced therapist attention makes them feel like they are a deer in the headlights of an oncoming motor vehicle at night. They feel immobilized and unable to break free of what feels like impending disaster. As reported by one OC client, "It feels like I am unable to look away when my therapist looks me in the eyes and starts asking questions. I just freeze up and can no longer hear what she is saying. Her words sound all jumbled together, and inwardly I'm beating myself up. I can't tell her about what's happening, because I can barely speak. My jaw feels like its been wired shut. I just try to nod and smile and agree with whatever she says. I am desperate for the conversation to end and hate myself for being so weak."

The apparently prosocial nature of "deer in the headlights" responses (smiling, nodding, or agreeing) can lead the therapist to conclude that the client is engaged with what is happening. On the contrary; inwardly, the OC client is experiencing overwhelming anxiety and most often silently chastising herself: *I'm such an idiot—I don't know what to say. He must think I'm a fool.* Interestingly, the appeasement smile seen in primates most closely resembles the "deer in the headlights" facial expression seen in humans (see the right side of figure 6.4).

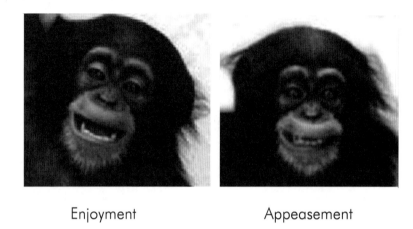

Enjoyment   Appeasement

Figure 6.4. Enjoyment and Appeasement Smiles

Photos courtesy of Dr. Lisa Parr, National Primate Research Center, Emory University

A "deer in the headlights" response is posited to most often begin as an unconditioned or classically conditioned anxiety response to therapist eye contact. Persistent and prolonged eye contact is experienced as threatening by most people (Ellsworth et al., 1972). What makes prolonged eye contact so powerful is when it is unresponsive to the reactions of others or violates social norms (for example, staring at a waiter to attract his attention is considered okay, but staring intently at a fellow passenger while riding the subway is not okay). Plus, top-down executive control processes and prior learning can exacerbate defensive responses to prolonged stares; for example, many OC clients dare not break eye contact with a therapist because they believe it will be seen as a sign of weakness or disrespect. The entire process can occur in seconds, escalating into panic and intense urges to flee. The dilemma for OC clients is that their desires for escape clash with their core values for dutifulness and obligation (to behave properly, to do the right thing, to comply with therapist requests), and their strong desires to appear self-controlled, combined with their superior capacities for inhibitory control, make it possible for them to grin and bear it and sit tight.

The end result of OC clients' self-control is a series of ambiguous social signals that are difficult to interpret because they contain mixed messages (polite smiles or head nods suggesting engagement or agreement may be combined with wide-eyed staring or frozen and tense body postures suggesting nonengagement, shutdown, or intense fear). Plus, the ambiguous nature of these signals makes it likely for therapists to similarly begin to feel anxious, albeit at a lower level, reflecting evolutionarily hardwired responses initiated at the preconscious or sensory receptor level of processing. Thus the dilemma for therapists is that their visceral responses are in conflict with their professional training. For example, a therapist might suddenly find herself feeling increasingly uncomfortable with the eye contact that she herself therapeutically initiated with her client. Her bodily discomfort reflects normal brain-body reactions to nonverbal ambiguous social signals (blank stare, frozen posture, forced smile), yet her training tells her to maintain eye contact at all costs or risk invalidating her client or communicating disinterest, disapproval, or fear if she were to look away.

Lacking an alternative model, most therapists err on the side of their prior professional training by maintaining eye contact and expressions of concern, despite continuing to feel uncomfortable. What was intended as a prosocial therapeutic encounter can quickly begin to feel like a stare-down contest that neither person knows how to stop. If not managed properly, panic-driven urges to flee can evolve into client avoidance of therapy (for example, missing or showing up late for sessions), therapist relief when a client doesn't show up for an appointment, and premature dropout. Plus, as mentioned, overlearned tendencies to mask inner feelings make it less likely for OC clients to disclose their discomfort (especially early in treatment), even when asked directly. Yet the real conundrum for the therapist is how to attend to a problem that has been triggered by therapist attention in the first place. The answer, described next, underlies one of the most important social signaling strategies in RO DBT, known as *taking the heat off*.

Heat-Off Strategies

When sensing a "deer in the headlights" response, therapists should take the heat off (that is, remove the cue) by diverting eye contact away from the client. Breaking direct eye contact removes the "headlights," allowing the client the personal space needed to downregulate. A simple break in direct eye gazing, for only a few seconds, is usually sufficient to interrupt a "deer in the headlights" response and allow the client sufficient time to downregulate (recall, OC clients are experts in self-control). When diverting eye contact away from a client, therapists should avoid staring at the floor (this signals shame, sadness, or lack of confidence); instead, therapists should break eye contact in a manner that does not call attention to it (for example, looking briefly upward or to the side while leaning back, as if in contemplation, or downward at a clipboard while writing a note). Following this, therapists can then feel free to reestablish eye contact and continue to manage the session as they would normally.

Especially in the early stages of treatment, therapists should avoid highlighting to a client in session when they are using a heat-off strategy (that is, making it a big deal). Although well intentioned, most often this only serves to place the heat back on hyperperfectionistic OC clients and trigger further shutdown. Thus heat-off strategies are most effective when they are delivered as anonymous gifts. The good news is that after a strong working alliance has begun to emerge (around the fourteenth session), therapists can begin to specifically discuss the "deer in the headlights" phenomenon (the initial discussion should not immediately follow a "deer in the headlights" response). Therapists can introduce the topic by saying, "You know, I have noticed when we discuss a hot topic, or perhaps when I am too attentive—say, with my eye contact—that you sometimes appear to shut down or freeze up. Have you ever noticed anything like this?" Therapists can read aloud the description of a "deer in the headlights" (see the client example earlier in this chapter) in order to help a client understand that he is not alone in experiencing this problem and to facilitate a more frank discussion of how it manifests for him.

It should be explained to clients that a "deer in the headlights" response is an automatic anxiety response, secondary to prolonged eye contact, that is most likely to occur between strangers or people just getting to know each other. Indeed, direct eye contact has been shown to increase defensive arousal (for example, increased heart rate, elevated skin-conductance responses) compared to gaze aversion (Coutts & Schneider, 1975; Nichols & Champness, 1971). Anxiety responses to eye contact vary widely across people and contexts (for example, as a function of differing biotemperaments, cultural backgrounds, or relationship histories). Following commitment by an OC client to target "deer in the headlights" responses in treatment, RO DBT uses four overlapping strategies to help facilitate change:

1. Monitoring the frequency of "deer in the headlights" responses (for example, on a diary card) and incorporating them into individual therapy chain analyses as needed

2. Encouraging clients to mindfully observe "deer in the headlights" responses as normal brain-body reactions to eye gaze that evolved to facilitate social connectedness and prevent intraspecies conflict, and that are both transitory and opportunities for self-enquiry

3. Using in-session exposure to eye contact or other "deer in the headlights"–eliciting cues while simultaneously practicing social safety activation skills

4. Encouraging clients to practice giving themselves permission to divert their eye contact away from the person they are interacting with whenever they begin to experience a "deer in the headlights" response, without completely avoiding eye contact

Heat-off strategies are a core part of repairing an alliance rupture. When sensing that an alliance rupture may be present, an RO DBT individual therapist is taught to briefly take the heat off by redirecting her eye contact away from the client (for example, upward) or by writing on a clipboard placed on her lap while simultaneously leaning back in her chair (away from the client), if possible. In addition, as already suggested, knowing how and when to take the heat off is particularly important during the early stages of therapy, when a strong working alliance is less likely to have been fully established. Finally, heat-off strategies are essential when wanting to reinforce new or adaptive behavior. Thus, following honest and candid expressions of emotion or vulnerability by an OC client (for example, admitting to a therapist that he disagrees or is angry with her), the therapist should briefly thank the client for his candid disclosure, link his disclosure to the client's valued goals for improved interpersonal relationships, and then be willing to move away from the topic rather than dig deeper in order to reinforce self-disclosure (that is, OC clients strongly dislike the limelight; thus, further exploration may function to aversively punish self-disclosure).

Heat-On Strategies

Heat-on strategies in RO DBT are essentially the opposite of heat-off strategies. Heat-on strategies have many guises, yet all involve some form of directed attention whereby clients feel they are being evaluated, examined, scrutinized, or in the limelight. Examples of what OC clients commonly perceive as heat-on stimuli include direct eye contact, giving a compliment or praising them, repeating a request for information, or unexpected teasing (for example, playful irreverence). Heat-on strategies help OC clients locate their edge or area of growth and deepen self-enquiry. Rather than explaining or telling an OC client how her behavior is ineffective, an RO DBT therapist is more likely to ask the OC client a question with open curiosity instead. For example, during a chain analysis of an interaction with her husband, a therapist might ask a client, "Do you think you might have assumed that you already knew what your husband was going to say, and this might have made you less likely to actually listen openly to what he actually said?"

When heat-on strategies are applied, most OC clients respond in three ways:

1. They may join with the therapist by directly answering the question in a manner that signals a willingness to openly explore the issue.

2. They may delay or pause before responding, quickly defend, change the topic, push back, or behave helplessly (see the material on "pushback" and "don't hurt me" responses in chapter 10), suggesting possible nonengagement.

3. They may exhibit behavior that is in between the preceding two (that is, it appears they are genuinely trying to reply or engage with the discussion, and at the same time their manner appears to have changed after being queried, or during the subsequent discussion; for example, a "deer in the headlights" response is possible).

Therapists should use these moments as opportunities for the client to practice more direct communication. Both heat-on and heat-off strategies can also function to reinforce adaptive behavior. For example, frequent and brief exposure to social attention that is not overwhelming (putting the heat on), combined with strategic removal of social attention following candid or vulnerable disclosures (taking the heat off), can function as a powerful incentive for open expression of emotion, thereby indirectly enhancing social connectedness.

Therapeutic Use of Cooperative Social Signaling

Across cultures, smiling signals social acceptance and friendly interpersonal intentions to others, happiness, and other positive emotions (Horstmann & Bauland, 2006; Lundqvist & Öhman, 2005; Parkinson, 2005). Smiles are powerful social signals; we emotionally respond to a smile before conscious awareness is even possible (that is, within milliseconds; see L. M. Williams et al., 2006). We are adept at knowing whether a smile is genuine or phony (Ekman, 1992), and we use smiles to quickly form reliable impressions of strangers' personality traits and trustworthiness—for example, whether they are warm (kind, friendly) or cool (aloof, prickly; see L. M. Williams et al., 2006). Research shows that smiles can function as a social reward for both adult and infant humans (Niedenthal, Mermillod, Maringer, & Hess, 2010). They are also highly contagious—people find it hard not to automatically return the genuine smile of a person smiling at them.

Smiles can also signal positive or nonaggressive intentions that may not involve pleasure or enjoyment (Cashdan, 1998; Fridlund, 1991, 2002). For example, the inhibited smiles that are a core component of embarrassment displays may reflect social status evaluations that combine an appeasement signal (averted eyes) with a friendly signal (coy smile), and that function to communicate both a hope of forgiveness and a desire to affiliate (see the prototypical expression of embarrassment shown in figure 6.3). Embarrassment displays are difficult to fake because they involve several coordinated movements (for example, averted gaze, head tilted down and away, compressed smile) and are often accompanied by blushing. Interestingly, most people prefer to spend more time with people who reveal intense embarrassment than with people who inhibit it (Feinberg, Willer, & Keltner, 2012), and people who blush are trusted and liked more than nonblushers (De Jong, 1999; Dijk, Voncken, & de Jong, 2009). Thus expressions of embarrassment may also function to authenticate or verify the prosocial intentions of a sender.

Another example of the prosocial signaling functions of smiling can be seen in what is often referred to as the *appeasement smile*. Among most primates, a silent bared-teeth display (see the right side of figure 6.4) occurs whenever the smiler intends no harm, resulting in a forced smile that is intended to signal nonaggression, nondominance, or desire to affiliate, and it shares similar musculature with human smiles of affiliation (Parr & Waller 2006; see also Niedenthal et al., 2010) and human smiles associated with anxious expressions of appeasement and nondominance ("deer in the headlights" responses), whereas the enjoyment smile on the left side of figure 6.4 shows a "play" face believed to be analogous to human expressions of genuine laughter and smiles of enjoyment (Parr & Waller, 2006). Thus, as social signals, smiles are more than just expressions of inner happiness. They represent evolutionarily prepared social signals that can function to communicate prosocial intentions essential for creating, maintaining, or repairing close social bonds.

Genuine Smiles

Genuine smiles (also known as *Duchenne smiles*, *enjoyment smiles*, and *pleasurable smiles*; see the right side of figure 6.5) reflect feelings of amusement, pleasure, contentment, or joy. They are characterized by a slightly slower onset and longer duration relative to social smiles or polite smiles and may not involve eye contact when exhibited in the presence of others (see the prototypical expression of amusement shown in figure 6.3). Thus, genuine smiles may not always represent a social signal. Yet smiles of pleasure, when observed by others, are highly contagious; it is hard not to laugh or smile when another person expresses genuine amusement. The genuine smile, or Duchenne smile, involves simultaneous activation of two sets of facial muscles—the *zygomaticus major*, which controls the corners of the mouth, and the *orbicularis oculi*, which encircles the eye socket—whereas activation of a single muscle, the *zygomaticus major*, characterizes the social or polite smile (see the left side of figure 6.5).

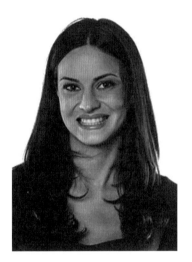 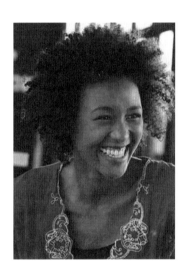

Polite Smile   **Genuine Smile**

Figure 6.5. Polite Smile vs. Genuine Smile

Polite or Social Smiles

Polite or social smiles are prosocial signals that can occur in the absence of pleasure and rarely occur outside of a social context (unless we are practicing our smile in front of a mirror). Unlike the slowly building and slowing fading smile associated with spontaneous genuine or pleasurable smiles, polite smiles are easily recognized by their quick onset and quick offset (for example, the quick flash of a smile displayed during a chance encounter with an acquaintance is likely to disappear just as quickly upon the acquaintance's departure). They are highly associated with self-conscious self-presentations designed to avoid social disapproval, mask inner feelings, flatter superiors, or appease dominant others. They are characterized by a conspicuous lack of *orbicularis oculi* activation and are appraised as inauthentic (or as "dead-eye smiles") by recipients when they are sustained or frozen (with teeth exposed) and are nonresponsive to what is happening in the moment, similar to the appeasement smile seen in chimpanzees (see the right side of figure 6.4).

OC clients, particularly the overly agreeable subtype (see chapter 9), are likely to overuse polite smiles during interactions. Unfortunately for OC clients, despite strong attempts to hide their negative feelings (such as envy, anger, or sadness) by increasing the duration and intensity of their prosocial signaling (for example, grins or wide smiles that display both upper and lower teeth), most often their attempts fail because most people are adept at differentiating between a genuine smile and a polite smile (L. M. Williams et al., 2006). The inauthenticity experienced by both the smiler and the recipient of a prolonged polite smile is analogous to the self-conscious discomfort that arises when we are asked to "hold that smile" by a fiddling photographer. Our original spontaneous smile of genuine enjoyment freezes and then quickly fades, replaced by what we inwardly recognize as a weak approximation of our former happiness (which is why we ask our fumbling friend to hurry up and take the picture). Thus deliberate attempts by OC clients to pretend that everything is fine, when it is not, elicit from others the very thing their effortful control hopes to avoid—that is, people find their overly prosocial behavior off-putting and as a consequence are more likely to avoid interacting with them in the future.

Yet not all polite or social smiles are problematic. Polite smiles can be altruistic—for example, smiling at a friend who is dying of cancer, and who you know would dislike displays of sad emotions, is an act of kindness. They represent important means for signaling positive social intentions and oftentimes function as a social lubricant during the initial stages of forming a close social bond with another. For example, when first meeting a new person, chitchat and polite smiling represent building blocks for greater intimacy; they signal positive intentions while allowing each person the space and time to deepen the relationship without feeling overtly pressured. Polite smiles can also de-escalate conflict (lighten the mood during a tense negotiation) or signal nonaggressive intentions (when one is approached by a police officer).

Closed-Mouth Cooperative Smiles

The solution to the dilemma is the closed-mouth cooperative smile. Contrary to other consciously produced smiles, the closed-mouth cooperative smile can be held static for relatively long periods of time without feeling contrived or phony. It avoids the problems associated with flat, neutral, or concerned expressions while blocking automatic tendencies by OC clients to be hyperserious during discussions of problem behavior or during repair of an alliance rupture. Plus, the closed-mouth smile is more likely to be experienced by both the sender and the receiver as a genuine smile of pleasure and, as a consequence, to trigger reciprocal smiling and social safety responses (Porges, 2003a). A closed-mouth cooperative smile (see figure 6.6) involves turning both corners of the mouth upward and stretching the lips over the teeth but keeping the mouth closed so that the teeth are not exposed. It almost always is accompanied by direct eye contact, a slight constriction or narrowing of the eyes, and the crow's-feet wrinkles that characterize genuine smiles of pleasure (that is, orbicularis oculi muscle activation).

The closed-mouth cooperative smile differs from the averted gaze and bowed head that characterize the closed-mouth appeasement smile or smile of embarrassment (Sarra & Otta, 2001; see also figure 6.3). It also differs from what is known as the *half smile* (Linehan, 1993a). The half smile is less expressive—that is, it does not involve stretching the lips, it is less wide, and it is less likely to be associated with crow's-feet wrinkles around the eyes. Instead, the half smile is more physically similar to a burglar smile (described later in this chapter) and as a consequence can be easily misread. Half smiles and burglar smiles are associated with a wide range of differing emotions and intentions, from contentment to strong dislike and feeling pleasure in another's misfortune. For example, the intimidating nature of the high-dominance half smile (burglar smile) shown in figure 6.7 becomes most apparent when the mouth is ignored (cover the mouth with your hand). The world's best-known half smile—in Leonardo da Vinci's painting known in English as the *Mona Lisa* (see figure 6.8)—is intriguing precisely because the elusive smile on the woman's face is so subtly shadowed that the exact nature of the smile cannot be determined, with interpretations ranging from pleasure to disdain (Livingstone, 2000).

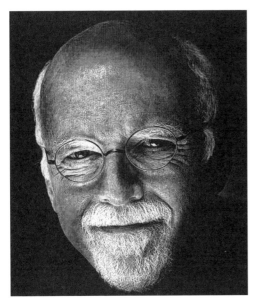

Figure 6.6. Closed-Mouth Cooperative Smile

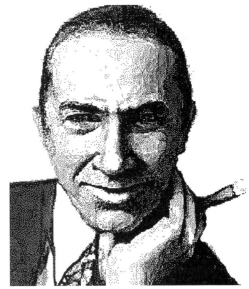

Figure 6.7. High-Dominance Half Smile (Burglar Smile)

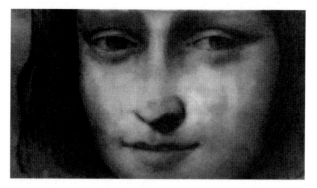

Figure 6.8. Enigmatic Half Smile

Therapists may need to practice closed-mouth cooperative smiles (for example, using a mirror) in order to naturally apply them in session. Indeed, analysis of video-taped therapy sessions has revealed that some therapists find it extremely difficult to break overlearned emotion expression habits or prior professional training emphasizing the importance of appearing calm, neutral, or concerned during therapeutic encounters and interpersonal interactions. In an attempt to go opposite to these overlearned habits, therapists can overcorrect by smiling too much or too intensely. Most often this translates into frozen and nonresponsive open-mouthed smiles that display the upper teeth. The therapist's aim is to communicate genuine affection and cooperation; however, smiles involving displays of teeth that are held constant (that is, nonresponsive) are quickly experienced as contrived by both the sender and receiver. The feeling is similar to what happens when we are asked to smile for the camera but the picture is delayed by a fumbling cameraperson—our candid smile of genuine pleasure quickly fades into a frozen polite smile that feels increasingly phony the longer we hold it.

The good news is that there are several automatic indicators that can help verify the genuineness of a smile. For example, it is common for an automatic deep breath or sigh of contentment to arise almost immediately after engaging a closed-mouth cooperative smile, implicating PNS-VVC activation. The PNS-VVC regulates not only our social signaling muscles (head and face) but also the neuroinhibitory vagal fibers that deepen and slow breathing and reduce cardiac output essential for signaling genuine warmth and calm friendliness during interactions. Social safety responses can often be enhanced when the smile is accompanied by a simultaneous upward movement of both eyebrows (see "The Eyebrow Wag," later in this chapter). Thus, when learning the closed-mouth cooperative smile, therapists can use their visceral or bodily experience of social safety to guide how big to make the closed-mouth smile. Plus, the presence of an unconscious deep breath or sigh can be used as convergent evidence that the smile successfully activated the therapist's social safety system, making it more likely for the client to feel similarly (via activation of the mirror neuron system).

The Therapist as Tribal Ambassador

Rather than fixing, correcting, restricting, or improving a hyperperfectionistic OC client, RO DBT prioritizes social connectedness by encouraging therapists to adopt a stance likened to that of a tribal ambassador. A tribal ambassador models kindness, cooperation, and affection to socially ostracized OC clients, saying, "Welcome home. We appreciate your desire to meet or exceed expectations and the self-sacrifices you have made. You have worked hard and deserve a rest." Yet ambassadors also recognize that sometimes kindness means telling a good friend a painful truth in order to help him achieve his valued goals, in a manner that acknowledges one's own potential for fallibility.

Ambassadors are also face savers—they allow a person (or country) to admit to some fault without rubbing anyone's nose in it. Plus, they learn the language and customs of a foreign country without expecting the people in the foreign land to think, feel, or behave the way they themselves do. They are able to make self-sacrifices in order to repair a damaged relationship, without always expecting something in return. Thus ambassadors recognize that when we lend a hand, we also simultaneously transmit a powerful message of social connectedness to the person we are helping, one that essentially says, "You don't owe me." This simple act of kindness underlies one of the core strengths of our species—that is, we are better together.

An ambassador talks to people from another country as if they were good friends. When among friends we feel naturally less self-conscious; we relax and drop our guard. In the context of therapy, dropping one's guard means dropping one's professional role (at least to some extent). Research shows that when we are with our friends we are likely to stretch out, lie back, and lounge around; our body gestures and facial expressions are more expansive and our use of language is less formal; we are less polite and likely to use slang or curse words to color our speech. For example, friends don't try to change each other; they trust each other to do the right thing and they respect their individual differences. Thus, by adopting a manner most often reserved for close friends or family, we signal to OC clients that we consider them to be part of our tribe (recall that OC is a disorder characterized by loneliness). Without saying a word, an easy manner communicates, "I like you. I trust you to do the right thing. I believe in your competence. I am interested in what you have to say. I am not out to cause you harm. I am no better than you, and I am open to being wrong."

Yet signaling an easy manner can go opposite to how a therapist has been professionally trained. Some therapists find it difficult or awkward to lean back in a chair, temporarily avert their gaze, or raise their eyebrows during a session with an OC client. This often reflects prior training emphasizing the importance of sitting upright and maintaining eye contact. It can also reflect a therapist's personality; for example, research shows that the majority of therapists lean toward an overcontrolled personality style or have overcontrolled family, culture, or environmental influences (for example, "Don't slouch"). Fortunately, our research and experience training therapists in RO DBT has shown that the vast majority of therapists who initially struggle modeling an easy manner can learn how to apply it with a little practice.

Importantly, an easy manner does *not* mean walking on eggshells or treating the client as fragile by immediately jumping in to validate, soothe, regulate, or find a solution for a problem. Instead, it places the responsibility back on the client by not assuming it is the therapist's job to make the client feel better or solve the client's problems while signaling a willingness to lend a hand. Thus the nondirective nature of an easy manner allows the client the space needed to recognize that, on some level, she chooses how she responds emotionally to events in her life (for example, no one can force a person to feel angry or sad) and begin the sometimes painful but mostly liberating process of taking responsibility for her life without falling apart or harshly blaming the world.

The Eyebrow Wag

The eyebrow wag or eyebrow flash is a universal social acceptance signal involving a simultaneous upward movement of both eyebrows, most often accompanied by a genuine smile, kind or happy eyes, and melodic tones of voice. Eyebrow wags are nature's way of saying, "I like you" or "You are in my tribe." The eyebrow wag occurs in a wide range of social situations, including greetings, flirting, approving, seeking confirmation, and thanking; it is a powerful social signal that occurs across cultures, most often without conscious awareness (Grammer, Schiefenhovel, Schleidt, Lorenz, & Eibl-Eibesfeldt, 1998). It is a friendly gesture that is posited to have evolved as a nonverbal signal of cooperation among nonkin, signaling prosocial desires for reciprocal altruistic exchanges (R. H. Frank, 1988). Plus, it is conspicuously absent when we are greeted by someone who dislikes us or during interactions with rivals, albeit lack of an eyebrow wag should not be assumed to be definitive proof of dislike. For example, the other person may be in pain or distressed (both pain and threat turn off social safety responses and prosocial signaling), or the person may rarely exhibit eyebrow wags with anyone, a social signaling deficit that is common among many OC clients.

Eyebrow wags not only signal cooperative intentions, they also facilitate openness and receptivity to new information or critical feedback by activating the social safety system (via micromimicry and the mirror neuron system). Thus an RO DBT therapist who is challenging an OC client, rather than adopting an expression of concern, is much more likely to adopt an eyebrow wag (see figure 6.9), both when speaking and when listening. This signals affection, interest, and openness while simultaneously making it more likely for both therapist and client to viscerally experience the interaction as an opportunity for new learning.

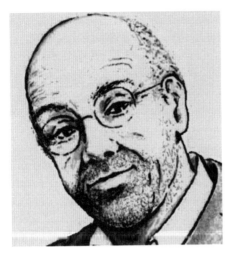 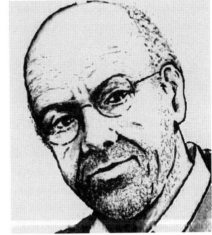

Eyebrow Wag   Expression of Concern

Figure 6.9. Eyebrow Wag vs. Expression of Concern

Signaling Openness and an Easy Manner

OC clients are biologically predisposed to react to minor discrepancies and uncertainty as potential threats; that is, they tend to be uptight internally and yet report they are fine externally. Unfortunately, attempts to suppress or mask emotional expression, either by the therapist or the client, negatively impacts the relationship even when such attempts occur outside of conscious awareness (recall that we react to facial affect or lack of affect within milliseconds; see L. M. Williams et al., 2004). Thus, if the therapist is pretending to be laid back, playful, or easygoing when inwardly feeling uptight, the client is likely to viscerally sense that something is not quite right and will become wary and hesitant: "If my therapist can't do it, then what chance do I have?" The good news is that the body postures, gestures, and facial expressions associated with an easy manner function to automatically trigger social safety responses (via PNS-VVC activation; see chapter 2) in both the therapist and the client (via the mirror neuron system), thereby making feelings of genuine ease and social engagement seem more attainable for both.

Socially signaling an easy manner in RO DBT (see figure 6.10) requires therapists to nonverbally adjust their posture, eye contact, and facial expressions, most often by doing what follows:

- Leaning back in the chair in order to increase distance from the client

- Crossing the leg nearest the client over the other leg, in order to slightly turn the shoulders away

- Taking a slow deep breath

- Briefly disengaging eye contact

- Raising the eyebrows

- Engaging a closed-mouth smile while returning eye gaze back toward the client

Finally, when using an easy manner strategically in therapy with OC clients (for example, to help take the heat off), therapists should resist the urge to explain to clients what they are doing, mainly because this places the heat back on clients or may prompt attempts by clients to justify or defend their behavior.

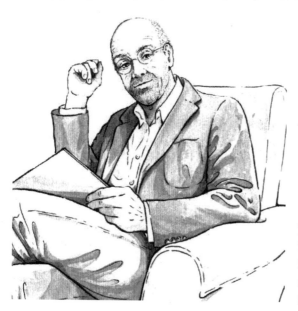

Figure 6.10. Signaling an Easy Manner

All of what was just described happens in seconds. Additional elements that can further augment signaling an easy manner include slightly pausing after each client utterance in order to allow the client time to say more, slowing how fast one is speaking, and speaking with a softer tone of voice. If the therapist is already leaning back in her chair, she should move her body rather than remaining frozen in the same posture (especially when tension is in the room). The best way to manage this, without calling undue attention to what is happening, is for the therapist to always have something to drink nearby (for example, a cup of coffee; don't forget to ask your client at the start of the session if he would like something to drink, too). Essentially, the therapist should make use of this simple prop by leaning forward and taking a sip from her drink. This breaks up a frozen body posture while signaling normality. After taking a sip from her drink, the therapist can begin again by leaning back in her chair and then reinstitute the same steps again (only this time, the therapist is likely to find that leaning back in her chair actually feels more relaxed than it did a moment before).

Finally, therapists should also be careful to not overcorrect when first learning how to signal an easy manner (for example, by smiling regardless of what the client is saying, or never leaning forward). There are a few general principles that can help minimize such problems. First, when struggling with signaling an easy manner, especially when first learning RO DBT, a therapist can use his inner discomfort as an opportunity for self-enquiry. He should out himself regarding his struggle to his consultation team, supervisor, or another therapist and practice being radically open to any feedback that results from this. Second, avoid taking an easy manner too seriously or applying it regardless of what might be happening in session. When a client is engaged in the session—freely answering questions, remaining on topic, actively listening, and revealing inner experience—nonverbal signals are likely less important (for example, leaning forward or engaging eye contact doesn't matter, because the client is not feeling threatened).

Connecting Gestures and Touch

Connecting gestures involve the use of smiles and head nods that are displayed without interrupting the speaker, signaling that the listener considers the speaker in the listener's tribe. Gestures of social connectedness and verbal statements of affection or sympathy are even more powerfully communicated when they are combined with touch, such as a comforting hand on a shoulder. In general, touching is reserved solely for those we are most familiar or intimate with (for example, friends, family, lovers, and pets). When used appropriately, touch can function as a powerful means for enhancing a positive therapeutic alliance. A simple touch to the elbow of a struggling client may be all that is needed to communicate genuine caring.

Yet when working with OC clients, therapists should not assume that touch of any kind will be received as intended. For one thing, heightened temperamental threat sensitivity makes it more likely for OC clients to have greater needs for personal space, and they may react negatively to relatively minor violations of their personal space (albeit they are unlikely to voice their discomfort). Personal space is the region surrounding a person that she regards as psychologically hers, and most people experience discomfort, anger, or anxiety when their personal space is violated (unless circumstances make nonintrusion impossible, such as a crowded subway). Moreover, past trauma (for example, sexual abuse or physical trauma) can further heighten fears or create strong aversions to being touched. Recall, too, that when the PNS-VVC-mediated social safety system is downregulated (as it often is for most OC clients), the desire to touch or be touch is diminished. Plus, most OC clients have less experience touching or being touched by others (for example, hugging, hand-holding, kissing, and stroking), making them more likely to be unsure how to respond when another person initiates touch (for example, gives them a hug at a party).

Thus OC clients may be more likely to misinterpret touch from a therapist as confusing, invasive, threatening, or even sexually provocative (especially early in treatment). A conservative approach most often works best when deciding when and how to use therapeutic touch when working with OC clients. For example, when unsure about whether touch might be received positively (for example, the therapist desires to hug a client at the end of a particularly difficult session), the therapist should err on the side of not touching. Sometimes simply telling an OC client "I am so happy about what you have just told me that I feel a strong urge to give you a hug" is all that is needed to get a positive affiliative message across. This also allows the client to take the lead when it comes to increasing physical proximity or engaging in touch. Interestingly, research has shown that client ratings of liking and connectedness increased with social touch by a therapist up to a point but decreased when touching was done in a manner that was experienced by the recipient as excessive (Montague, Chen, Xu, Chewning, & Barrett, 2013).

Despite these caveats, therapists should not avoid discussing the topic of touch when working with OC clients. Like other potentially sensitive topics (for example, sexuality and trauma), discussions about touch should be conducted in a matter-of-fact manner that signals to the client that difficulties pertaining to touch are common and nothing to be ashamed about. Some OC clients may need instruction on how to touch someone (for example, how to hug, how to shake hands, what type of touch is appropriate depending on the relationship) or even how to touch themselves (for example, they can practice hugging themselves by wrapping their arms across their chests, stroke their own faces or necks, or hold hot water bottles against their stomachs; see the skills training manual, chapter 5, lesson 3). Finally, touch can represent a core means of signaling caring. Therapists should be careful to not overcorrect by making it a rule to never touch an OC client. Instead, therapists should recognize that issues surrounding touch will vary considerably across clients and, as a consequence, should tailor their actions accordingly.

Connecting gestures also include what are often referred to as *big gestures* or *expansive gestures* in RO DBT. Expansive and open gestures signal receptivity, safety, and willingness and are most often associated with positive mood states. They are not learned, nor does their expression vary across cultures. For example, blind athletes who have never in their lives seen another person's facial expressions or gestures have been shown to exhibit the same expansive facial expressions and gestures when they win or lose as athletes who are not blind (Matsumoto & Willingham, 2009). In contrast, when we distrust someone or experience a loss, we automatically tighten up our gestures and body movements; our gestures are smaller, and we defensively hold our arms closer to the body. Therapists should get in the habit of engaging bigger or more expansive gestures when working with OC clients, particularly when there is tension in the room.

Teasing, Nondominance, and Playful Irreverence

The very first laugh exhibited by an infant occurs when a safety signal (such as a smiling mother) is combined with a danger signal (such as a game of peekaboo). Similarly, friendly teasing involves a combination of danger and safety signals, most often accompanied by displays of mutual laughter and light touching. Friends playfully and affectionately tease each other all the time. Research shows that teasing and joking are how friends informally point out flaws in each other, without being too heavy-handed about it. Learning how to tease and be teased is an important part of healthy social relationships, and kindhearted teasing is how tribes, families, and friends give feedback to each other. Plus, being able to openly listen and act upon critical feedback provided a huge evolutionary advantage because our individual survival no longer depended solely on our personal perceptions. This helps explain why we are so concerned about the opinions of others.

A good tease is always kind. Most often it starts out with an unexpected provocative comment that is delivered with an unsympathetic (expressionless or arrogant) tone of voice or intimidating facial expression (such as a blank stare), gesture (such as finger wagging), or body posture (such as hands on hips) that is immediately followed by laughter, gaze aversion, or postural shrinkage. Thus a kindhearted tease momentarily introduces conflict and social distance but quickly reestablishes social connectedness by signaling nondominant friendliness. The nondominance signal is critical for a tease to be taken lightly (that is, as a friendly poke; see Keltner et al., 1997). When teasing is playful and reciprocal it is socially bonding. In fact, teasing is an important component of flirting (Shapiro, Baumeister, & Kessler, 1991). People who are okay about being teased have an easy manner; they don't take themselves or life too seriously and can laugh (with their friends) at their personal foibles, gaffes, and mishaps.

> A good tease is always kind.

In RO DBT, playful irreverence represents the therapeutic cousin of a good tease between friends. Playful irreverence is part of a dialectical strategy in RO DBT that challenges the client's maladaptive behavior while signaling the therapist's affection and openness. Most often playful irreverence begins with the therapist's nonverbal or verbal expression of incredulity or amused bewilderment after a discrepant, odd, or illogical comment or behavior by the client (for example, the client verbally indicates that he is unable to speak, or he reports complete lack of animosity toward a coworker he has admitted lying about in order to get her fired), and it is accompanied by a nondominant signal of openness and affection. Nondominance body postures and facial expressions accompanied by or immediately following playful irreverence communicate that we intend no harm; that is, our actions are not to be taken too seriously. Such postures and expressions are especially important when the person teasing or playing irreverently is in a power-up position (as in the therapist-client relationship) because they signal that the person in the power-up position desires an egalitarian relationship and is open to feedback from the other person. Nondominance signals combine appeasement signals (slight bowing of the head, slight shoulder shrug, openhanded gestures) with cooperative-friendly signals (warm smile, eyebrow wags, eye contact; see figure 6.11).

An example of playful irreverence occurred when a highly committed OC client arrived at her third RO DBT session with a typewritten list of 117 novel activities she had done in the prior week, whereupon her therapist responded by saying, "Wow— 117 new things! That's fantastic! Okay, now—time for a power nap. Let's both put our heads down and catch a few z's!" The therapist then mimicked a sleeping position for only a brief moment before he smiled warmly and then sat back in his chair (that is, he moved from playful irreverence to compassionate gravity); following this, the therapist slowed down his rate of speech and lowered his tone of voice and then asked the client, after a closed-mouth smile and eyebrow wag, "So…why do you think I said that?" The power nap represents a playfully irreverent (or friendly) tease, whereas the question about the nap tells the client that the therapist is using metaphor to help the client recognize that her well-intentioned attempts to fix her overcontrol may actually represent another form of the OC problem itself.

Therapists should also combine nondominance and cooperative-friendly signals when encouraging OC clients to practice candid disclosure. For example, when a client appears to be nonengaged, a therapist might say (after dipping her head down and engaging a prolonged shoulder shrug that is combined with a warm closed-mouth smile, raised eyebrows, and direct eye contact in order to nonverbally signal that she is open to hearing whatever the client may have to say, even if it's critical of the treatment or the therapist), "I've noticed something seems to have changed. Can you let me know what's going on with you right now?" Similarly, when making a difficult request of a client (for example, asking him to role-play in session), the therapist should signal respect and positive regard by combining friendly signals with low-level nondominance signals.

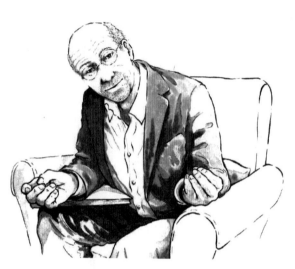

Figure 6.11. Signaling Nondominance

Nondominance signals are also a core feature of RO DBT confrontation strategies. Confrontation in RO DBT most often begins with a topic-relevant question designed to encourage an OC client to discover her own potential stuck-point(s) rather than telling the client what her problem is or how she needs to do something different. The use of confrontation varies according to the stage of treatment an OC client is in (that is, early versus late). As mentioned previously, during the early stages of therapy (that is, before the ninth session), therapists are encouraged to adopt a stance that models how they might manage similar behaviors exhibited by a person whom they are just getting to know outside of therapy. For example, most people would not immediately confront a new friend who, when asked how he feels about something, reports feeling fine or okay, even though we sense he is not actually fine. Instead, we are likely to discuss our concerns only after this pattern has occurred on multiple occasions over multiple interactions. Therapists should reflect back their perplexity or confusion regarding an indirect social signal only after it has occurred repeatedly, giving the client the benefit of the doubt and reserving judgment until having robust evidence to the contrary—for example, by saying, "I've noticed that on multiple occasions, whenever I've asked about how you are feeling, especially about difficult topics, you seem to always respond by saying that you are fine. My question is, are you always really fine?" The idea is to signal trust and respect to clients as we learn who they are, similar to the grace we give to others we are just getting to know.

Nondominance postural signals help facilitate in-session RO DBT confrontation by signaling equality, openness, and friendliness.

Appeasement, Submission, and Embarrassment

When threatened we can flee, hide, attack, call on the aid of nearby others, or appease. Universal signals of submission among humans include lowering the head, covering the face with the hands or hiding the face from view, slackened posture, lowering the eyelids, casting the eyes downward, avoiding eye contact, slumping the shoulders, and postural shrinkage. Appeasement gestures evolved to de-escalate aggression, elicit sympathy, and regain entry into the tribe after making a grievous error that threatened the well-being of another tribe member or the tribe as a whole (Keltner & Harker, 1998; Tsoudis & Smith-Lovin, 1998), whereas minor social transgressions (for example, exhibiting poor table manners or forgetting the name of a person you have known for a long time) call for displays of embarrassment, not submission. Embarrassment displays differ from appeasement and submissive displays linked to shame (see figure 6.3). Both involve downward head movements and gaze aversion. Embarrassment displays involve compressed smiles and face touching; in contrast, appeasement expressions involve frowning and sometimes covering of the face with the hands.

Research shows that appeasement gestures must be present when a person is attempting to repair a transgression. People distrust expressions of guilt (such as saying, "I'm sorry") if they are not accompanied by bodily displays prototypical of shame (postural shrinkage, lowered gaze, blushing; see Ferguson, Brugman, White, & Eyre, 2007). Nonverbal displays of shame or embarrassment during an apology signal that the violator values the relationship because he is viscerally distressed by his actions, making it easier for the person who has been wronged to trust he will not commit them again. Thus appeasement gestures are essential whenever a therapist is attempting to repair an alliance rupture, especially when the rupture was the result of something the therapist did (recall that repair of an alliance rupture is the responsibility of the therapist).

Therapeutic Sighs

Sighs are common phenomena that are most often ignored or considered irrelevant when it comes to socioemotional well-being. Frequent sighing has been linked with chronic anxiety and post-traumatic distress (Blechert, Michael, Grossman, Lajtman, & Wilhelm, 2007; Tobin, Jenouri, Watson, & Sackner, 1983) and negative affect (McClernon, Westman, & Rose, 2004). Sighing has also been linked to relief of stress (Soltysik & Jelen, 2005). Yet few have linked sighing to the communicative function of emotions.

RO DBT posits that the sounds stemming from a sigh function as a social signal when displayed in the presence of others. Under distress or despair, a sigh can signal

"Help me" or "I'm fed up" or "I'm exhausted," whereas sighs that accompany the relief that occurs following the termination of a stressor may signal to other tribe members that all is well. During interactions between people who have a close bond (for example, therapist and client), a sigh might also signal contentment, satisfaction, or a desire to see the world from the other person's point of view. Thus therapists can use a sigh to signal to a client a desire for affiliation or a desire to not engage in conflict.

Managing Maladaptive OC Social Signaling

The key to treatment targeting with OC is to continually ask oneself in session, *How might this client's social signaling impact social connectedness?* Thus, rather than targeting maladaptive cognition, internal emotion dysregulation, or avoidance coping as primary, RO DBT considers social signaling deficits and low openness the core factors maintaining OC isolation, loneliness, and psychological distress. Yet to target social signaling deficits, therapists must know what they are. The sections that follow provide an overview of some of the more common means of observing aloud and asking about social signaling discrepancies occurring in session.

Burglar Smiles

The burglar smile, or high-dominance half smile (see figure 6.7), involves a quick upturn of the corners of the mouth into a slight smile that is not easily controlled and most often occurs without conscious awareness. This type of smile is most likely to occur whenever a secretly held belief, desire, or knowledge about oneself has been exposed or highlighted that would otherwise be considered improper, bad-mannered, or inappropriate to overtly display or take pleasure in. For instance, if you consider yourself intelligent, you are unlikely to boast about it, because you are aware that your self-assessment is subjective and that there are many types of intelligence. Even if you have recently won the Nobel Prize for being particularly clever, you are likely to recognize that bragging about your accomplishment to your peers is more likely to trigger feelings of envy, and secret desires on their part for you to encounter misfortune in the future, than admiration. Thus, when a colleague unexpectedly reveals that she admires your brilliance, you may express your gratitude with a slightly low-intensity but genuine smile that may be barely detectable (a burglar smile). A burglar smile in this context is prosocial because it avoids appearing conceited.

However, not all burglar smiles are prosocial. For example, many OC clients have secret pride about their superior self-control abilities, an attitude that can sometimes lead them to believe they know better or are better than others (see "The Enigma Predicament," chapter 10), which can function to exacerbate their sense of difference and isolation. Therapists can test for the possible presence of secret pride by praising an OC client for possessing superior abilities in self-control and watching to see if a burglar smile appears. Burglar smiles are also likely whenever we find ourselves hearing about a rival's misfortune, when we are successful at manipulating circumstances for personal gain, or have escaped punishment or disapproval that would be warranted if our crime were discovered (such as cheating or lying). For example, an OC client might exhibit a burglar smile after having successfully diverted a topic away from something he did not want to discuss or after his apparently innocent question upset a person he dislikes or wants to punish. Rather than being experienced positively by nearby others, this type of dominance smile has been shown to be associated with the triggering of negative affect in recipients rather than positive (Niedenthal et al., 2010).

The problem for the OC client is that burglar smiles are more than low-level emotional leakage; despite their low intensity and short duration, they are powerful social signals that impact how others feel toward us. Recall that our brains are hardwired to react emotionally within milliseconds to the slightest smile or frown. Thus, if a burglar smile stems from desires to see another fail, secret pride, or similar nonprosocial behaviors, it is highly likely that others are aware of the smiler's nefarious intentions and may want to avoid him, albeit they are unlikely to tell the smiler about this because they no longer trust him.

Teaching OC clients about burglar smiles is the first step toward reducing those behaviors that may be unhelpful for a client's well-being, especially for clients who may pride themselves on being able to control others or have frequent envy. Clients can increase their awareness of burglar smiles by recording on their diary cards when, with whom, and how often such smiles have occurred, and what triggers them. Values clarification can be used to help a client, and sometimes simply being aware of burglar smiles when they occur is sufficient to reduce their frequency; it is hard to secretly gloat about another person's misfortune when you recognize that gloating goes against a core value to be fair-minded. Therapists can begin targeting burglar smiles around the fourteenth session (that is, when a genuine working alliance is more likely to be operative).

Ambiguous, Low-Intensity, and Indirect Social Signals

OC clients are experts at indirect communication. Indirect or disguised social signals are powerful because they allow the sender to influence others without having to admit it; that is, they contain plausible deniability. For example, many OC clients are expert at using indirect communication to avoid revealing personal information. They may change the topic, answer a question with a question (for example, "What do *you* think?"), provide a vague response (such as "I'm not sure" or "Maybe" or "It depends"), report they don't know, or provide long rambling explanations that never get around to answering the question. Unfortunately, indirect communication frequently leads to misunderstanding or distrust because it is hard to know what the true meaning or intentions of the sender are.

For example, it is not uncommon for an OC client to report "I'm fine" when asked whether she might feel distressed or unhappy about something. This is called the "I am fine" phenomenon. Habitual minimization of personal needs and stoicism are common coping strategies among OC clients. Yet direct confrontation about this early in therapy, prior to establishing a working alliance, may lead to premature dropout because it is experienced by the client as disrespectful, critical, or socially inappropriate.

Yet indirect communication is not the core OC difficulty. For example, telling a friend who is dying of cancer that she looks great may represent an act of kindness, or discreetly changing the topic during a heated discussion may prevent an argument. Instead, the negative social consequences of indirect speech may be less about what a person does and more about what he fails to do. A conspicuous lack of prosocial signaling is often interpreted to mean disapproval, dislike, or deception by most people. Here are some examples of indirect or absent prosocial signals that can be interpreted as social rejection by others:

- Not smiling during greetings or interactions

- A conspicuous lack of prosocial touching (for example, refusing to shake hands)

- Lack of affirmative head nods

- Absence of eyebrow flashes or wags during greetings or conversations

- Low frequency of openhanded or expansive gestures

- Lack of eye contact

- Lack of facial affect or emotional expression during interactions

- Failure to reciprocally respond or match the level of emotional expression exhibited by others (for example, not laughing when they laugh)

Subtle, low-intensity signals can also reflect expression habits or emotional leakage never intended as disapproving (for example, the sender has a habit of closing his eyes when someone is talking, or the sender has a painful toothache; see figure 6.12).

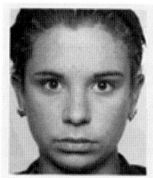 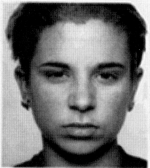 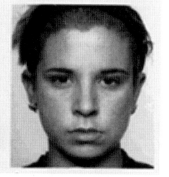

Fear	Disgust	Anger
Eyelids raised	*Nose wrinkled*	*Jaw thrust forward*

Figure 6.12. Subtle, Low-Intensity Social Signals Are Powerful

The silent treatment represents another good example of a powerful yet indirect social signal that is experienced as punitive by those on the receiving end and is damaging to relationships (K. D. Williams, Shore, & Grahe, 1998). It most often occurs following a disagreement with someone, or when a person fails to conform to expectations. It signals disagreement or anger without overtly disclosing it, involving a sudden reduction in verbal behavior, a flattened facial expression, and avoidance of eye contact. If asked by the recipient about the sudden change in social signaling, the sender will usually deny the change and, with a blank face and unemotional tone of voice, say, "No, I'm fine" or "Everything's okay." The sudden nature of the silent treatment and its plausible deniability are what make it so infuriating to those on the receiving end and so damaging to interpersonal relationships.

Addressing indirect communication (that is, disguised demands) in RO DBT involves a three-step process:

1. The individual therapist introduces the problem of masking inner feelings during the orientation and commitment phase of treatment (ideally in the third session). This functions to introduce an often difficult or sensitive subject in therapy, during a time when most OC clients are highly committed.

2. The RO skills training class explicitly teaches clients about the most common types of maladaptive OC indirect communication and the skills needed to change them. Explicit skills training makes what was previously a well-kept secret become public knowledge. This makes it harder for socially conscientious OC clients to continue pretending (to others and themselves) that a maladaptive style of indirect signaling either does not exist or is an appropriate way to behave. Essentially, clients lose their plausible deniability, and their sense of social obligation is likely to compel them to practice more prosocial and direct means of communication.

3. The individual therapist looks for patterns of indirect communication that likely negatively impact rejoining the tribe and achieving valued goals. As with the "I am fine" phenomenon, in general the individual therapist highlights a potentially maladaptive form of indirect communication only after having observed it multiple times and over multiple sessions rather than rushing in to address a potential problem the first time it occurs. This makes it less likely for the client to feel that she is being unfairly criticized while simultaneously making it more difficult for the client to deny the behavior's occurrence.

Prosody and Voice Tone

The term *prosody* refers to the nonverbal components of speech, such as rate (how fast or slowly a person talks), pitch (the relative sound frequency—high or low), intonation (emerging pitch movements during speech), rhythm (how speech is organized into regular time intervals), and loudness (voice volume; see Reed, 2011). A person's rate of speech and tone of voice can tell us much about her current emotional state and about the type of person she is (warm or cool, fearful or calm, dominant or submissive). For example, research shows that people can accurately detect tension in the voice of a person (Pittam & Scherer, 1993), even over the telephone. One way we evaluate whether a person is trustworthy is whether what he is saying matches what he is expressing. For example, a person who says he is having a good time at a party in a flat, monotonic voice is likely to be disbelieved.

Research shows that depressed patients are more likely use a flat, monotonic, and expressionless voice when speaking; to talk more slowly than others; and to exhibit longer pauses during conversations (a pattern of speech commonly observed in OC clients). Depressed clients are also more likely to end a sentence with a downward rather than upward inflection, which can signify low mood, boredom, or disinterest. Unfortunately, OC biotemperamental heightened threat sensitivity makes a monotonic and expressionless voice more likely. In an effort to compensate for this, some OC clients have developed an overly singsong or hypermelodic tone of voice that does not reflect inner experience (such as a happy singsong voice when feeling resentful) or is context-inappropriate (such as a happy singsong voice when reporting that one's husband is having an affair).

Interestingly, empathic responses have been shown to be accompanied by prosodic matching; that is, the recipient of a verbal communication mirrors back the same voice qualities that were present in the speaker (Couper-Kuhlen, 2012). Yet prosodic matching can sometimes inadvertently reinforce maladaptive behavior. RO DBT teaches therapists to purposely use tone of voice, rate of speech, or voice volume contingently in order to modify their OC clients' behavior. For example, rather than engaging a concerned or sympathetic tone of voice after a client reports being unable to get out of bed, an RO DBT therapist is much more likely to engage an incredulous tone of voice and facial expression (playful irreverence) as he says, "Really? That's surprising, because somehow you are here talking to me now, and from what I can tell, you don't seem to be in a bed." And then, with a gentle smile and eyebrow wag, he says, "What do you think this might tell us?"

Atypical prosodic responses (tone of voice, rhythm, rate, and volume) characterize OC verbal behavior. For example, some OC clients launch into an overlearned pattern of speech involving long-winded explanations that never seem to answer a question or ramble on without an apparent point or ending. This pattern ignores prosodic rhythm and turn-taking conventions during conversations, whereby a speaker pauses occasionally to allow a listener an opportunity to speak. Long-winded monologues by OC clients are rarely (if ever) driven by appetitive affect or high reward states (as commonly seen in undercontrolled disorders, such as narcissistic personality disorder or bipolar disorder). Instead, for OC clients, not taking turns in conversations most often reflects anxiety-driven attempts to control a conversational topic ("Please don't interrupt me—let me finish") or desires to not appear anxious ("Only anxious people are quiet"). Long pauses and delays in responding to questions or requests for information represent another atypical OC prosodic response, most often linked to defensive responding and anxiety. This can sometimes be excruciating for therapists (and others), since the client often combines long delays with a barrier gesture (for example, a quick upward movement of the hand, with palm facing outward, that effectively signals "Come no closer" or "Don't interrupt"). Therapists should use the same principles for managing the "I am fine" phenomenon outlined earlier in this chapter as a guide for when and how to target OC prosodic deficits.

Tribe Matters

Compared to other animals, humans are hypercooperative. We are able to share resources, work together, and form strong bonds with genetically dissimilar others in a manner that is unprecedented in the animal world. To accomplish this, our species is posited to have developed a highly sophisticated social signaling system that allowed us to communicate intentions and feelings (an angry glare linked to a desire to attack) without having to fully express the actual propensity itself (hitting someone). Signaling intentions from afar (for example, via facial expressions, gestures, or vocalizations) reduced unnecessary expenditures of energy and provided a safer means to resolve conflicts or initiate collaborations with others without having to fully commit oneself. Plus, revealing intentions and emotions to other members of our species was essential to create the type of strong social bonds that are the cornerstone of human tribes. When we reveal our true feelings to another person, we send a powerful social safety signal that most often functions to increase trust and social connectedness, thereby making it more likely for the other person to make self-sacrifices for our benefit or collaborate with us in order to accomplish tasks and overcome obstacles that would be impossible if attempted alone. Yet our hypercooperative nature was also accompanied by some downsides.

For example, for our very early ancestors living in harsh environments, the cost of not detecting a true disapproval signal was too high to ignore, since tribal banishment was essentially a death sentence from starvation or predation. As a consequence, we are constantly scanning the facial expressions and vocalizations of other people for signs of disapproval and are biologically predisposed to construe the intentions of others as disapproving, especially when social signals are ambiguous. This means we are essentially a socially anxious species. Blank expressions, furrowed brows, or slight frowns are often interpreted as disapproving, regardless of the actual intentions of the sender (for example, some people frown or furrow their brow when intensely listening). Plus, being rejected by a tribe hurts; research shows that social ostracism triggers the same areas of the brain that are triggered when we experience physical pain (Eisenberger & Lieberman, 2004). Thus we fear the pain of social exclusion, and our emotional well-being is highly dependent on the extent to which we feel part of a tribe.

Moreover, humans are not always prosocial. As a species, we can be ruthlessly callous and deceptive to those we dislike, or to rival members of another tribe. Yet, as individuals, we cannot simply decide not to play the social signaling game. We are constantly socially signaling when around others (via microexpressions and body movements), even when deliberately trying not to. For example, silence can be just as powerful as nonstop talking. Indeed, effective social signaling is always a two-way street, requiring both accurate transmission of inner experience or intentions and accurate reception and openness to the transmissions of others.

Finally, the social signaling recommendations outlined in this chapter are not meant to be applied as rigid rules. For example, therapists should avoid temptations to overcorrect (for example, concluding that expressions of concern should never be expressed when working with OC clients). Therapists should use contextual cues to help guide how and what they socially signal in session. Plus, when OC clients are engaged in therapy, the social signaling behavior displayed by a therapist may matter less. Yet, at the same time, RO DBT social signaling strategies are principle-based. Loosely translated, an RO DBT therapist is encouraged to stop behaving like a therapist and start behaving like a friend, in order to teach emotionally lonely and isolated OC clients how to make genuine connections with others (often for the first time in their lives). This is why RO DBT therapists are likened to tribal ambassadors. Ambassadors interact with other cultures in a manner that most others reserve solely for interactions with close friends or family. When a therapist adopts this stance, she automatically signals to OC clients that she considers them part of her tribe. Without a word spoken, clients receive a gift of kindness that essentially says, "I trust you, I believe in you, and I am the same as you."

Now You Know...

► The great number and variety of verbal and nonverbal social signals available to our species increases the likelihood that our social signals will be misinterpreted, especially when their meaning is ambiguous.

► The social signaling deficits of OC clients leave them uniquely vulnerable to being misunderstood and even ostracized. OC clients also tend to experience intense social engagement, including therapists' expressions of concern, as overwhelming, intrusive, or threatening.

► RO DBT therapists teach OC clients the social signaling skills that have been shown to enhance social connectedness. Therapists also modify their in-session nonverbal behavior in ways that enhance treatment outcomes for OC clients by facilitating their clients' engagement in therapy and by activating experiences of social safety in their clients as well as in themselves.

CHAPTER 7

Radical Openness and Self-Enquiry: Personal Practice, Therapeutic Modeling, Supervision, and Team Consultation

Radical openness is the core philosophical principle and core skill in RO DBT. Radically open living is posited to impact not only how we see the world (we are more receptive to critical feedback) but also how others see us (people like people who are open-minded). Thus it is considered both a state of mind and a powerful social signal that influences personal and other perception. The primary aims of this chapter are as follows:

- To provide an overview of core RO concepts

- To highlight the rationale for therapist practice of RO skills and describe how to develop a personal practice of self-enquiry

- To describe principles for modeling RO with clients and how to integrate self-enquiry into therapy

- To outline ways to enhance supervision using videotape and how to structure, conduct, and integrate RO and self-enquiry principles into therapist supervision and team consultation meetings

The chapter begins with tribal glue. [Editor's note: Careful, Dr. Lynch—our attorneys have advised us that this is a sticky proposition.]

Openness Is Tribal Glue

Why do we like open-minded people? As a species, we instinctively recognize the value openness brings to relationships. For example, we tend to trust open-minded people because they are more likely to reveal than hide their inner feelings during conflict. We desire to affiliate with open-minded people because they are humble—they are more likely to give others the benefit of the doubt during interactions and don't automatically assume that their way is the best, right, or only way. RO DBT considers open-mindedness both a state of being and a prosocial personality trait (see "Characteristics of Trait Openness" for other advantages of open-minded living). Thus openness, according to RO DBT, is both a transitory state of being and a habitual way of coping.

Essentially, openness is a powerful social safety signal. It helps ensure that cooperative intentions are perceived as intended, especially during times of potential conflict. It is the cure for arrogance, selfishness, and lack of empathy, and it helps curb our ego by placing the needs of others on an equal footing to our own. Without a word being spoken, openness allows the recipient of this social signal the luxury of dropping his guard because it acknowledges the sender's inherent potential for fallibility and signals the sender's willingness to learn from what the world has to offer. As recipients, we are able to viscerally recognize (in our bodies) open-minded behavior during an interaction, even when the person we are interacting with speaks a different language or comes from a differing culture. Indeed, openness does not have to be loud, articulate, or specific to be heard; there are many ways to express openness. Nonverbally, open-minded behavior is most often associated with expressions and gestures universally associated with friendliness, curiosity, and nondominance—eyebrow wags, smiling, openhanded gestures, shoulder shrugs, affirmative head nods, a musical tone of voice, and taking turns during conversations.

> We tend to trust open-minded people because they are more likely to reveal than hide their inner feelings during conflict.

Plus, by openly revealing our opinions, feelings, and thoughts to others, we create reciprocal learning opportunities or dialogues with others that can further refine ideas, improve coping strategies, and enhance social connectedness, not only for the individuals involved but also for the tribe as a whole. Thus RO DBT considers openness a type of tribal glue—it evolved in our species as a core means for establishing strong collaborative relationships with genetically dissimilar individuals, and it represents the cornerstone of all new learning.

Characteristics of Trait Openness

The term *trait openness* refers to an individual's habitual way, across context and over time, of responding to new or discrepant information and tolerating chaos or ambiguity—that is, the extent to which a person is receptive to new ideas, novel situations, and unexpected information. Individuals high in trait openness can be considered open-minded people, as indicated by the following types of behavior and attitudes:

- Open-minded people are able to listen to disconfirming feedback and modify their behavior, when necessary, in order to learn, live by their values, or adapt to changing circumstances.

- Open-minded people state their opinions in a manner that acknowledges their imperfection. They don't assume that their way of thinking is the only one or the correct one.

- Open-minded people don't take themselves or life too seriously. They can laugh at personal foibles, quirks, and habits without harshly blaming themselves or others.

- Open-minded people are willing to engage (and reengage) in conflict in order to learn, resolve a problem, or improve a relationship. They view conflicts as opportunities for growth rather than threats.

- Open-minded people are able to admit when their actions have caused harm to others, and to apologize when an apology is warranted.

- Open-minded people are excited to learn new things and are likely to exhibit high curiosity in novel situations.

- Open-minded people celebrate diversity.

- Open-minded people give others the benefit of the doubt during interactions.

- Open-minded people don't need to prove that they are right (even when they are).

- Open-minded people take responsibility for their reactions to the world rather than automatically blaming others, falling apart, or expecting the world to change.

- Open-minded people openly express, with humility, what they feel or think.

- Open-minded people allow the other person (and themselves) the grace of not having to understand, resolve, or fix a problem or issue immediately.

Openness, Collaboration, and Compliance

The benefits of collaboration for our species can be seen everywhere. For example, as I write this I am aboard a nighttime ferry crossing the English Channel. I'm gazing out the window of our cabin berth toward a line of brightly illuminated cargo ships, each unique in size, shape, type of cargo, country of origin, and style of lighting. Despite these differences, their movements appear coordinated, cooperative, and purposeful as they await permission from the harbormaster to enter the Port of Caen in France. There are no physical barriers forcing these ships to take turns, yet every ship complies, presumably because each captain recognizes the value for doing so over the alternatives (such as being a pirate). Thus compliance matters. Indeed, compliance is so important that most societies use aversive contingencies such as shaming rituals or imprisonment to enforce it. Yet what's good for society may not always be good for the individual. Plus, blind compliance can lead to disastrous consequences (see "The Milgram Experiment," in the skills training manual, chapter 5, lesson 30), and sometimes noncompliance is needed to prevent a moral wrong or stop an injustice.

From a social signaling perspective, compliance is a nondominance signal. It requires the complier to give in or submit to the wishes, desires, expectations, or requests of another (or at least appear to be doing so). Yet social signaling an intention to comply represents only part of the story. It is also important to understand what motivates us to comply, especially since our motivations or actions are not always prosocial. In RO DBT, four broad functions or motivations are posited to underlie compliant responses:

1.   We comply out of fear. Fear-based compliance is most often motivated by one of two possible contingencies: we fear punishment from powerful others not in our tribe (such as border police, an invading army, a rival gang, a mugger with a gun), or we fear punishment (social disapproval, social exclusion, shaming rituals, solitary confinement, a sentence of death) from powerful others within our tribe.

2.   We comply in the moment, in order to dominate later. Dominance-based compliance always involves some type of purposeful deception or pretending. We concede defeat while secretly planning revenge. We compliment a rival to hide our envy. We ingratiate ourselves to get someone to like us, only so we can use that person later. We attempt to appear similar to another or to appear more attractive in order gain favor. We drop names of famous people to enhance our status. We smile (not in agreement) or physically touch someone in order to get that person to trust us.

3.   Our compliance is logical, reason-based, or rule-governed. We capitulate to superior reasoning, we concede a chess match when we realize that there is no way for us to win, or we nod in agreement because it is the polite thing to do.

4. We comply out of kindness, passion, or love. Love-based compliance is posited to emerge in three differing ways, the second and third of which are posited to be linked with radical openness. First, compliance may be motivated by faith, admiration, or respect for another person or system of belief. In this situation, we are not required to understand why compliance is needed; we blindly accept promises, predictions, or directions from a charismatic leader, or we concede an argument because we have faith in the other person's supposedly better judgment or superior intellect, or we sacrifice ourselves for a cause or out of devotion. Second, compliance may be motivated by curiosity or love of learning. In this situation, we relinquish our worldview in order to understand a new culture, purposefully seeking new ways of thinking or behaving in order to enhance self-growth. This component of love-based compliance is closely aligned with the practice of radical openness in that it requires us to relinquish our perspective in order to be open to a new one. And, third, compliance may be motivated by a desire for intimacy, closeness, or mutual understanding—a desire to be one with another. This component of love-based compliance is closely aligned with the practice of radical openness in that it requires us to be kind—to make sacrifices for another person, without always expecting something in return.

RO DBT posits healthy compliance and genuine openness as prosocial sides of the same coin, with compliance representing the overt social signal and openness the underlying mechanism.

Openness, Tribes, and Learning

We are tribal by nature. Our species' survival depended on our being able to form long-lasting social bonds, share valuable resources with unrelated others, and work together in tribes or groups. For example, tribes provide instrumental support for individual members (as when tribe members help a neighbor repair her roof after a storm) as well as for the tribe as a whole (as when tribe members collectively build a wall to keep out enemies). Plus, tribes provide opportunities for individuals to acquire vast amounts of knowledge and skill that would be impossible for individuals to acquire on their own. There are two types of social learning—passive and active—and both require openness on the learner's part. Passive (or observational) learning involves didactic instruction (going to a lecture), modeling (observing someone riding a horse), and feedback (criticism or praise). Active (or interactive) learning takes observational learning one step further: in interactive learning, the individual, rather than solely being a passive recipient of information, is required both to openly observe and to openly reveal his observations to others in order to stimulate further feedback. Revealing to others our observations about the world ("This mushroom looks tasty—maybe just a little nibble") and then receiving (or not receiving) verification of our perceptions from another member of our tribe ("No, it's deadly—spit it out") provided a huge evolutionary advantage because our individual survival no longer depended solely on our personal perceptions. This helps explain why we are so concerned about the opinions of others.

Indeed, the capacity to benefit from the collective wisdom of the tribe, without the necessity of personal experience, may be a core defining feature of our species. Yet our unprecedented capacity to learn from others did not just appear overnight. It required our early ancestors to develop increasingly sophisticated ways to *signal intentions* (via facial expressions and gestures), *communicate observations about nature* (via gaze direction, pointing, and pantomime), and *imitate complex actions* (as in toolmaking), all behaviors posited as evolutionary precursors of human speech (Arbib, 2012). Social discourse, stories, myths, advice, and feedback increasingly became our primary sources of learning, and with the advent of spoken and written language we could pass on our accumulated knowledge to the next generation (what time of year to plant corn, caribou herds' migration patterns, how to make bread or build a water aqueduct). Our survival no longer depended solely on trial-and-error learning. Social learning became our evolutionary solution, manifested most often in the following ways:

- Observational learning, or modeling of successful others (watching or imitating someone who is throwing a spear)

- Explicit instruction (being told how to throw a spear)

- Direct feedback (being corrected on throwing a spear: "You missed the target because you were gripping the spear too tightly")

Yet our ability to learn from others also arrived with some downsides. As our capacity to symbolically represent and communicate our inner experience, intentions, and observations developed, it moved from pantomime to cave drawings, from regional specific gestures to coded gestures, from spoken language to written language, and from mathematical equations to computer programming. The sheer amount and availability of potentially important new information became too much for any one person to ever fully grasp, let alone master, eventually leading to the frequently heard complaint of information overload in contemporary society. Plus, social learning requires a person to drop his perspective (at least momentarily) in order to absorb a new one while simultaneously trusting the source of the new information or collective wisdom (a friend's opinion, a tribal elder's memory, a written document). The worry is that the source may be wrong ("When it comes to accuracy in spear throwing, your grip is less important—what matters most is keeping the shaft close to your body at all times during the throw") or intentionally deceptive ("My so-called friend is giving me the wrong advice on purpose so he can win the tribal spear-throwing contest").

Moreover, when it comes to treating problems of overcontrol, not only do most OC clients find it difficult to trust—they prefer passive learning (studying alone) to interactive learning (asking for help and seeking feedback)—they are also likely to experience interactive learning as exhausting or frightening. It is exhausting because it requires collaboration, open listening, and taking another person's point of view seriously. It is frightening because it requires not just open dialogue (and sometimes debate) but also dependence on others to achieve a desired outcome. In addition, interactive learning almost invariably involves receiving some form of disconfirming feedback, which can sometimes lead to disagreement or conflict. Most OC clients would rather abandon a relationship than deal directly with interpersonal conflict, making it less likely for them to experientially learn that disagreement often leads to new discoveries and that conflict can be intimacy-enhancing.

RO DBT posits that there is a way forward. It involves the creation of a temporary state of self-doubt, which does not necessitate a validity check on every source of new information or a character reference for every person who gives us some advice. This temporary state of mind is referred to in RO DBT as *healthy self-doubt*. It begins with the assumption that we don't see things as they are but instead see things as we are, and it is based on the notion that it is impossible for us to ever fully rid ourselves of our personal backgrounds or biogenetic predispositions (see table 7.1).

Table 7.1. Healthy vs. Unhealthy Self-Doubt

When We Operate From Healthy Self-Doubt…	When We Operate From Unhealthy Self-Doubt…
We are in a temporary state of openness to disconfirming or unexpected stimuli, with the aim of learning.	We fear self-examination.
We are able to consider that our way of behaving or thinking may be inaccurate or ineffective, without falling apart or harshly blaming others.	On the surface we may appear willing to question ourselves or admit a mistake in order to grow, but underneath we're convinced that we're right.
We don't take ourselves too seriously, and we have a sense of humor. We can laugh at our own foibles, strange habits, or unique quirks with a sense of kindness. We can acknowledge that all humans are fallible.	We may feel unfairly accused or singled out and may harbor secret anger or resentment toward people or events we believe are responsible for triggering uncertainty in us or forcing us into unwanted self-examination.
We take responsibility for our actions and emotions by not giving up when we're challenged.	We have a secret desire not to change and not to be challenged.
We signal our willingness to learn from the world and others, and thus we enhance our relationships.	We may express our unhealthy self-doubt in a passive manner (by sulking, pouting, walking away, giving up, or behaving helplessly), but we are still sending a powerful social signal, one that often blocks further feedback and thus has a negative impact on our social relationships.

One Secret of Healthy Living Is the Cultivation of Healthy Self-Doubt

A core RO tenet is that we need to be open only when we are closed. Though in principle this sounds simple, the actual task of determining whether our current state of mind is closed can be extremely difficult. For example, have you ever noticed that you often think you are open, only to discover later that you were actually closed—and that your friends always seem to notice this before you do? [Editor's note: Not *our* friends.] Sometimes our way feels so right that it almost feels wrong to question it. I have come to realize that when I find myself trying to convince others (or myself) that I am open, most often I am not. Our belief systems are so much a part of us that we often don't even recognize them as beliefs; it's a bit like asking fish to notice the water they are swimming in. Plus, we tend to pay attention to things that fit our beliefs and ignore or dismiss things that don't, and we don't know what we don't know, thereby making it doubly hard for us to notice our closed-minded thinking because our way of thinking feels so right. Here is an example of how an OC client's worldview biases how he interprets the behavior of his son:

> I expect my son to call every two weeks, on Sunday at exactly 2.00 p.m. What's important in these calls is that we catch up on the latest family news. So I go through my list of what I have been doing and then ask him to report his news. But he usually doesn't have a prepared list and instead rambles on about trivial things. So after he finishes talking, I double-check to see if there is anything I have forgotten and then finish with "I think I have told you everything." Recently my son asked me how I feel about some of the news I report. I told him that I feel it is important for us to keep each other up to date on what is happening. He seemed agitated in his response. He told me that my answer wasn't a feeling, and then he complained that he didn't feel close to me. I just don't understand what he wants. After all, he knows everything that is going on with me. What more is there?

In general, we are more likely to be closed-minded when we encounter a novel or uncertain situation, when we feel invalidated or criticized, or when our expectations and beliefs about the world, ourselves, and other people are challenged. Yet closed-mindedness is not always about feeling threatened; as in the example just cited, closed-mindedness for many OC clients can be rule-governed and relatively nonemotional. Indeed, OC biotemperamental superiority in detail-focused processing, though primarily nonemotional, may function to exacerbate OC clients' closed-mindedness. The reason this occurs is that individuals with a superior eye for detail are not only faster than most others at noticing minor changes and patterns in the environment but also more likely to be correct in what they have observed, and thus naturally prone to trust their own personal observations over those made by others. Indeed, most societies depend on individuals with superior detail-focused brains to find the errors that others may have overlooked—the seemingly innocent missing word in a trade agreement, the loose stone on a footbridge, or the frayed wire in a jet engine.

What is infuriating for the detail-oriented person is not only that other people frequently fail to notice an error or a minor discrepancy but also that, even when they do notice it, they may question its relevance.

What is important to remember is that superior detail-focused processing does not equate to being effective or even correct. Plus, it impacts not only what is seen but also what is *not* seen. For example, a detail-focused individual might accurately note the exact number of mixed metaphors or dangling participles in a page of writing but be relatively clueless about what the writer is actually saying. [Editor's note: All resemblance between the author's example of a detail-focused individual and any real person, living or dead, is purely coincidental, especially with respect to the allegation of cluelessness.] Thus the challenge for OC clients learning open-minded living is multifold: not only must they learn to overcome their biotemperamental tendencies to prefer detail-focused processing over global processing when contextual clues suggest that it would be more effective to see the big picture, they also need to be alert for misplaced self-confidence or arrogance after they are proven right.

> When I find myself trying to convince others (or myself) that I am open, most often I am not.

Closed-mindedness can also occur during positive mood states linked to overcoming obstacles, defeating a rival, or successfully attaining a long-term goal. According to the RO DBT neuroregulatory model (see chapter 2), when we are excited, elated, or proud of an accomplishment, our sympathetic nervous system (SNS) excitatory approach/reward system is activated, and, because of neuroinhibitory relationships between the parasympathetic nervous system (PNS) and the SNS, the excitatory approach/reward system functions to downregulate or impair the social safety system mediated by the ventral vagal complex of the PNS (the PNS-VVC). Excitatory reward mood states are energizing and associated with feelings of joy, self-confidence, and agency. When we are in positive mood states, we are more likely to be assertive, arrogant, and opinionated. Despite feeling on top of the world, we lose our ability to empathically read the subtle social signals displayed by others and also are less aware of how our behavior may be impacting them. For example, we may fail to notice that the person we are speaking to is in pain, that he is embarrassed by what is being said or by what is happening, and that he would like to make a comment or change the topic. During a conversation, we may be unaware that we are speaking more rapidly, failing to provide time for the other person to speak, or frequently talking over or interrupting the other person, and we are more likely to overestimate our own capabilities and underestimate the capabilities of others. If challenged, we may begin to feel irritable or attempt to convince the other person or dominate the conversation by repeatedly giving our point of view. Essentially, during high excitatory reward states, we are likely to be more expressive but less empathic and open-minded (via downregulation of the PNS-VVC social safety system and upregulation of SNS excitatory reward system).

But let's think about this for a moment. If maladaptive overcontrol is characterized by low reward sensitivity, as posited in RO DBT, then is the closed-mindedness that can result from SNS excitatory reward states likely to be much of a problem for OC clients? The quick answer is yes. OC clients do have biotemperamental predispositions for low reward sensitivity, but they can still have high reward experiences. Remember, however, that their superior capacity for inhibitory control and their overlearned tendencies to mask inner feelings make it likely that they will automatically inhibit expansive and dramatic expressions most others display when feeling highly excited or happy. Thus, instead of grinning from ear to ear or dancing with abandon when experiencing joy, an OC client is more likely to display a burglar smile. Remember also that OC clients' excitatory reward experiences are most often associated with resisting temptation, achieving long-term goals, or defeating a rival—for OC clients, in other words, rewards must be earned (and deserved). This helps explain why most OC clients are less likely to be thrilled or excited by rewards that arise by chance or without any effort on their part—rewards like winning a door prize, observing a beautiful sunset, or receiving an unexpected compliment. Indeed, most OC clients believe that, given the choice, it would be better for them to choose the most difficult path—in order to test their mettle and prove their worth (most often to themselves)—than to take the path of least resistance. In short, closed-mindedness is not always about feeling threatened; it can just as easily be due to the excitatory reward states secondary to attaining success, achieving a long-term goal, overcoming an obstacle, or vanquishing a rival. Thus radical openness is useful, not just when experiencing defensive arousal but also when feeling highly self-confident, self-assured, calm, in control, or wise (overconfidence was a major factor in the sinking of the *Titanic*). The good news is that even though it's difficult to recognize when we are closed, there are some things we can do to improve our detection rate (see "How Can You Know You're Closed, Especially When You Think You're Not?," page 188).

What Is Radical Openness?

The term *radical openness* represents the confluence of three core capacities posited to underlie emotional well-being:

1. Receptivity to new experience and disconfirming feedback, in order to learn

2. Flexible self-control, in order to adapt to changing environmental conditions

3. Intimacy and connectedness with at least one other person

Thus radically open living requires a person to be open to disconfirming feedback and adapt her behavior in a manner that also accounts for the needs of others. For example, she might strive for perfection (but stop when feedback suggests that striving is counterproductive or damaging a relationship), be rule-governed (except when breaking the rules is needed—for example, to save someone's life), or be polite and cooperative (yet be bad-tempered if the situation calls for it, as when safety concerns are overriding).

Radical openness can trace its roots to a spiritual tradition known as Malâmati Sufism. Malâmati Sufism originated in the ninth century in the northeast of Persia, in an area called Khorasan (what is now Iran), and in the present day it has a strong following in Turkey and the Balkan States. The name Malâmati comes from the Arabic word *malamah*, meaning "blame" and referring to the Malâmati practice of sustained self-observation and healthy self-criticism in order to understand one's true motivations (Toussulis, 2011). Malâmatis believe that one cannot achieve heightened self-awareness in isolation; as a consequence, emphasis is given to spiritual dialogue and companionship (in Arabic, *sohbet*). The Malâmatis are not interested so much in the acceptance of reality or in seeing "what is," without illusion; rather, they look to find fault within themselves and question their self-centered desires for power, recognition, or self-aggrandizement.[43]

A core principle in RO DBT is that innate perceptual and regulatory biases make it impossible for a person to achieve heightened self-awareness in isolation; we need others to point out our blind spots. Truth in RO DBT is considered real yet elusive; thus, for example, "If I know anything, it is that I don't know everything, and neither does anyone else" (M. P. Lynch, 2004, p. 10). It is the pursuit of truth that matters, not its attainment. Rather than assuming we could ever know reality just as it is, radical openness assumes that we all bring perceptual and regulatory biases into every moment, and that our biases interfere with our ability to be open and to learn from new or disconfirming information.[44]

Yet simply being frank or forthright with our opinions, observations, feelings, or beliefs is not sufficient to create the type of open dialogue and equal status that characterize experiences associated with optimal interactive learning. As such, RO DBT contends that it is essential not only to reveal our inner experience or opinions to others but also and simultaneously to acknowledge our own potential for fallibility. Rather than automatically assuming that the world should change ("You need to validate me because I feel upset") or automatically prioritizing regulation or acceptance strategies that function to reduce arousal or lead to a sense of peace, RO DBT posits that the *truth hurts*. That is, often reaching the place of most personal self-growth involves coming to grips with (attending to) the very place we don't want to go. Thus radical openness means developing a passion for going opposite to where we are. It is more than mindful awareness. It means actively seeking those areas of our lives that we want to avoid or may find uncomfortable, in order to learn. It involves purposeful self-enquiry and a willingness to be wrong, with an intention to change if we need to change. It is humility in action.

A practice of radical openness involves three sequential steps:

1. Acknowledging the presence of a disconfirming or an unexpected event that triggers a feeling of tension, resistance, dislike, numbness, or desires to attack, control, or flee

How Can You Know You're Closed, Especially When You Think You're Not?

The short answer to that question is that you can't, at least not without a little help from your friends. The longer answer has to do with research suggesting that your peers will often be more accurate than you are at assessing your personality quirks (Oltmanns, Friedman, Fiedler, & Turkheimer, 2004; John & Robins, 1994), and that if you think you have fewer problems than others, your peers probably think you have more (Oltmanns, Gleason, Klonsky, & Turkheimer, 2005). Therefore, to find out whether you're closed-minded, practice these skills.

- When you find yourself striving to convince either yourself or someone else of how open you are, consider your insistence on your openness as evidence of your being closed.

- Don't always trust your gut. In the heat of the moment, when you're in the middle of an argument, and when you're convinced that you are being open-minded, don't automatically assume that you are right. Instead, stop and ask the person you're interacting with for his opinion about how open you are being. To do this, briefly disengage eye contact (to take the heat off) while taking a slow, deep breath, and then say, "You know, I've got a question for you." Pause, make direct eye contact, and offer a closed-mouth smile. "How open-minded do you think I am being right now? I'd really like to know because it is something I have been working on lately. I know it's a bit off topic, but I'm curious. So what do you think?" Allow the other person time to answer fully before you respond. It's important when you ask that you not try to feel or appear calm but instead communicate an earnest desire to openly hear what the other person might have to say. This is a fantastic practice because you get feedback right in the moment, and yet the very act of asking is a powerful social safety signal.

- Don't automatically assume that you are closed. After the interaction is over, use the other person's feedback as an opportunity to practice radical openness skills. For example, take out your skills training manual, turn to chapter 5, lesson 22, handout 22.2, and practice Flexible Mind ADOPTS, using the handout's twelve questions to help you determine whether you should accept or decline the feedback.

- When you're *not* in the heat of the moment—when the other person is not around—you can still get a sense of how open or closed you might be in your interactions. For example, ask yourself how willing you would be to find out or admit that you're wrong, that you're not open, that you're holding a grudge, or that you're feeling envious. The more energy or resistance you feel when asking this question, the less likely it is that you are genuinely open.

- Practice self-enquiry (see "Practicing Self-Enquiry and Outing One-self," later in this chapter). Ask yourself, *Is there something here for me to learn?*

- Remember that asking for feedback is anxiety-producing for all humans. Self-consciousness, fear of disapproval, and social anxiety reflect our tribal nature and our fundamental dependence on other people; as we've seen before, exclusion from the tribe was essentially a death sentence for our primordial ancestors, so don't assume that the presence of anxiety means you are necessarily closed. Practice self-enquiry (*What might my anxiety tell me? Is there something here for me to learn?*) while blocking quick answers. It is the very act of asking, not the actual feedback itself, that may be what is most important when it comes to close social bonds. The simple act of allowing yourself to consider the possibility that your perspective may be wrong, and then communicating this possibility to another person by asking for candid feedback, sends a powerful message of friendship, openness, and equality. It allows the recipient of your message the luxury of dropping his guard because he can viscerally sense that you are open-minded enough to listen to his point of view.

Thus openness, despite its energy-depleting downsides (openness requires cognitive effort), is posited to be a core part of a uniquely human evolutionary advantage that allowed for unprecedented cooperation among genetically unrelated individuals. In other words, open-minded-ness is tribal glue—it binds together differences and creates new and previously unimagined accords.

2. Practicing self-enquiry by temporarily turning toward the discomfort and asking what we might need to learn, rather than automatically regulating, distracting, explaining, reappraising, or accepting

3. Flexibly responding with humility by doing what's needed in the moment to effectively manage the situation or adapt to changing circumstances in a manner that accounts for the needs of others

Plus, being open to learning new things does not mean that we must reject our prior learning. Instead, it recognizes that most often there are many ways to get to the same place (numerous roads lead to London) or do the same thing (there are countless ways to cook potatoes); and, because the world is in constant change, there is always something new to learn. For example, the best scientists are humble because they realize that everything they know will eventually evolve or change into greater knowledge. Practicing self-enquiry is particularly useful whenever we find ourselves strongly rejecting, defending against, or automatically agreeing with feedback that we find challenging or unexpected. Yet it can be painful because it often requires sacrificing firmly held convictions or self-constructs. The good news is that openness frees up energy that in the past was used to protect ourselves. It is the opposite of pretending, complacency, passivity, or resignation. Although it does not promise bliss, equanimity, or enlightenment, what it promises is the possibility of genuine friendship and dialogue.

Radical openness does not mean approval, naively believing, or mindlessly acquiescing. Sometimes being closed is what is needed in the moment, and sometimes change is unnecessary. For example, being closed-minded about eating cottage cheese when one dislikes its taste is fine, assuming there is something else to eat. Closed-mindedness is highly useful when being attacked by a mugger or tortured when captured in war. Being closed-minded might help protect certain family or cultural traditions that help bind tribes together—for example, doggedly celebrating Christmas despite no longer being religious. Openness is a behavior. Finally, radical openness is not something that can be grasped solely via intellectual means—it is experiential. It requires direct and repeated practice, and one's understanding evolves over time as a function of continued practice.

Practicing Self-Enquiry and Outing Oneself

RO DBT considers defensive arousal, tension in the body, or unwanted emotions helpful because they can alert us to areas in our lives where we may need to change or grow. Rather than automatically assuming that the world needs to change so we can feel better, radical openness posits that we often learn the most from those areas of life that we find most challenging. Thus RO DBT considers an unwanted emotion, thought, or sensation in the body a reminder to practice self-enquiry by redirecting our attention to the challenging or threatening experience and asking, *Is there something to learn here?* Self-enquiry might eventually lead a person to the conclusion that there is nothing to learn, or that being closed is what is needed at a particular time or in a particular situation. However, radical openness means retaining a willingness to revisit the issue and practice self-enquiry again—say, when circumstances change, or if tension in the body keeps reemerging around the same issue.

Radical Openness Is Not the Same as Radical Acceptance

It is important to note that the skills associated with radical openness differ from the radical acceptance skills taught as part of standard DBT (Linehan, 1993b). Radical acceptance means letting go of the *fight with* reality, and turning intolerable suffering into tolerable pain, whereas radical openness challenges our *perceptions* of reality. Radical openness posits that we are unable to see things as they are but instead see things as we are. Thus RO encourages the cultivation of self-enquiry and healthy self-doubt in order to signal humility and learn from what the world may have to offer.

The RO DBT practices of outing (revealing) oneself share similarities with the concept of *parrhésia*, defined today as boldness or freedom of speech, and by the ancient Greeks (such as Plato, Socrates, and Diogenes of Sinope) as the practice not only of speaking boldly and candidly but also of speaking the truth for the common good. The practice of outing oneself most often begins with awareness of tension in the body, followed by openly describing what is happening (thoughts, feelings, sensations) regardless of how silly, inarticulate, or judgmental it may sound, in order to locate one's edge—that is, the point where personal growth can occur. Most often one's edge involves feelings of embarrassment, discomfort, desires to avoid, or thoughts and images that one would prefer not to acknowledge in public. Self-enquiry practices do not have to be about big issues or big emotions. In fact, sometimes we learn more about ourselves when we enquire into a relatively small event (for example, feeling annoyed by a question asked by a subordinate, feeling unappreciated when our spouse fails to notice that we rearranged his or her desk, or feeling happy when a colleague tells us about a misfortune).

Self-enquiry seeks self-growth by turning toward the very things one wants to avoid and then outing what one has discovered to a fellow practitioner (or friend) in order to locate one's blind spots. Thus self-enquiry practice often results in embarrassment or feelings of shame (though not always). Despite this, the practices associated with outing oneself go opposite to the unwarranted shame or embarrassment that may arise when self-enquiry reveals parts of our personality we are not proud of or might wish to deny. Shame is unwarranted because acknowledging fallibility, after resisting that acknowledgment or being afraid of others' reactions, is a courageous and noble pursuit. By outing yourself, you are telling your brain that there is nothing to be ashamed of, whereas hiding your fallibilities or personality quirks from others says to your brain that having a personality quirk or being fallible is bad (shameful). All humans are flawed, and radical openness celebrates our quirky habits as opportunities for self-discovery, not opportunities to get down on ourselves.

The good news is that outing ourselves helps us take responsibility for our perceptions and actions. It blocks habitual avoidance and denial. For OC clients, this can be an important process in self-discovery. Many OC clients avoid revealing personal feelings or opinions because it means they could be criticized or that they may then be expected to change. Outing oneself enhances relationships because it models humility and willingness to learn from what the world has to offer. Revealing personal information to another person is a powerful prosocial signal; it essentially says, "I trust you" (we don't reveal vulnerability to those we distrust) and "You and I are the same" (meaning we share a bond of fallibility). Thus, in many ways, outing oneself is the foundation of true friendship. For example, friends take responsibility for their own emotions rather than blaming them on each other. Friends are open to feedback even when it hurts. Friends protect each other yet are also willing to tell each other a painful truth in order to help each other achieve valued goals, in a manner that acknowledges their own potential for fallibility. Thus true friends (people with close bonds) know things about each other that could hurt, but they don't use these things against each other.

Finally, self-enquiry is able to question self-enquiry itself. It recognizes that every query (or answer) emerging from a practice of self-enquiry, regardless of how seemingly profound, wise, or discerning it may appear, is subject to error. Plus, self-enquiry means having the courage to admit our faults to others or acknowledge how we may have contributed to a problem, without getting down on ourselves, and yet it is suspicious of quick answers. Quick answers to self-enquiry questions often reflect old learning, rigid rules or beliefs to the effect that everything should be fixed immediately, or compulsive desires to avoid social disapproval by coming up with a solution or explanation that justifies one's behavior. This tendency to quickly fix or answer is one of the core reasons behind the emphasis in RO DBT on revealing our self-enquiry insights and observations to caring others (as in outing ourselves to a fellow practitioner). Outing one's personality quirks or weaknesses publicly goes opposite to OC tendencies to mask inner feelings and can become a powerful means for OC clients to rejoin the tribe; therefore, the importance of this when treating OC cannot be overemphasized.[45] The steps for conducting formal self-enquiry and practices for outing oneself in consultation teams are outlined in the following section as well as in the skills training manual.

RO DBT Team Consultation and Supervision

A central premise in RO DBT is that both therapists and clients bring perceptual and regulatory biases into the treatment environment, and that these biases impact outcomes. Plus, RO DBT posits that the technical aspects of psychotherapy are not independent of the person delivering them or of the relational context they are delivered in. Thus therapists using RO DBT ideally build into their treatment programs a means to support their own practice of radical openness in order to effectively deliver the treatment. This most often translates into a weekly therapist consultation team meeting that can be held in person or via the internet. Consultation team meetings serve several important functions; not only do they provide a platform for therapists' practice of radical openness, they also help reduce therapists' burnout, enhance empathy in therapists, and promote therapists' adherence to the treatment. RO is experiential; it is not something that one can grasp solely via intellectual means, and it requires a fellow practitioner to reflect our blind spots. This requires therapists to bring self-enquiry and radical openness into their own lives. Similar to mindfulness, self-enquiry requires direct and repeated practice; plus, one's understanding of RO evolves over time as a function of continued practice. Finally, OC clients are unlikely to believe that it is appropriate for an adult to relax, play, or express vulnerability unless their therapists model such behavior first, and therapists' practice of RO helps facilitate this type of growth in OC clients.

Therapists Working with OC Problems Need Support

Most OC clients struggle to reveal vulnerable emotions, openly admit fault, and candidly disclose their inner thoughts, making it difficult for therapists to understand or feel connected to their clients. Indeed, this lack of information can be vexing for therapists, triggering interpretations that a client may be deceptive or manipulative, uncertainty about how to respond, or feelings of frustration and anger at what is perceived as stubbornness, hostility, or lack of commitment on the part of a client. Research shows that therapists treating chronic forms of depression (characterized by high OC) are likely to perceive their chronically depressed clients as more hostile and less friendly than their clients who are not chronically depressed (Constantino et al., 2008). Social signaling deficits in OC may help explain this.

In addition, OC clients can subtly block exploration of important topics, and this behavior can lead to therapist burnout or uncertainty about what may be important to target in treatment (see the material on "pushback" and "don't hurt me" responses in chapter 10). For example, a therapist might sense that his client is less engaged, basing his sense of the situation on his observations of the client's nonverbal behavior (for example, the client slightly rolls her eyes and looks away after a comment by the therapist). However, if the client is queried about this behavior and consistently denies it or dismisses the therapist's question as irrelevant, the therapist can begin to feel a nagging sense of demoralization. One of the most commonly reported dislikes or frustrations reported by therapists is feeling deskilled, or uncertain about how to conceptualize a case or manage a clinical situation. In RO DBT, feeling uncertain, demoralized, or confused is an opportunity to practice self-enquiry. Therapists are encouraged to first turn toward their angst (before attempting to regulate or accept it) and ask what their sense of demoralization might be trying to tell them, and then, if possible, reveal what they have learned to a consultation team. The following questions can be used to facilitate self-enquiry:

- Does my experience of demoralization emerge only when I am working with this particular client?

- Am I feeling demoralized in general—with other clients, at home, or with colleagues? What is it that I need to learn or do in order to help manage these outside issues?

- If my demoralization occurs primarily with my OC client, is it pervasive or episodic? If it is not always present, then what triggers it? For example, what am I doing or thinking just before it happens?

- Is my behavior different when working with this client? For example, am I speaking faster than I normally do? Do I feel compelled to explain or justify my questions or comments when working with this client? Is there something here to learn?

- Do I look forward to my next session with my client? How often do I think about my client outside of our therapy sessions? Do I ever purposely try *not* to think about my client outside of session? What might my answers tell me about my relationship with my client?

- Is it possible that my demoralization represents an unrecognized alliance rupture? Has there been a recent alliance rupture? Is it possible that the rupture was never fully repaired?[46]

- Do I find it hard to feel positive toward my client? If the answer is yes or maybe, then what might this tell me about my client's style of social signaling, or about my own worldview?

- To what extent is my client engaged in therapy? How does my client socially signal engagement? How does my client signal nonengagement?

- Am I afraid of my client? If the answer is yes or maybe, then what am I afraid of?

- To what extent do I feel it is my responsibility to fix my client or make my client feel better? What might this tell me about my beliefs about my professional role, my client, or myself?

- Do I feel guilty, ashamed, or humiliated when working with my client? If the answer is yes or maybe, are my feelings justified? What is it that I might need to learn or do differently?

- If I were not a therapist for my client, would I enjoy spending time with him or her? Do I like my client? If the answer is no or not particularly, then what might this tell me about my client's social signaling? What might this tell me about myself?

- Am I feeling annoyed or angry with my client? If the answer is yes or maybe, then have I shared my distress with a supervisor or colleague?

- When I am working with this particular client, do I behave or feel differently from how I behave or feel when working with other clients? What do I find easy to talk about when working this client? What types of discussions or topics do I find more difficult? Are there any topics or issues that I am avoiding or afraid to bring up? What might this tell me about my client or myself?

- To what extent am I blaming myself for my demoralization? How might my beliefs about my role as a therapist, health care provider, or doctor impact my expectations about therapy when working with my client? What is it that I might need to learn?

- To what extent does my demoralization stem from perplexity on my part because my client has not responded as quickly or in the same way as my other clients have responded in the past? Do I pride myself on being an extraordinarily competent or understanding counselor, therapist, or doctor? What might this tell me about how I am reacting to my client? What is it that I might need to learn?

- To what extent am I blaming my client for my demoralization? What might this tell me about myself? About my relationship with my client? About my worldview?

Therapists' demoralization can occasionally stem from OC clients' compulsive desires to fix or solve problems, achieve mastery, or dominate other people or situations. For example, some OC clients are so keen to fix their problem of overcontrol that they not only do what is expected of them, such as completing diary cards or homework assignments, but also memorize, word for word, every RO skill (to the point where they know the skills better than the therapist does), or they independently create new assignments in order to quicken or enhance treatment progress. Such clients' diligence and commitment to change are admirable, and yet their hyperdiligence represents maladaptive overcontrol in disguise (that is, compulsive fixing). Therapists can become demoralized working with supermotivated OC clients because therapy can start to feel a bit like a reality TV competition called *Who's the Best Fixer?*

Who will come up with the best task, assignment, insight, or challenge and finally change overcontrol, once and for all? Will it be the therapist? Will it be the client? Will the client vote the therapist off the case? Stay tuned for next week's session!

The therapist can start to feel increasingly inadequate if he is unable to recognize that he can never win—not only does the client know herself better than the therapist ever will, the entire premise of the competition is that overcontrol can be cured by working harder. The therapist can help himself and his OC client by not competing in the first place and by helping the client recognize that her hypermotivation to change her overcontrolled coping most likely represents another way in which her maladaptive overcontrol is sneaking into her life. From here, the therapist and the client can decide how they might want to proceed—for example, "Instead of fixing, maybe we should practice how to take a nap."

The main point is for therapists to remember that most OC maladaptive behaviors are not necessarily obvious. Plus, OC clients are often expert at blocking unwanted feedback suggesting change (for example, by bringing up an apparently important new topic of discussion), and when this goes unrecognized, treatment progress slows, and the therapist may find himself losing his normal sense of self-efficacy, may feel that the client is in charge, or may find himself bored or experiencing a sense of dread whenever he works with a particular client. Moreover, since the emotional displays of an overcontrolled person are often understated (particularly in public), therapists can wrongly assume that work with OC clients may be less demanding or less distressing than work with other clients. However, the opposite is often true. Despite their relatively unobtrusive nature, OC clients' behaviors strongly impact their social environment (albeit usually with plausible deniability), and therapists are not immune to these effects. Working with a nonexpressive and closed-minded OC client can be highly distressing and oftentimes perplexing. Consequently, RO DBT therapists are encouraged to bring their personal emotional reactions to their consultation teams (even if these reactions are of low intensity) and practice self-enquiry, both to enhance their own personal growth and to help their clients make the changes they need to in order to reach valued goals (see "Signs of Possible Burnout in a Therapist Working with an OC Client").

Transactions Between Clients' and Therapists' Personality Styles

OC clients (like most of us) prefer their own way of coping. As such, clients can subtly shape a therapist to behave in an overcontrolled manner, even when the therapist's personal style normally leans toward undercontrol. For example, therapists are often subtly reinforced to prepare, plan, and behave cautiously when working with OC clients. Plus, since OC clients are highly rule-governed, they often have developed rules about what should occur during therapy and how the therapist should behave. OC clients, for instance, may believe that a therapist should exemplify self-control, never express vulnerable emotions, or never disclose personal information during sessions, and they may signal their disapproval in subtle ways (a slight frown, avoidance of eye contact, apparent lack of interest, an abrupt change of topic). If not recognized, these reactions can condition the therapist to avoid certain topics, to be less genuine, or to be less inquisitive; this conditioning leads to poor outcomes for OC clients and demoralization for the therapist. Moreover, because OC clients frequently find the expression of emotion (by anyone) difficult, the therapist may, without conscious awareness, begin to match the OC client's emotionally constrained style of expression. This can subtly reinforce the client's belief that emotion inhibition and self-control are always best.

Thus it is important for therapists to find a way to examine their own personality styles or coping habits and how they impact therapy. Most often this is best accomplished via supervision or team consultation. For example, some therapists find silence during interpersonal interactions (a common OC response) unnerving or difficult to tolerate. But if this discomfort is not addressed, it can lead to iatrogenic effects, or to the therapist's demoralization. Moreover, our research suggests that most therapists lean toward an overcontrolled style of coping, which can make it more difficult for a therapist to recognize a maladaptive OC behavior in session, or it can mean that the therapist may inadvertently reinforce, defend, or normalize a client's behavior because it appears similar (on the surface at least) to how the therapist behaves. For example, one OC client reported to her OC-leaning therapist an elaborate strategy that she had come up with in order to visit a local bar. First she approached the bartender and said, "I'm supposed to meet some friends here later. If anyone comes in looking around for someone, can you direct them to my table?" Then she ordered a drink, pointed to an empty table, and said, "In the meantime, I'll just wait over here. Thanks." And then she went to the empty table, sat down, and began reading a book. The therapist working with the client praised the client's non-avoidance of social environments (getting out of her house and going to a bar) but failed to assess whether she actually ever socialized with anyone (other than the bartender) or to highlight the potential downsides of using a false pretense when she arrived at the bar (telling the bartender she was waiting for friends). During the consultation team meeting, the possible disadvantages of the client's behavior were discussed. The therapist challenged the discussion, saying, "Why does she have to relate to people in the bar? She might just want to sit there and have a quiet drink, without anyone bothering her." Further discussion by the team revealed that the therapist herself was uncomfortable in many public situations and had a number of rituals and strategies, including harmless deceptions that were designed to help her avoid feeling exposed and anxious. The therapist admitted to feeling uncomfortable challenging a client to change a behavior that she herself would find difficult to change. This discussion helped the therapist work with the client in later sessions on recognizing the pros and cons of this type of low-intensity deception around others. The client was then able to recognize that while her white lies helped make her feel safe, they also functioned to reinforce her secret belief that she was a social misfit (because she had to make up excuses or lie in order to participate in social events).

Signs of Possible Burnout in a Therapist Working with an OC Client

- Feeling relieved when an OC client doesn't show up for a session or reports wanting to drop out of treatment

- Sounding irritated, frustrated, flat, or unexpressive when talking about a particular client

- Engaging in more planning, preparing, or rehearsing before sessions with an OC client than is usual before sessions with other clients

- Avoiding supervision, discussion, or consultation about a particular OC client

- Being less directive or less playfully irreverent with a particular OC client than is usual with other clients (a possible indication that the therapist is behaving toward the OC client as if the client were fragile)

- Not targeting emotional expression or improved relationships with the client (a possible indication that the client subtly punishes the therapist for bringing up emotional topics or interpersonal issues)

- Finding it difficult to reach out to or feel warmth for the client (as when the therapist is reluctant to call if the client does not show up for a therapy appointment)

Using a Consultation Team to Enhance Supervision and Treatment Outcomes

As mentioned earlier, a core defining feature of our species is our capacity to benefit from the collective wisdom of the tribe. Similarly, therapists can benefit from the collective wisdom of their colleagues via peer consultation and outside supervision. Moreover, since effective delivery of RO DBT requires therapists to practice radical openness skills themselves, the use of outside consultation is one of the most effective ways to make this a reality. A well-functioning consultation team provides not only support but also corrective feedback, with an open mind. However, considering the inconspicuous nature of most OC problems, it is rarely sufficient for therapists to simply talk about their struggles or verbally describe what they believe to be the problem during peer supervision. Instead, therapists should get into the habit of demonstrating or showing what they are struggling with via role playing and videotaped recordings of actual sessions, particularly since most OC problems are problems of social signaling. Thus RO DBT consultation team meetings prioritize showing over telling when it comes to understanding an OC client or planning treatment. In addition, the treatment's emphasis on nonverbal social signaling highlights the importance of watching videotapes of individual sessions (or skills classes) during consultation team meetings and supervisory sessions.

Ideally, each team meeting should allocate fifteen minutes for watching video-recordings of actual therapy sessions. The team should practice stopping the videotape during the consultation whenever someone on the team notices something that seems to represent a maladaptive (or adaptive) behavior on either the client's or the therapist's part. For example, the team member observing the behavior can simply shout out "Stop!" to the person controlling the playback and then label or describe what has been observed (for example, an eye roll, a gaze aversion, or a sudden change in tone of voice). Team members should focus on describing the problem as a social signaling excess (a hostile stare), a social signaling deficit (avoidance of a direct answer to a question), or a problem with stimulus control (presentation of a flat face regardless of the situation). Team members watching videotapes should pay attention to two types of behavior on the client's part:

1. The team should attend to the client's verbal behavior, or the language the client uses during the interaction. Specifically, this means attending to idiosyncratic uses of language (describing feelings as "plastic"); set responses or repetitive use of particular phrases ("I'm fine," "It's okay," "I can't," or pet phrases like "It's only common sense"); the degree of the client's verbosity (one-word sentences, short and clipped answers, vague and rambling or overly verbose answers, or storytelling); and the degree to which the client actually answers the therapist's question (changing the topic, answering a question with a question, talking a great deal but never answering the question, answering a question about feelings with a report about thoughts, or frequently saying, "I don't know").

2. The team should also attend to what is *not* said—that is, the nonverbal social signals of the client. These involve the voice (monotonic or musical); the rate of speech (very slow or very fast, or changes from normal to slow or from normal to fast); changes in voice volume (for example, the client starts whispering); microexpressions of emotion (eye rolls, burglar smiles); changes in eye contact; delayed response in answering certain questions, or overly quick responses; shifts in body posture; the degree to which the client matches the therapist's body movements; and the frequency and degree of cooperative prosocial signals (nodding the head in agreement, smiling) as well as whether prosocial signals are context-appropriate. Sometimes team members can become more adept at noticing subtle social signals if the volume is turned off and the team simply watches the nonverbal behavior of both client and therapist.

It can be helpful to reverse a tape and replay a particular segment that either the therapist or the team has identified as difficult, particularly when the potential problem involves a subtle social signal. However, it is equally important for team members to avoid assuming that their observations about a client's nonverbal behavior represent the truth; instead, they should consider their observations to be working hypotheses. It is also important for teams watching videotapes to take the therapist's verbal and nonverbal social signals into account. Often the difficulty or the problem is transactional and occurs at the sensory receptor (preconscious) level of emotional processing. For example, one therapist reported a vague sense of discomfort about working with a particular client and was able to discover its source only while she and her consultation team were reviewing a videotaped recording of the problematic session and it was observed that each instance of the therapist's defensiveness was preceded by a nonverbal microexpression of contempt by the client. This observation, which came to form an essential contribution to the client's treatment and eventual recovery, would not have been possible without a videorecording.

Finally, one simple way to practice increasing therapists' skill in recognizing subtle and indirect OC social signals is to simply stop the tape every thirty seconds and ask team members, "At this point, is the client engaged or nonengaged in therapy?" The emphasis in RO DBT on noticing OC clients' engagement (or lack thereof) is twofold: first, OC clients struggle (especially early in therapy) to openly reveal disagreement, dislike, or nonengagement to their therapists because they feel socially obligated to try hard; and, second, when OC clients are feeling nonengaged, they are much more likely to drop out of therapy or not show up for sessions, without ever directly revealing their reasons. By watching videotaped sessions, therapists can become increasingly astute at picking up subtle social signals that impact the therapeutic relationship and, most important, the client's sense of well-being.

Thus, if sessions are not already being taped, therapists working with OC clients should institute videorecording of sessions as a normal part of clinical practice. Although at first this may be anxiety-producing for both the therapist and the client, the importance of the information gleaned from taped sessions cannot be overstated, as already noted. Clients' consent should be obtained, ideally in the first session or during a pre-first-session assessment. The therapist can explain that because the types of problems the client has sought help for (anorexia nervosa, for example, or chronic depression) are complex in nature, the videotaped sessions will enable the therapist (and the client) to benefit from an outside perspective from other professionals, who may notice something important or help the therapist deliver the treatment at its optimal "dose." This approach also smuggles concepts of radical openness early in treatment because the therapist is signaling that she is fallible and depends on a community of fellow therapists to ensure that she provides the best possible care for her clients.

Most clients recognize videorecording as an important and appropriate way to ensure high-quality care, and they easily give consent. However, success in obtaining consent often depends on how the therapist goes about asking for it. A therapist who is anxious about being videorecorded can inadvertently communicate his anxiety to his client nonverbally (for example, by adopting an overly apologetic or solicitous attitude when asking for consent, thus implying that there may be something wrong or potentially dangerous about recording sessions). Essentially, any implication on the part of the therapist that videotaping is odd, embarrassing, or not the norm makes it more likely for the client to refuse consent. That said, regardless of how competently a therapist asks for consent, some clients will still refuse to grant it. When this occurs, the therapist can reintroduce the idea of videotaping at a later stage in therapy, after a strong working alliance has been established.

Once consent for videotaping is obtained, the therapist should arrange the room in such a way that the camera is not particularly obvious (for example, by placing it on a bookshelf) and is positioned so that both the therapist and the client can be taped. If for some reason this is not possible, the camera should be placed to tape the client. The camera should be started before the client enters the room, and in general the therapist should avoid referring to the camera or to the fact that the session is being videotaped. Over time, since taping occurs during every session, both the therapist and the client become habituated to it. Audiotaping, for those clients who refuse to allow videotaping, can also be done; however, audiorecordings fail to capture nonverbal expressive behaviors, which often are extremely useful in identifying stuck points in therapy. Finally, clients should be encouraged to bring into session their own audiorecording or even videorecording equipment and to record sessions themselves for playback, in order to enhance memory and learning.

The RO Self-Enquiry Journal

As outlined in earlier chapters, RO DBT expects therapists to apply radical openness skills in their personal and professional lives in order to model to their OC clients core concepts that can only be grasped experientially (they cannot be grasped solely by rational thought or logic). This expectation includes an ongoing practice of self-enquiry. The skills training manual provides a number of handouts that include self-enquiry questions and helpful hints for practicing self-enquiry that therapists should be familiar with and be able to incorporate into their personal practices of self-enquiry on an as-needed basis. An additional structural feature that facilitates the development of a practice of self-enquiry involves journaling, or recording in writing the thoughts, images, sensations, and emotions that arise during self-enquiry practices. Since RO DBT therapists must practice what they preach, they must also journal, not only in order to understand from the inside out their OC clients' experience of recording daily self-enquiry experiences but also to enhance their own personal understanding of self-enquiry.

In the beginning, an RO self-enquiry journal is like a *tabula rasa*, or blank slate. All that is needed physically is something that is able to retain a record of one's insights and thoughts, is sturdy enough to stand the test of time, and is aesthetically pleasing to the eye of the practitioner (for example, a blank leather-bound book). The pages await the writings of each self-enquiry practitioner, and the book's physical appearance will vary with the aesthetic or practical preferences of different practitioners. Often journaling is important in RO DBT because it serves as a reminder of personal discovery. It is a positive reminder of repeated themes, continued struggles, and occasional triumphs in self-discovery, and most often the manner of writing or recording evolves over time, as a function of continued practice. It is similar to a personal diary, but with a specific purpose. The aim of an RO self-enquiry journal is not to record life's daily events and stop there; instead, the self-enquiry journal is a record of personal questions about oneself, for oneself, and to oneself, so as to cultivate a sense of self that is able to challenge the self in order for one to actively seek out the things one wants to avoid or may find uncomfortable, for the purpose of learning. An RO self-enquiry journal is a private matter, meaning that its contents need not be shared with anyone, including a client's therapist. OC clients should be encouraged not only to record what emerges from brief practices of self-enquiry but also to use the self-enquiry journal to record individualized targets and client-specific skills. The following example shows entries made in a self-enquiry journal by a therapist on three consecutive days (notice how on each day a new self-enquiry question emerged):

January 13: Silent practice. Picked an interaction I had with the contractor we hired two weeks ago to design and build a deck extension to our lovely house. However, I've noticed a growing sense of tension throughout the week because every couple of days our contractor kept informing me of this little added expense and that additional cost. I noticed that I had some energy around this, and so today I decided to give him some feedback about this, and it didn't go well. So what is it I need to learn? I definitely felt anger in my body: How dare he challenge me? Doesn't he know the customer is always right? *I used this for my practice today. My first self-enquiry question to myself was* Where did I ever get the idea that the customer is always right? Who ever said that was an absolute truth? *An image of Dad showed up, just a flash—something about him working and telling me to do the right thing. I feel foggy about it. So where is my edge? How do I get back to it? Wow, it just showed up!* How dare he challenge me? Who is this "me" that does not want to be challenged? *Is it me? Wow—that hurt, or something. The last question—Who is this "me" that insists on not being challenged?—closer, maybe. I can feel some excitement in my body. What is it I need to learn about being challenged? I will stop here. I'm worried that I will fall back into trying to solve things.*

January 14: Silent practice. I was excited today about the practice. I started out with the question I discovered yesterday that seemed to generate the most energy in me: Who is this "me" that insists on not being challenged? *Nothing... then, suddenly, Why do I hate the word* insist? *Closer... INSIST! INSIST! How often in my life do I insist? I don't think I do it very much at all. I always feel like I'm the meek one. Wow—a question just popped:* But do I really? How meek am I really? Am I meek? *Or is this just a story I like to tell myself? What is it I need to learn? My first thought is that I need to learn that I am not meek, and to stop thinking I am. But since this sounds like an answer, I will stop here. But which question gets me to my edge? Hmmm. It seems to be something like this:* Am I meek? Am I meek?

January 15: Silent practice. Started my practice by repeating my question from yesterday: Am I meek? *First thing that came to mind was a shout of* No! *Then an image of myself as a young boy, maybe eight or nine. I feel suddenly afraid. Now...What's wrong with challenging someone? Where did that come from? What am I afraid of? Wow. I've never really thought of myself as meek. Could it be that I am actually afraid of the contractor and don't want to admit it, even to myself? When I am saying,* How dare he challenge me?, *is it possible that what I am really saying is* I dare not challenge him? *I suddenly feel like crying, or like tears might show up. Why am I afraid to challenge people? That seems close—but I think I am actually starting to move away from my edge. So what's my question for tomorrow? I think the one that seems the closest to my edge has to do with saying,* I dare not challenge him. *Ouch. That hurts. The word "coward" comes to mind. I think I should stop my self-enquiry practice—I am aware of a desire to extend the practice. Maybe tomorrow.*

The therapist in the preceding example kept with this line of self-enquiry for several more days. He reported that the end result was a powerful learning experience for him. He had always thought of himself as a caring person, but through this practice he was able to recognize two new insights about himself that became an important area of new self-discovery: *I'm not always caring* and *I attack others out of fear.* The therapist recorded that he was amazed at how often his "evil me" showed up, in places he had never expected it. The label "evil me" became an in-joke for his RO consultation team: "Watch out—his 'evil me' is coming around again." These insights also helped him recognize why he disliked loving kindness meditation, and this became an important source of a whole range of self-enquiry questions and insights over the months. What is important to notice in the preceding example is that the therapist was able to recognize when he was starting to move toward trying to find an answer (rather than a good question), and that he knew to stop the practice at that point and take it up again the following day. Plus, this is a good example of how one self-enquiry question often triggers another.

Consultation Team Practices of Self-Enquiry and Outing Oneself

RO DBT therapists are encouraged to practice what they preach, and participation in an RO consultation team is one way to ensure this. For example, ideally, each consultation team begins with an RO mindfulness practice taken directly from the skills training manual. However, well-functioning consultation teams take this a step further by providing opportunities for therapists to work on more personal issues that might be impacting their delivery of the treatment. The overall idea is to use the consultation team not just as a vehicle for supervision but also as an important means of therapists' self-growth. A team can facilitate this process by remembering the core principles underlying radical openness and self-enquiry. For example, bodily tension can signal that we have evaluated (often without conscious awareness) something as threatening, and this can automatically make us less receptive to perhaps truthful but uncomfortable or disconfirming feedback. Therapists should look for opportunities to incorporate brief practices of self-enquiry and outing themselves into their team meetings or supervisory sessions. The following questions can facilitate this process:

- When I feel tense during a team meeting, how willing am I to reveal this to my fellow team members? What might my answer tell me about myself? About my team? What is it that I might need to learn?

- Is it possible that my feelings of defensiveness or resistance, at least in part, signal that I do not want to fully listen to what is being suggested? Is it possible that I am operating from Fixed Mind?[47]

- Am I secretly blaming my team for not being supportive enough or validating? Even if this is true or partly true, what is it that I might need to learn? What might this tell me about myself? About my team?

- Am I quickly jumping to self-blame, shutting down, or wanting to give up? Is it possible I am operating from Fatalistic Mind?

Protocol for Practices of Self-Enquiry and Outing Oneself in Team Consultation

When a therapist reports feeling demoralized, frustrated, uncertain, guilty, or embarrassed, the members of the consultation team should encourage self-enquiry

203

rather than automatically soothing, validating, or regulating their distressed colleague. Mostly because of time constraints, a formal practice of self-enquiry is seldom possible when a therapist experiences or reports distress during a consultation team meeting. The good news, however, is that self-enquiry practices, by definition, are designed to be time-limited—no longer than ten minutes, since anything longer almost always means that practitioners are moving away from core self-enquiry concepts and are instead attempting to solve a problem or find a solution. The members of a well-functioning RO DBT consultation team will find a way to practice self-enquiry together on a regular basis. Here is a protocol for a therapist's practice of self-enquiry in the setting of a consultation team:

1. The therapist locates and reveals her edge to the team (that is, she practices outing herself). Outing oneself about difficulties in treating an OC client almost always involves some type of judgmental thinking about the client or oneself, or about emotions that are considered inappropriate for therapists to experience (such as anger or strong dislike of a client). The therapist should not feel compelled to reveal every private thought, sensation, or experience; the goal is to reveal what she can and recognize that "editing" is not only unavoidable but also appropriate.

2. The team asks the therapist what she needs to learn from her edge. The primary question is "What question do I need to ask myself in order to get myself to my edge?" There is no right question; plus, when asking questions (either self-directed or provided by the team), the goal is not to solve the problem. The team actively blocks (without judgment) anti-self-enquiry behaviors from other team members that function to move the therapist away from her edge. Examples of anti-self-enquiry behaviors include soothing ("Don't worry—everything will work out"), validating ("I would have found that hard, too"), regulating ("Let's all take a deep breath"), assessing ("You must have learned this somewhere—do you know where?"), cheerleading ("Remember, you are a really excellent therapist"), problem solving ("You need to confront the client about this"), or encouraging acceptance ("You need to accept that you cannot fix this problem"). The therapist responds aloud to the team's self-enquiry queries, and the team listens without comment to the therapist's responses.

3. The team helps the therapist stay in contact with her edge. This most often involves simply asking, at sixty-second intervals, "Are you still at your edge, or have you regulated?" The therapist can use her visceral experience as a way to know how close to her edge she is (one's edge is never peaceful).

4. After approximately three to five minutes, the practice ends, and the team asks the therapist whether there was any question that emerged from the practice that she found most likely to elicit her edge. The team encourages the therapist to use this question for further self-enquiry practice by (ideally) committing to ask it once per day in three- to five-minute minienquiry

practices during the coming week and then noticing what arises when she does so. The therapist should record the images, sensations, emotions, or thoughts that are triggered by the question, along with any observations of her attempts to regulate or avoid the practice or question, in her RO self-enquiry journal. Each day of self-enquiry usually elicits some new awareness.

The team should block attempts to summarize or interpret, since most often these actions function as "answers" or "resolutions" to the self-enquiry dilemma. That is, quick answers to self-enquiry questions are often avoidance masquerading as wisdom. This is why most self-enquiry practices in RO DBT are encouraged to continue over days or weeks. The goal of self-enquiry is not to find a good answer but to find a good question and then allow an answer—if there is one—to be discovered by the practitioner and later, ideally, shared with the team. A resolution or answer that emerges can be anticipated to become the next area of self-growth.

Recommended Structure for RO DBT Consultation Team Meetings

Consultation team meetings occur weekly and, depending on the size of the team, should last from ninety minutes to two hours. A therapist who does not already belong to an established team should work to establish connections with other RO DBT therapists and form a virtual team, using web-based technologies. Our experience has been that these can work very well and are particularly useful in enhancing self-enquiry practice. Before attending a consultation team meeting, a therapist should briefly conduct a self-enquiry practice around whether she is experiencing any emotion toward a particular client, is worried about an alliance rupture, or is struggling with particular treatment issues where a client is concerned. A summary of RO DBT's core assumptions about OC clients and about therapy (see chapter 4) should be prepared and made available for reference during team meetings.

Setting the Agenda and the Team Leader's Responsibilities

As mentioned earlier, each team meeting begins, ideally, with a brief RO mindfulness practice taken directly from those that are recommended in the lesson plans found in chapter 5 of the skills training manual. After this, the team leader for the day (a role that can be rotated) assigns the other team roles (observer, notekeeper, and timekeeper). The leader then uses the RO DBT treatment target hierarchy to help organize the agenda (see "Hierarchy of Treatment Targets in Individual Therapy," chapter 4). Discussion of any important business items or clinical organizational issues occurs at the end of the team meeting and should not be a major element of the meeting. Issues related to general clinic business are best discussed outside the team meeting. Client issues involving life-threatening behavior are given the highest priority, followed by alliance ruptures and OC behavioral themes. Agenda setting is facilitated by the leader asking four key questions:

1. Does anyone have a client dealing with imminent or serious life-threatening behavior?

2. Does anyone have a problem associated with an alliance rupture?

3. Does anyone need consultation related to social signaling targets or OC behavioral themes?

4. Are there any important issues to discuss about skills training classes?

The team leader should also be alert for other issues not related to the four key questions just listed. Here are some additional important questions that are useful to consider:

- Does anyone have a client who is threatening to drop out of therapy?

- Does anyone have a client who is disengaged from therapy—missing sessions, or not doing homework?

- Is anyone feeling strong emotion or demoralization about working with a client?

- Is anyone worried about a client for any other reason?

- Does anyone have an issue that requires consultation and hasn't already been mentioned it?

Notekeeper's Role

The notekeeper ensures that brief records are kept of decisions and actions. This notetaking is not the same as recording minutes. Team notes are much briefer than what might normally be considered minutes because the primary goal is simply to record major decisions (for example, action points regarding the next steps a therapist will take with a suicidal client) or important issues that will need to be followed up in the next meeting. Taking notes should not interfere with the ability of the notekeeper to fully participate in the team meeting.

Monitoring Team Functioning

The team should also be alert for how it may, as a consultation team, be out of balance. Here are some signs that a team is unbalanced:

- The team avoids discussing a client, or members spend a great deal of time discussing only one issue or one client.

- The team focuses on clients who have not yet committed to RO DBT therapy, with little time left for discussion of clients who are already committed and working.

- A team culture develops that emphasizes the imperative of fixing clients. As a result, the team focuses on solutions, with less time spent on therapeutic relationship issues or therapists' feelings.

- The team rarely questions consensus-driven decisions or understandings of client-related problems or rarely evaluates the pros and cons of the team's recommendations.

- Team members fail to discuss secretly judgmental thoughts about clients ("The client is lying about not feeling any emotions").

- The team is overly serious. For example, team members find it difficult to laugh at their personal foibles.

- A culture of equanimity develops, with therapists' expressions of negative emotions or judgmental thoughts covertly frowned on, or with a permeating expectation that team members should remain calm.

- Vulnerable emotions are rarely expressed.

- Team members spend a great deal of time making sure that rules and protocols are adhered to.

- Covert competition develops among team members over who is the most radically open.

Now You Know...

- ▶ Radical openness is both the core skill and the core philosophical principle of RO DBT.

- ▶ Therapists must practice radical openness and self-enquiry themselves if they hope to model radical openness and self-enquiry for their OC clients.

- ▶ It can be difficult to know when one is open and when one is closed.

- ▶ Therapists who work with OC clients but don't normally and regularly receive team-based consultation and support are encouraged to seek out or create and develop this resource.

CHAPTER 8

The Therapeutic Alliance, Alliance Ruptures, and Repairs

The aim of this chapter is to describe in detail the strategies in RO DBT that are designed to enhance OC clients' engagement in therapy. OC clients inwardly experience themselves as outsiders. To help correct this, the role of the RO DBT therapist is to welcome the emotionally lonely OC client back to the tribe. The chapter is organized according to four broad topics:

1. The RO DBT therapeutic stance

2. The therapeutic alliance

3. Alliance ruptures and repairs

4. Prevention of premature treatment dropout

The RO DBT Therapeutic Stance

Rather than focusing on what's wrong with hyper-detail-focused OC perfectionists who tend to see mistakes everywhere (including in themselves), RO DBT begins by noticing what's healthy (about all of us) and uses this to guide treatment interventions. Psychological health or well-being in RO DBT is hypothesized to involve three core transacting features:

1. Receptivity and openness to new experience and disconfirming feedback, in order to learn

2. Flexible control, in order to adapt to changing environmental conditions

3. Social connectedness (with at least one other person), based on premises that species survival required us to form long-lasting bonds with unrelated others and work together in groups or tribes

OC clients, like a lot of other people, struggle with all three. Yet the feature they need the most is the one they struggle with the most—feeling socially connected.

Indeed, RO DBT posits that the primary downsides of maladaptive overcontrol are social in nature. For example, both low openness and pervasive constraint of emotional expression have been repeatedly shown to exert a negative impact on the formation of close social bonds, leading to an increasing sense of isolation from others. OC clients suffer from emotional loneliness—not lack of contact, but lack of *intimate connection* with others. Thus, rather than focusing on how to do better or try harder, the primary aim in RO DBT is to help the OC client learn how to rejoin the tribe and establish strong social bonds with others. Consequently, the role of the therapist in RO DBT can be likened to that of a tribal ambassador who metaphorically encourages the socially isolated OC client to rejoin the tribe by communicating, "Welcome home. We appreciate your desire to meet or exceed expectations and the self-sacrifices you have made. You have worked hard and deserve a rest."

As ambassador, the RO DBT therapist adopts a stance that models kindness, cooperation, and playfulness rather than fixing, correcting, restricting, or improving. Plus, ambassadors don't expect people they interact with in other countries to think, feel, or act the way they do, or speak the same language. They celebrate diversity and recognize that as a species we are better when together and don't automatically assume that their perspective is the correct one. They reach out toward those who are different and learn their customs and language, without expecting anything in return. Ambassadors build bridges. They are face savers—they allow a person (or country) to admit to some fault, without rubbing anyone's nose in it (that is, without publicly humiliating anyone). For example, RO DBT therapists recognize that it would be arrogant to assume that they could ever fully understand their clients and, as a consequence, are more likely to use qualifiers in session ("Is it possible that…" or "Perhaps…") rather than absolutes ("I know…" or "You are…"). Ambassadors take the heat off when things get extremely tense during negotiations by allowing the other person (and themselves) the grace of not having to understand, resolve, or fix a problem or issue immediately. Yet they also recognize that sometimes kindness means telling good friends painful truths in order to help them achieve their valued goals, and they tell these painful truths in a manner that acknowledges their own potential for fallibility. The overarching goal of RO DBT is to help the OC client create a life worth sharing, based on the premise that our individual experience of well-being is highly dependent on the extent to which we feel socially connected or part of a tribe.

The Therapeutic Alliance

RO DBT does not consider treatment compliance, declarations of commitment, or lack of conflict as indicators of a strong therapeutic relationship. Indeed, alliance ruptures (those that are repaired) are considered working proof of a solid therapeutic relationship in RO DBT. Alliance ruptures provide the practice ground for learning that conflict can be intimacy-enhancing and that expressing inner feelings, including those involving conflict or disagreement, is part of a normal healthy relationship. Consequently, RO DBT considers a therapeutic relationship relatively superficial if by the fourteenth session a therapist-client dyad has not had several alliance ruptures and successful repairs. Yet getting to that point can be difficult because OC clients are not only expert at masking inner feelings but also more inclined to abandon a new relationship (for example, therapy) than to deal directly with a potential conflict.

The difficulty of establishing a genuine working therapeutic relationship with an OC client should not be underestimated. OC biotemperamental predispositions, combined with an avoidant or dismissive attachment style and overlearned tendencies to mask inner feelings and avoid conflict, make the development of a genuine working therapeutic alliance not only difficult to establish but also difficult to recognize. Plus, most OC clients dislike being labeled or pigeonholed; they pride themselves on their uniqueness and psychological complexity, and are more likely to see themselves as different rather than the same as other people in most situations. This difficulty should be anticipated regardless of how skilled a therapist is in delivering adherent RO DBT, the therapist's number of years of experience, the therapist's prior training, or the therapist's special or unique talents (such as high empathic intuition).

Plus, a significant proportion of OC clients (usually without conscious awareness) share a worldview or premise about themselves that impacts therapy. It can be translated broadly as "I do what I do because that's the way I am; ergo, I cannot be held responsible for my actions or mood states, because I am what I am." Although rarely verbalized explicitly or necessarily even consciously acknowledged, the underlying premise is "Don't expect me to change, because I can't." This can be hard to recognize, particularly because most overcontrolled individuals are adept at providing a range of seemingly plausible and logical explanations for why they cannot make important changes—for example, "I can't go on a date with anyone because I have no money." If the therapist accepts this as a reasonable explanation, then he is likely to shift his treatment target from the client's learning how to date to the client's finding more money, neglecting the fact that poor people around the world go on dates all the time. RO DBT therapists are trained to be alert for plausible yet fundamentally illogical reasons for not making changes and to use these as self-enquiry opportunities for the client.

RO DBT joins other interpersonally focused therapies as well as contentions by Rogers (1959) that certain features of the therapeutic relationship are curative alone, with empathy being the most likely mechanism (Miller, Taylor, & West, 1980; Najavits & Weiss, 1994; Miller & Rose, 2009). Thus RO DBT considers the development of a strong working alliance during individual therapy an essential component of the treatment, an emphasis that is shared by a number of differing psychotherapeutic approaches, such as functional analytic psychotherapy (FAP; see Kohlenberg & Tsai, 1991), the cognitive behavioral analysis system of psychotherapy (J. P. McCullough, 2000), standard DBT (Linehan, 1993a), motivational interviewing (Miller, 1983), client-centered therapy (Rogers, 1959), and brief relational therapy (BRT; see Safran & Muran, 2000), to name just a few. RO DBT also overlaps with the therapeutic stance in motivational interviewing (Miller, 1983; Miller & Rose, 2009). Similar to motivational interviewing, RO DBT promotes a collaborative rather than authoritarian (directive) therapeutic stance, encourages clients to discover their own motivations rather than using external contingencies to force such discovery, and honors clients' autonomy (Miller & Rose, 2009).[48]

Despite being developed independently, RO DBT and brief relational therapy share similar hypotheses regarding the potential benefits of using alliance ruptures and subsequent repairs to enhance positive outcomes. BRT was developed from principles derived from relational psychodynamic theory (Ferenczi & Rank, 1925; Greenberg & Mitchell, 1983). It considers recurrent maladaptive patterns of interpersonal behavior as key to the development and maintenance of psychopathology, and the therapeutic relationship as a crucial element of treatment success (Safran & Muran, 2000). Both RO DBT and BRT include an intense focus on the here and now of the therapeutic relationship; a collaborative, ongoing exploration of how therapist and client jointly contribute to interactions; an examination of subtle changes in the client's experience of therapy and interactions; and a focus on the importance of the therapist's modeling open expression of emotions and thoughts (Satir et al., 2011). With respect to how rupture repairs are managed, the major differences between RO DBT and BRT have to do with RO DBT's emphasis on accounting for biotemperamental biases as they are linked with inhibited emotional expression and overlearned tendencies to avoid vulnerable self-disclosure. For example, RO DBT explicitly outlines specific sequential steps and nonverbal social signaling strategies designed to facilitate conflict-avoidant OC clients' engagement during rupture repairs. RO DBT also encourages therapists to keep repairs time-limited (shorter than ten minutes) in order to shape OC self-disclosure (OC clients dislike the limelight). In contrast to motivational interviewing (Miller, 1983), which prioritizes de-escalating a client by not confronting him when "resistance" occurs, and to standard DBT (Linehan, 1993a), which conceptualizes alliance ruptures as behaviors that interfere with therapy and require the use of change, validation, or regulation strategies, RO DBT considers alliance ruptures and interactions aimed at rupture repair to be opportunities for growth and self-enquiry, not problems. This perspective overlaps to some extent with principles of functional analytic psychotherapy (Kohlenberg & Tsai, 1991) that consider it important for therapists to evoke problem behaviors in session in order to create opportunities for change. The overall idea in FAP is that if the behavioral problems causing difficulty outside the therapeutic relationship are not occurring in session, then progress is less likely, an idea that parallels the notion in RO DBT of considering alliance ruptures as opportunities for growth. What is important is for therapists to learn to see alliance ruptures and subsequent repairs as proof of therapeutic progress.

In summary, RO DBT is more conservative or pessimistic about how easy it is and how long it takes to establish a genuine therapeutic alliance in work with OC clients, by comparison with other, less aloof client groups. Indeed, RO DBT teaches therapists not to expect a strong working alliance until approximately midway through treatment (about the fourteenth session), even if they have evidence suggesting that such an alliance already exists (such as client reports of admiration, respect, or fondness and strong proclamations of commitment to therapy). This is partly strategic in that it encourages therapists to use RO DBT self-enquiry principles to question the depth and genuineness of their interpersonal encounters with their OC clients rather than assuming that compliance (as indicated by dutifully completed diary cards), expressions of commitment, or lack of conflict indicate the presence of a strong therapeutic relationship. On the contrary, from an RO DBT point of view, a strong working alliance is present when resistance, disagreement, strong opinions, or ambivalence are openly expressed and the OC client remains willing to open-mindedly engage in resolving such issues, without walking away.

Alliance Ruptures and Repairs

Recognizing an Alliance Rupture

RO DBT defines an alliance rupture according to either or both of two criteria:

1. The client feels misunderstood by the therapist.

2. The client experiences the treatment as not relevant to his unique problems or issues.

Both of these issues are the responsibility of the therapist to manage (that is, a client is not blamed for creating an alliance rupture). Alliance ruptures are like the tides of the ocean: not only are they inevitable, they are growth-enhancing because they may be, in the words of the thirteenth-century poet Mewlana Jalaluddin Rumi (ca. 1230/2004, p. 109), "clearing you out / for some new delight." Fortunately, when it comes to repairing an alliance rupture, therapists can remind their OC clients to relax, since the management of an alliance rupture is not the client's responsibility (at least in RO DBT).

The first step in repairing an alliance rupture is noticing that there is one going on (with OC clients, this is harder than you might think). The primary reason why ruptures can be hard to detect is that most OC clients, most of the time, tend to communicate indirectly. Indirect communication is often used to avoid taking responsibility, deceive or manipulate others, or hide inner feelings ("No, you didn't wake me—I had to get up to answer the phone"), albeit sometimes an indirect communicator is just being polite. Indirect communication is also much more likely to be misinterpreted, making alliance ruptures (and interpersonal conflict or misunderstandings) more likely.

An alliance rupture can be triggered by almost anything—a facial expression, a tone of voice, or, for many OC clients, a simple compliment. Fortunately, there are a number of verbal and nonverbal indicators that suggest the possibility of an alliance rupture. Therapists should be alert for sudden changes that suggest nonengagement, as in the following examples involving clients' verbal behavior (see also "Statements Possibly Indicating an Alliance Rupture," page 217):

- The client suddenly shifts the mood or tone of the conversation.

- The client quickly changes the topic being discussed.

- The client's rate of speech suddenly slows, an indication that she may be editing what she reveals.

- The client suddenly becomes less talkative.

Shhh! I've Got a Secret… Relationships Matter! Pass It On

Therapists should look for opportunities to orient clients to the importance of the therapeutic relationship in RO DBT, including how alliance ruptures (and repairs) are considered a core mechanism of change. Most of the time, these teaching points can be woven into the fabric of existing session activities (during a chain analysis, for example, or following successful repair of an alliance rupture). Regardless of how these mini-teaching moments manifest, their primary aim is to build trust. Yet establishing trust

> A strong therapeutic alliance cannot be rushed; trust takes time.

with a hyper-detail-focused, overly cautious OC client, one who secretly prides herself on being hard to impress, can sometimes feel like a daunting task. Plus, for most OC clients, trust is something that is earned, and when it comes to the therapeutic relationship, the person responsible for earning it is the therapist (sorry, therapists—it's your job). Plus, to add fuel to the fire, many OC clients are skeptical about psychotherapy in general, psychotherapists in particular (often for good reason), and anything in particular that sounds too good to be true (such as a genuinely caring therapist or the notion that love is possible).

Thus overly enthusiastic proclamations or prolonged explanations about the benefits of the therapeutic relationship or the importance of repairing alliance ruptures can often be viewed with suspicion. As one OC client put it, "If it's really so good, then why is my therapist working so hard

- The client suddenly starts to use one-word responses, such as "Okay" or "Sure."

- The client changes from unprompted talk to prompted talk (that is, he answers questions but does not elaborate).

- The client begins to say "Hmmm" instead of "Yes," a change that may signal disagreement.

- A previously verbose or eager client suddenly begins to qualify her responses ("I suppose" or "I guess so" or "Yeah, but…" or "I'll try").

Here are some nonverbal signals that an alliance rupture may have occurred:

- The client suddenly averts his gaze or turns away from the therapist.

- The client slightly rolls her eyes (a disgust reaction).

- The client suddenly hides or covers his face (a shame response).

to convince me?" Fortunately, everyone can relax: a strong therapeutic alliance cannot be rushed; trust takes time.

Similarly, therapists should orient clients to the value of alliance ruptures as opportunities for growth, whereas successful rupture repairs are proof of a strong therapeutic alliance. Yet this does not mean that therapists should attempt to artificially create an alliance rupture (for example, by purposefully misunderstanding a client). Not only is this unkind, it is also unnecessary. Plus, it sends the wrong message to an OC client—namely, that it's okay and effective in intimate relationships to be phony or manipulative. Fortunately, therapists don't have to worry about trying to create alliance ruptures—like magic, they happen all by themselves.

Yet most OC clients, despite being armed with the new revelations just mentioned, still find it difficult to admit to the existence of interpersonal conflict (that is, an alliance rupture), let alone talk about it. OC clients' natural tendencies to mask inner feelings and walk away from conflict can exacerbate this. They may struggle to imagine conflict with a therapist or may consider a discussion about a possible alliance rupture as implying that they are not fully committed to treatment (the latter response suggests that they are not feeling understood and, as a consequence, are already experiencing a first alliance rupture). Therapists should also explain that a strong therapeutic alliance in RO DBT does not mean that the therapist believes that clients will (or need to) become personally close to therapists; rather, what is most important is that clients feel understood and that they experience their treatment as relevant.

- The client suddenly becomes immobile or frozen or exhibits a blank face or a rigid stare (the "deer in the headlights" response; see chapter 6).

- The client suddenly furrows his brow.

- The client displays unusual movement of the hands or feet.

- The client suddenly displays an apparently out-of-context smile.

- The client's eyes momentarily flick away in a central or downward direction ("I'm not sure"), in an upward direction ("You're wrong"), or to the side ("You may be right, but I'm not going to do what you suggest").

- The client's lips tighten ("I'm angry at you, but I'm not going to tell you").

- The client offers a burglar smile, a subtle nonverbal indication of a possible alliance rupture when it occurs repeatedly during a session or over many sessions, and when it seems to be at the therapist's expense.

Therapists must train themselves to become adept at noticing these small changes in verbal and nonverbal behavior.

Finally, an alliance rupture is often—perhaps *most* often—the consequence of a simple misunderstanding. For example, during a discussion of valued goals, one therapist shared an example of a valued goal from her own life ("It is important for me to write"), but the client heard something else entirely ("It is important for me to be right"). The alliance rupture that was triggered by this exchange did not become apparent to the therapist until the next session, when the client reported that he had been ruminating during the past week and had almost decided not to come to the session; indeed, the only reason he had come back was that he had committed to do so in person and to talk about any urges to quit therapy before actually doing so. He reported feeling confused and angry about his therapist's "hypocrisy," and he said, "How can a therapist ethically preach the value of not being right when the therapist herself doesn't believe it?" Fortunately, in this instance, the therapist and the client were able to collaboratively identify the source of the rupture (that is, "write" doesn't mean "right"), and the client was able to use this experience as a reminder of a core RO skill—namely, the skill of recognizing that mere belief in something doesn't make that thing true. In this example, the therapist was skillfully able to identify the trigger—but, fortunately, you don't have to know the trigger before you can repair an alliance rupture. Finally, the best way to tell whether there has been an alliance rupture is to check in with the client frequently during the session and ask for information about the client's experience in the current moment in order to monitor the client's engagement. Examples of check-ins include asking, "Does that make sense?" or "Are you with me?" or "What is it that you would like to tell me?" Essentially, check-ins work because they give a client permission to complain, thus making it easier for the therapist to get to know who the client is (and, hopefully, as a consequence, help the client).

Statements Possibly Indicating an Alliance Rupture

Noncommittal Responses, Denials, or Subtle Signals of Disagreement

- Repeatedly being nonspecific, vague, or noncommittal: "I guess so" or "Maybe"

- Repeatedly denying distress: "No, I'm fine" or "It's okay" or "No, I'm not upset"

- Hostile compliance and insincere capitulation: "If you think so" or "Sure, let's do it your way"

- Repeatedly correcting the therapist: "You don't know me" or "Not exactly" or "No, that's not it" or "You're mistaken"

- In a context of earlier agreement, saying, "Hmmm..." or "Not really..."

"Pushback" Responses

- Answering questions with a question: "Why are you asking that?" or "Why does that matter?" or "How could this help?" or "Why should I do that?"

- Sarcastic comebacks: "I'm sure it's my fault" or "You wouldn't want an entirely positive session, would you?" or "Let's do it your way" or "What would you suggest?"

- Proclamations and personal attacks: "This sounds more about you than me" or "Perhaps you should consider using skills yourself" or "I think you are starting to sound like my other therapist" or "Your enthusiasm is part of the game plan"

"Don't Hurt Me" Responses

- Using painful emotions to avoid responsibility: "This is too painful" or "I'm too anxious" or "I'm too depressed" or "I've got a headache" or "I feel overwhelmed" or "I can't..." or "It's just not possible"

- Blaming outward: "You don't understand my suffering...I just can't do what you want" or "It's not fair" or "If you don't stop, I will fall apart—and it will be your fault!"

"Enigma Predicament" Responses

- Vague answers: "I don't know" or "Probably" or "It just depends"

- Indirectly disagreeing: "I'll try, but..." or "Yeah, but..." or "I guess so..."

- Secret pride: "I'm not like other people" or "How could you possibly understand?" or "Labels don't apply to me"

It is not uncommon for an OC client to ignore, suppress, or disguise an alliance rupture, as in the following scenarios:

- A client who has always completed her diary cards suddenly begins arriving without a card, or with an incomplete diary card.

- A client who used to follow instructions to the letter reports that he forgot to do his homework.

- A client who has always been timely shows up late.

- A client who has never missed a session fails to show up.

- A client who is proud of never having called in sick at work leaves a voice message saying that she is too ill to come to the session.

- Without warning, a client who has always reported enjoying contact with his therapist begins to screen calls from the therapist or fails to respond to the therapist's emails and text messages.

The examples just listed have a common feature—they all involve social signals (whether the client intends these signals or not), which is to say that they all send a powerful message. The question for the therapist is, for example, *What is my client trying to tell me by not completing his homework?* Regardless, when these behaviors are present, they should first be viewed as signals of potential nonengagement and understood as suggesting the presence of a possible alliance rupture.

The following report from a therapist offers a clinical example that illustrates the importance of being awake to subtle in-session behaviors:

> *Early in therapy, during the seventh session, prior to the establishment of a full working alliance, my OC client described himself as experiencing a pervasive lack of joy in his life. I pointed out to him that, despite this lack, he still retained a sense of humor, and as proof I pointed to his occasional expressions of laughter during our sessions. Unbeknownst to me, my client experienced this statement as extremely invalidating, and yet during the session he kept his feelings tightly controlled. During the following session, I observed that he appeared less engaged in our discussion, and I asked whether something might have happened to trigger this, whereupon my client reported that he had almost dropped out of therapy because of what I had said during the session before, about his having retained some joy through humor.*

In the situation just described, the therapist thanked the client for his willingness to return to therapy and reveal his true feelings about what had happened the week before. The therapist pointed out that this represented therapeutic progress and a genuine commitment to change. She then used this disclosure by the client to model radical openness and flexibility. She took a moment to slow down and reflect aloud with the client about how she might have been off the mark during the previous session. She solicited feedback from the client about how to manage similar issues in the future, including encouragement for the client to feel free to let her know, in the moment, whenever he disagreed with a statement she had made. Finally, the therapist checked in with the client about his experience of this discussion, and she asked him how relevant the therapy was at this point to the unique problems he faced.

Repairing an Alliance Rupture

The idea of repairing an alliance rupture is not to fix the client but to repair the relationship. Thus, when an alliance rupture is suspected, the therapist should first drop his agenda (such as conducting a chain analysis or teaching a new skill) and turn his attention toward understanding his client (see "Using Open Curiosity to Repair an Alliance Rupture," page 220). Typically this involves slowing down the pace of the interaction and asking the client what is happening in the moment. The basic idea in addressing a potential alliance rupture is to briefly take the heat off the client, most often by taking one of the following actions:

- Leaning back in one's chair in order to increase one's distance from the client

- Crossing the leg nearest the client over one's other leg in order to slightly turn one's shoulders away

- Taking a slow deep breath

- Briefly disengaging eye contact

- Raising one's eyebrows

- Engaging a closed-mouth smile while turning one's gaze back toward the client

The therapist should then nonjudgmentally enquire, highlight, or notice aloud what he has observed in session that he believes may be related to an alliance rupture. At the same time, the therapist should privately practice self-enquiry by asking himself what he may have done to contribute to the rupture. During the discussion of an alliance rupture, the therapist should allow the client time to reply to queries and should let go of desires to jump in and immediately start fixing problems. The idea is for the therapist to realize that dealing with an alliance rupture and the subsequent repair is at least equal to and perhaps even more important than any other skill he might teach the client during the course of treatment. This also means that the therapist must practice radical openness himself by not blaming the client.

The following transcript provides an example of repairing an alliance rupture with a client during the fourteenth session (that is, midway through treatment):

Therapist: So I noticed that you slightly changed the topic. Is that because you were done with what we were discussing, or is it that you wanted to work on something else? (*Notices sudden change in direction and hypothesizes presence of a possible alliance rupture.*)

Using Open Curiosity to Repair an Alliance Rupture

1. Drop your agenda.

2. Take the heat off the client by briefly (1-2 seconds) disengaging eye contact.

3. Signal cooperation (and activate personal social safety) by leaning back, taking a slow deep breath, and offering a closed-mouth smile and an eyebrow wag.

4. While signaling nondominant friendliness (slight bow of the head, slight shoulder shrug, openhanded gestures combined with a closed-mouth smile, an eyebrow wag, and eye contact), ask about the change you've observed. Say, for example, "I noticed that something just changed." Describe the change, and then ask, "What's going on with you right now?"

5. Allow the client time to reply to questions, slow the pace of the session.

6. Reflect back what is said, and confirm his or her agreement.

7. Reinforce the client's self-disclosure, and practice radical openness yourself.

8. Keep the repair short—spend less than ten minutes repairing the alliance rupture.

9. Check in with the client, and confirm his or her reengagement.

Client: I changed the topic? From what?

Therapist: Well, we were talking about relationships and being alone. And I shared that I have found this very difficult, too, particularly after my mother died.

Client: There's tremendous resistance on my part. (*Pauses.*) You didn't want a completely positive session, did you? (*Chuckles slightly.*)

Therapist: Do you have a sense as to what the resistance is about? Is it something about my suggestion that we have had similar experiences? (*Asks about the possible source of the alliance rupture.*)

Client: Yeah, I suppose. I think…you just don't know me.

Therapist: Something along the lines of not ever having experienced the type of pain you've had? (*Extends client's comment and asks for confirmation.*)

Client: Yeah, something like that. (*Nods.*)

Therapist:	You're right. I can't know what it's like to have your pain or life. *(Pauses.)* Does it help to know that I'll try to understand?
	(Client nods in agreement.)
Therapist:	Plus, it seems to me that your telling me about this, or any other time you don't feel understood, is actually an important step in getting better. What do you think? *(Validates client's willingness to reveal inner feelings and links this to therapeutic progress.)*
Client:	It's not something I'm used to doing. I usually figure people either don't care or couldn't understand anyway, but I can see that it might make a difference. *(Engages more actively in discussion, a change suggesting that the alliance rupture is being repaired.)*

Alliance ruptures can also be triggered by clients experiencing therapy as not relevant to their unique problems. It is up to the therapist to make the therapy relevant to the client, which is most often and best achieved by ensuring mutual agreement on individualized treatment targets and via frequent check-ins to confirm that agreed-upon targets remain relevant. The only exception is life-threatening behavior, which always takes precedence. It is especially important for therapists to realize that targets are expected to change as the client grows. Treatment targets may also need to be adjusted in order to address what might be relevant for the client in a particular moment (see the material on individualized treatment targets in chapter 9).

> The idea of repairing an alliance rupture is not to fix the client but to repair the relationship.

When assessing and repairing an alliance rupture, the therapist should avoid overly long discussions about the rupture itself. Essentially, the therapist should assume that if she has not successfully repaired a rift in a relatively short period of time (within ten minutes), she may somehow be exacerbating the rift via her attempts at repair itself. Belabored discussions of alliance ruptures can inadvertently result in a client's feeling pressured or manipulated to reveal inner feelings that he is not yet ready to share with his therapist. Such a discussion may also elicit harsh self-blame from a client who considers a long discussion as representing yet another example of his failure to communicate with others. It may trigger additional anger or heighten anxiety, or it may simply suggest that attachment to the therapist is considered mandatory in RO DBT. Regardless of the underlying reasons, overly intense discussion of an alliance rupture may reinforce a client's overlearned tendencies to abandon relationships and may punish an early attempt on his part to openly and directly discuss inner feeling with others. Thus, although open discussion of conflict should not be avoided, long-drawn-out discussions should be because they punish open disclosure. Instead, the therapist should take the heat off the client. The therapist should consider it highly possible that she may be bringing some form of personal perceptual bias, past learning, or assumption with her into the therapy session, which makes it difficult for her to fully understand her OC client's perspective or behavior.

When a repair is proving difficult, the therapist can take the heat off by sharing his observations with the client and asking permission to return to the discussion about the rupture in the next session. Thus the therapist should be prepared to admit to his client how his own actions or perceptions may have damaged the relationship, and to apologize if an apology is warranted. Taking responsibility for our actions signals openness, nonarrogance, and commitment to the relationship. This models radical openness while taking the heat off the client:

Therapist: I'm not sure if this makes sense to you, but I am aware of imagining that somehow, for whatever reason, I am not fully grasping what you are trying to communicate to me or how you are feeling right now. On the one hand, I am aware of thinking that this is okay because getting to know anyone well always involves some type of missed communication. And yet, at the same time, understanding you is my job. So what I am thinking is that it might be wise for us to simply take a short break from trying to sort out what might be going on. It may be a way for us to signal respect to each other and allow us some time for reflection, and then we can come back later and work further on this, with perhaps new insight. For example, we might just leave the issue until next session. How does that sound to you right now?

The therapist should then let the client know that he plans on practicing some self-enquiry in the coming week regarding the session and what he might be missing, and he should also suggest that the client might want to do something similar. Regardless of the actual words used, the therapist's manner should be easy, should signal a willingness to be wrong, and should clearly communicate that it is okay for the client to tell the therapist her true feelings or thoughts (even if they are judgmental). After this, the therapist should briefly check in with the client and then move the topic to a different area of discussion. The therapist should not simply end the session at this point, as this would reinforce abandonment as the solution to conflict. The therapist should ask for a commitment from the client to return to the next session in order to discuss the rupture again. As part of the orientation and commitment process (during the first four sessions), the client has already been asked to make a commitment not to drop out of therapy without discussing it first in person with the therapist. The client can be reminded of this earlier commitment whenever such a reminder is appropriate.

Finally, although a rupture repair can be considered successful only when the client says it has been, there are some external indicators that a repair has gone well. Probably the earliest signs are that an OC client starts to naturally reengage eye contact, uses more than one-word sentences, independently contributes to the discussion, stays on topic, and asks questions about a previously avoided or distressing topic, without prompting from the therapist.

Prevention of Premature Treatment Dropout

OC clients are likely to abandon a relationship when conflict emerges rather than directly dealing with the problem. The OC client's commitment not to drop out of therapy without first discussing her concerns in person with her therapist is essential to the prevention of her premature termination of treatment and allows an opportunity to repair an alliance rupture, if one has occurred. Usually this commitment is very easy to obtain because during the early stages of treatment most OC clients are highly motivated to change. In fact, the therapist should expect an OC client to protest or even suggest that she is offended by the therapist's suggestion that she might drop out without first discussing this decision in person with the therapist. Nevertheless, years of research and clinical experience in treating OC clients show that it is not uncommon for a seemingly highly committed client to suddenly abandon therapy, usually via an email or letter indicating that she has decided that the treatment is not for her. Sometimes written correspondence will explicitly refer to an alliance rupture (that is, the client will allude to having felt misunderstood or having experienced the treatment as not relevant to her specific problems). It is equally common, however, for a written explanation not to reference any problems with the therapist or the treatment. Instead, it may refer to plausible instrumental impediments—the client's new job or a change in work schedule will interfere with traveling to further appointments, or a physical illness makes it impossible to continue therapy, or the client feels "better" or has been "cured" and no longer requires therapy, or the client has decided to take a much needed vacation—and it may include expressions of gratitude for help received. The therapist must be careful not to automatically assume that an OC client's apparently plausible reasons, expressed in writing, represent the truth. Most often when a client terminates therapy by way of a written communication, and without openly discussing this decision in person with the therapist, the issue is avoidance, perhaps due to an alliance rupture, and only an in-person discussion is likely to confirm any other possibility. Since OC clients feel obligated to comply with prior agreements, this commitment can be highly influential in preventing premature dropout. Thus, prior to the end of the very first session, the therapist should obtain this commitment by saying, "The research with people with problems like those you are seeking help with shows that at some point during treatment you may wish to stop treatment, or that sometimes you might feel like not coming to therapy or may even feel like dropping out. This is entirely normal, but I would like to ask you if you could give me a commitment to come back in and discuss with me, in person, your concerns about therapy or your desires to drop out before you actually do so. Can you give me a commitment that you will be willing to do this?" The therapist should also anticipate objections such as:

- "I would never think of dropping out!"

- "I am really committed to this therapy."

- "I consider you to be a competent therapist, and so I believe it's highly unlikely that I would consider dropping out."

The therapist should note that none of these statements is actually responsive to the request for a commitment to return in person and discuss desires to drop out before actually doing so. As one OC client later reported to her therapist, "I knew that if I gave this commitment, I would be obligated to follow it, and so it was actually difficult to do, although at the time you were asking me about it, I dared not let you know this." When commitment clarity is lacking, the therapist should gently repeat the request, the goal being for the client to actually give a response. Most often the client will provide this commitment (albeit sometimes with reluctance, or by implying that it is unnecessary). Importantly, once the client's commitment has been obtained, the client can be reminded of it if and when the need arises. Plus, this commitment should be reobtained repeatedly, particularly prior to the end of a session that has involved repair of an alliance rupture, a confrontation of maladaptive behavior, or discussion of highly charged emotional material.

Three Key Commitment Principles in Working with Overcontrol

1. Prevent treatment dropout. Say, "Because you may sometimes feel like not coming to therapy or may even feel like dropping out, I would like to ask you to commit to coming back in person to discuss your concerns with me before you make the decision to stop treatment. Would you be willing to do this?"

2. Encourage candid disclosure. Say, "I just wanted to let you know that we should expect during our work together that you may sometimes feel ambivalent about treatment or uncomfortable for some reason. This is normal and not a bad thing. Instead, it often signals engagement in treatment because you are questioning things, or it shows that you may be working hard to do something different. What I would like to ask is for you to let me know whenever these feelings arise. Do you think you might be willing to do so?"

3. Encourage disagreement. Say, "I am aware of imagining that sometimes you may disagree with me. Dissent is not a bad thing. In fact, it often is a sign of therapeutic progress because it is the opposite of masking feelings and may help us make important adjustments in our work together. Do you think you might be willing to let me know when you disagree, even when it might be difficult or you are unsure whether it would be the right thing to do?"

When a client prematurely terminates treatment, the overall goal is to reengage him, if possible. This is done with respect and compassion, and the process follows similar principles whether the event involves a no-show for treatment or a formal indication of dropout. When a no-show occurs, either for individual therapy or for skills training classes, the therapist or instructor should immediately attempt to telephone the client. If the client answers the telephone, a brief assessment of the problem preventing him from attending can be done, with the goal of getting him to come back to the clinic without delay for a partial session (or back to the classroom). This is based on the principle that some therapy is better than none and on the importance of blocking avoidance. If the client cannot be reached in person, then a voice mail message can be left or a text message can be sent. Voice mail is preferred because it is more personal. Here is an example of a voice mail left by a therapist who was unsure why his client failed to show up for a session:

Therapist: Hi, Jayne. It's Chris from the RO DBT clinic. I couldn't help but notice that you didn't make it to session today. *(Pauses momentarily and then resumes, with an easy manner.)* Definitely something different for you! So I thought I might just give you a call and see if everything is okay with you…and I'd really appreciate a call back. My number is 555-555-5555. And, by the way, you should know that you were missed. So call me as soon as you get this. Thanks.

And here is an example of a voice mail left by a therapist after his client wrote to say that she wanted to discontinue therapy:

Therapist: Hi, Jayne. It's Chris from the RO DBT clinic. I wanted to let you know that I received your letter. I appreciate your letting me know about your concerns. *(Pauses.)* And I take them seriously. *(Pauses.)* I would really like to continue working with you, and at the same time I recognize that this may not reflect your experience. Clearly some adjustments need to be made. *(Pauses.)* I am hoping that you will be willing to honor our agreement that we would meet in person to discuss any issues or concerns you might have that could result in therapy ending early. *(Pauses.)* So please give me a call and let me know if our regularly scheduled session will work for you this week, or if we need to find another time. My number is 555-555-5555. And, by the way, you should know that I do care about what happens to you and really want to make this work. I look forward to hearing from you, hopefully soon. Thanks.

Dropout from treatment, whether expected or unexpected, should generally be considered an alliance rupture and should therefore automatically trigger use of engagement and attachment strategies. The best outcome is when the client agrees to come back to therapy or at least return for one last session. This provides an important opportunity to repair the alliance rupture. A wide range of factors can result in a desire to end treatment prematurely; here are some examples:

- A "wrong" word was used by the therapist.

- The client felt unappreciated or misunderstood.

- The therapist was experienced as too directive.

- The treatment was experienced as not relevant to the client's unique problems.

- The therapist or treatment was perceived as too impersonal or officious.

- Questions from the therapist were perceived as inappropriate or intrusive.

- The therapist broke a "rule" or expectation that the client had about therapy.

- The client experienced shame secondary to emotional leakage.

- The client became hopeless when depression or anxiety suddenly worsened.

- The client felt criticized, exposed, or overwhelmed during a session.

- The client became fearful of becoming intimate with the therapist.

Getting the client to talk about why she wants to drop out helps her learn how to successfully engage and repair conflict. The idea is to reach out and communicate to the client that she is cared for, that her concerns are taken seriously (as shown, for example, by her therapist's willingness to admit that he has done something unhelpful), and that she has done nothing wrong (for example, by letting her know that disagreeing or disliking something is not bad). Strict adherence to clinic protocols or quick acceptance of a client's request to terminate treatment and be referred elsewhere (frequently disguised as respect for a client's wishes) can sometimes reflect a therapist's or a team's wish to avoid dealing with a difficult-to-treat client. A compassionate pause to consider options invariably provides the space needed to repair an alliance rupture.

Alliance ruptures that lead to dropout cannot always be foreseen. It is not uncommon for a therapist to be surprised, perplexed, or confused when it occurs without apparent warning. When an impersonal dropout occurs—for example, when the client writes a letter or an email or leaves a voice mail indicating that he is discontinuing therapy but avoids talking to his therapist directly—it is probable that the therapist missed or ignored earlier warning signs of a possible alliance rupture or that a serious rupture occurred during the last session and was either left unaddressed or inadequately repaired. This can be shared with a client; that is, therapists model radical openness by explicitly revealing to a client that they are aware of imagining that they may have misunderstood something or failed to ensure that the treatment was experienced as relevant to the client's unique problems.

Regardless, an unexpected, personally hostile, or impersonally communicated dropout can be painful and demoralizing for a therapist. It can feel like a personal failure. As such, dropouts should always be discussed in the consultation team. The team should work to understand and validate the therapist's perspective (for example, a sense of betrayal or demoralization) and emotions (such as anger, humiliation, despair, or relief) while maintaining phenomenological empathy for the client. That is, the team should avoid becoming unbalanced by blaming either the therapist or the client for what has happened. Solutions designed to treat the therapist should focus on blocking or redefining harsh self-blame, going opposite to unjustified emotions, or deciding how to manage justified emotions, with the goal of finding a way for the therapist to reengage with the client. A wide range of creative attachment strategies should be entertained:

- Sending a postcard requesting a call, inquiring about the client's well-being, or expressing affection or caring

- Making creative use of text messages, email, or the internet

- Having someone other than the individual therapist make contact

- Sending a card or balloon that says, "Missing you"

The therapist can also remind the client, if possible, of the client's prior commitment to talk in person with the therapist prior to dropping out of therapy. It is crucial to remind the client that the therapist is strongly committed to working with her and understands that there is no one way to behave or talk about issues and that everyone is not the same. Finally, regardless of the therapist's or team's intensity in attempting to reengage a client, we have found that, rather than giving up, simply staying in contact with the client (usually over a period of many months) can serve as a powerful means to communicate caring, which leads to the client's eventual reengagement. The type of contact need not be complex—for example, it might involve simply handwriting a brief note every month that expresses a sincere desire for the client to feel better (see "Tips for Maintaining the OC Client's Engagement," chapter 5).

Now You Know...

▶ Alliance ruptures are both emotional and interpersonal.

▶ Small alliance ruptures are expected to occur frequently during treatment of OC; rather than being feared, they should be seen as important opportunities to practice skills.

▶ In RO DBT, if there have not been numerous alliance ruptures and repairs by the fourteenth session, the therapeutic relationship is assumed to be superficial.

▶ OC clients, experts at masking their feelings and not revealing vulnerability or anger, tend to abandon relationships when conflict emerges, and so alliance ruptures and repairs offer a core means of allowing them to successfully engage in and resolve conflict and thus practice the skills needed to form close social bonds.

CHAPTER 9

Treatment Targeting and Intervention: Prioritizing Social Signaling

In many ways, all of the prior chapters have prepared us for this one. The key to effective treatment targeting when treating problems of overcontrol is not to focus solely on inner experience (for example, dysregulated emotion, maladaptive cognition, lack of metacognitive awareness, or past traumatic memories) as the source of OC suffering. Instead, RO DBT targets indirect, masked, and constrained social signaling as the primary source of OC clients' emotional loneliness, based on robust research linking inhibited and constrained expressions of emotion to social isolation and treatment-resistant internalizing problems, such as refractory depression.

Starting as early as the fourth session and then continuing throughout treatment, the individual therapist remains alert for social signaling targets and collaborates with the client to individualize treatment targets linked to OC social signaling themes. This is the third-ranked priority in the treatment target hierarchy in RO DBT. Once identified and agreed upon, the targets begin to be monitored on the diary card. This chapter discusses how to individualize these targets and suggests treatment strategies for addressing them. Life-threatening behaviors and alliance ruptures, however, always take precedence. I begin by discussing how the concept of a life worth sharing guides targeting and how the treatment hierarchy is used to structure the session. I go on to look at the basic principles of targeting and the importance of social signaling when targeting and outline the targeting protocol. I take a look at the common pitfalls we have seen and elaborate on the use of the diary card in RO DBT. The chapter ends with a look at some of the treatment interventions, details of which can be found in the skills training manual.

Kindness First and Foremost

Selfishness is considered far from a virtue in most societies. Yet acts of generosity and kindness rarely make the headlines. Instead, we are bombarded with stories and gossip about moral failings, deception, greed, violence, and cruelty. However, there is a silver lining—the reason why antisocial acts are so newsworthy is that they are so rare (despite what the news media or certain politicians may wish you to believe). Every day throughout the world you can see examples of small acts of kindness being performed without thought of recognition or repayment (for example, people opening doors for each other, helping someone who appears lost, allowing a person waiting in line to go first, giving up one's seat on a bus, letting another win simply because it matters to him more, or offering food to a homeless person). Small acts of kindness are what unite us as a species. Plus, contrary to what is often depicted in Hollywood films, when a major catastrophe strikes (for example, the 9/11 attack in New York, the Fukushima nuclear power plant disaster in Japan) most people respond not with panic or aggression but altruistically (for example, by banding together and sharing resources; see Boehm, 2012). Indeed, generosity and kindness have been shown to occur as early as eighteen months of age (Warneken & Tomasello, 2006), and children between the ages of three and five years have been shown to provide a greater share of a reward to a partner who has done more work on a task, without ever being asked, even when it meant getting less of the reward for themselves (Kanngiesser & Warneken, 2012). Plus, our capacity for kindness can be so powerful that it overrides individual survival instincts (for example, the stranger who dives without forethought into an icy river to save a drowning child, the soldier who throws himself over a grenade to protect his unit, the whistleblower who risks all to expose an injustice), suggesting that it may be evolutionarily hardwired.[49] Indeed, our capacity for kindness may be rightly regarded as a preeminent human quality because it may be what makes all others possible.

Yet kindness differs from compassion, despite being used interchangeably to mean the same thing. Broadly speaking, compassion is a response to suffering; "it has but one direction, which is to heal suffering" (Feldman & Kuyken, 2011, p. 152). Compassion involves a feeling state of sympathetic understanding that can be directed either outward (empathy with another person's suffering) or inward (self-compassion). Interestingly, kindness entails affection or love, whereas compassion entails empathy, mercy, and sympathy; for example, judges reduce punishments because they feel merciful toward the accused, not affectionate. Kindness does not require the other person to be suffering for it to emerge; that is, we can be kind to happy people, not just to those who are suffering. Plus, although kindness is always caring, it is not always nice (sometimes the kindest thing a person can do is say no), whereas compassion is always nice (that is, rarely critical). Table 9.1 provides an overview of some other differences between kindness and compassion.

Table 9.1. Differences Between Kindness and Compassion

Kindness	Compassion
Social signal	Inner experience
Signal affection, warmth, playfulness	Feel sympathy, empathy, concern
Priorities are humility, openness, transparency, and willingness to publicly admit fault or wrongdoing	Priorities are acceptance, nonjudgmental thinking, and validation
Orientation is toward questioning oneself and signaling openness to others in order to learn and socially connect with others	Orientation is toward healing oneself and others via empathetic understanding, validation, and nonjudgmental awareness
Emphasis is on celebrating our differences as well as our tribal nature and on contributing to others' well-being without expecting anything in return	Emphasis is on alleviating suffering and acknowledging the universality of human suffering with tolerance, equanimity, acceptance, and generosity

Yet if kindness means telling a good friend a painful truth or helping someone without ever expecting anything in return, then why do we bother—or, perhaps more specifically, what would be the evolutionary advantage for our species? According to the RO DBT neuroregulatory model (see chapter 2), our stress-regulation systems evolved, at least in part, to connect us to others. They calm down when we are feeling close to people we care about, whether related to us or not, and spike during isolation and loneliness. Even short periods of solitary confinement can derange the mind and damage the body because of the stress they create. Feeling socially isolated from one's community can be as destructive to health as cigarette smoking (and is the most common predictor of completed suicide). Acts of kindness and generosity are powerful social safety signals that function to bind us together rather than tear us apart. Unfortunately, despite being highly conscientious, most OC clients are clueless about how to socially signal kindness. Thus treatment targeting in RO DBT is an iterative process whereby the OC client is incrementally shaped to both live by his values and learn how to prosocially signal to others (that is, to behave kindly). The strategies for accomplishing this form the basis of this chapter.

Radically Open Living: Developing a Life Worth Sharing

Radically open living means learning how to flexibly adapt one's behavior to ever-changing circumstances in order to achieve a goal or live according to one's values, in a manner that accounts for the needs of others. It's the last part of the prior statement—"in a manner that accounts for the needs of others"—that is posited to be most important when working with emotionally lonely and socially isolated OC clients (and perhaps for all people). Consequently, radically open living is learning how to create a life worth sharing (with others), based on the premise that our personal happiness is highly dependent on other people and the extent to which we feel part of a tribe.[50] Robust research shows that when we feel connected, we feel less agitated, less anxious, less depressed, and less hostile. A life worth sharing is worth sharing because it is lived in a manner that goes against older, "selfish" tendencies linked to survival of the individual in order to contribute to the well-being of another (without always expecting something in return). It is humility in action and the basis for all human acts of altruism. Yet radically open living recognizes that when I lend a hand, it is because I choose to, not because I have been forced. My self-sacrifices are freely chosen; therefore, those I help don't owe me. I alone am responsible for my decisions to help or not help. It also recognizes that one cannot achieve heightened self-awareness in isolation—that we need other people (hopefully, our friends) to point out our blind spots, and, as a consequence, a life worth sharing highlights open dialogue and companionship as a core means for personal growth but also a core means to contribute to the welfare of others. A life worth sharing is also courageous. It actively seeks to find fault in itself and question its motives without falling apart. On the other hand, it doesn't take itself too seriously—it can laugh at its own foibles and share the laugh with others. Plus, it can boast with the best of them, when boasting is needed (for example, to ensure that hard work is recognized), or it can be arrogant with the arrogant (for example, to stand up against injustice to protect others). Yet, fundamentally, a life worth sharing is humble because it recognizes that each of us is dependent on other people for our personal well-being and success. For example, it might mean giving the other person the benefit of the doubt during interactions because it acknowledges that our perceptions, beliefs, and convictions can be (and often are) invalid. Regardless, each of us must decide for ourselves what a life worth sharing means for us and how it might manifest (for example, whether it means improving a long-term relationship, establishing a new one, or enhancing our sense of belonging by contributing to the welfare of others).

Nevertheless, although a life worth sharing and social connectedness are posited as essential for human happiness, therapists should not expect every OC client to necessarily agree, especially during the earlier phases of treatment. Despite often secretly longing for social connectedness, the vast majority of OC clients have very little experience in knowing how to establish close intimate bonds or may fear they will lose their independence or sense of self. Some may attempt to convince the therapist that they are the type of person who just doesn't need other people, that they are unlovable, or that love is phony. The challenge for the therapist then becomes *How does one induce someone to approach something he would prefer not to do?* One common method is to exert pressure on the reluctant individual in an effort to force him to comply (for example, by increasing the intensity of the request, highlighting the dangers of noncompliance, or repeated badgering). This often works, but not with everyone.

> Despite often secretly longing for social connectedness, the vast majority of OC clients have very little experience in knowing how to establish close intimate bonds or may fear they will lose their independence or sense of self

Indeed, OC clients may be particularly resistant to active attempts at persuasion; for them, the harder you try, the more skeptical they become, but if you don't try, then it means either that you don't care or that you never believed in a life worth sharing in the first place. The important thing for therapists to recognize is that most of the time this type of mixed message is rarely intentional. OC clients are simply suspicious in general (not just when it comes to therapy). The good news is that they are much more likely to respond positively to interpersonal feedback that allows them time to consider the consequences and decide for themselves than to feedback that pressures them for an immediate answer or assumes that it knows what is best for them. Thus "foot in the door" techniques (Freedman & Fraser, 1966) that ask for little but hope for more are more likely to generate positive outcomes than are "door in the face" approaches that ask for a great deal but are willing (often secretly so) to accept less (the only exception to this is imminent life-threatening behavior).

Structuring Sessions with the RO DBT Treatment Target Hierarchy

Individual therapy treatment targets are organized hierarchically into three broad categories:

1. Severe and imminent life-threatening behaviors

2. Alliance ruptures

3. Maladaptive OC social signaling linked to five OC social signaling themes

This broad treatment target hierarchy provides a means for therapists to organize an individual therapy session and make adjustments as needed (see "Hierarchy of Treatment Targets in Individual Therapy," chapter 4). In general, individual therapy sessions follow a similar structure, yet within each session therapists may purposefully move between the hierarchy levels on more than one occasion in order to address issues emerging in the moment. Problem behaviors that are life-threatening behaviors are given top priority. Thus, when imminent life-threatening behavior is present, therapists should drop their agenda and prioritize keeping the client alive. The RO DBT protocol for assessing and addressing imminent life-threatening behaviors when working with OC clients can be found in chapter 5. The second-most important target in RO DBT is a rupture in the therapeutic alliance between the OC client and the therapist (see chapter 8).

Though life-threatening behavior and alliance ruptures take precedence, RO DBT posits that social signaling deficits represent the core problem underlying OC emotional loneliness, isolation, and psychological distress. Thus, ideally, the vast majority of therapy time is spent on these issues. Five OC social signaling themes are posited to be uniquely influential in the development and maintenance of OC social signaling deficits. They provide an evidence-based framework that allows therapists to introduce previously taboo or undisclosed topics and correct oftentimes long-held beliefs by an OC client that her difficulties are especially weird, odd, or abnormal relative to other people. This helps start the important process of helping the socially isolated OC client rejoin the tribe. Most important, the OC signaling themes function as the backdrop for the creation of individualized treatment targets that are essential for achieving a life worth sharing. The practical aspects of accomplishing this represent the core aim of this chapter. But before one can target a social signaling deficit linked to an OC theme, it helps to know what is meant by a social signal, which is the topic of the next section.

It Takes Two to Tango: Social Signaling Defined

RO DBT defines a *social signal* as any action, regardless of form, intent, or conscious awareness, that occurs in the presence of another person. According to this definition, even behaviors never intended as signals (such as a yawn), and those occurring outside of conscious awareness (a sudden sigh), function as social signals if they occur in the presence of another person or are observed remotely, as in a video-recording. Thus the words I am typing at this moment are social signals only if someone other than me ever reads them. Actions, gestures, or expressions delivered without an audience (that is, in private) are simply overt behaviors, not social signals. Even when rehearsing in front of a mirror what you might say to your boss, you are not social signaling; you are simply preparing your lines before you go onstage.

What's more, most people are highly adept at knowing when they are onstage (being observed) versus offstage (completely alone) and adjust their behavior accordingly (we are less likely to pick our nose when we think someone may be watching). Plus, research shows that we trust nonverbal expressions of emotion over what a person says. Thus the problem for the sender is knowing whether or not the actual intended message was received as intended, including times when nothing was intended at all (sometimes a yawn is just a yawn). Moreover, perhaps the most frequently misinterpreted and most powerful nonverbal social signal is less about what was said or done and more about what was *not* said or *not* done. For example, a conspicuous absence of expected or customary prosocial signals during interactions (not smiling during greetings, low rates of affirmative head nods) is almost always interpreted to mean disapproval or dislike, regardless of the actual intentions of the sender. We are constantly socially signaling when around others (via microexpressions and body movements), even when desperately trying not to (not saying anything can be just as powerful as a long speech).

Knowing What to Target: The Key to Successful Treatment

The difficulty in treatment targeting when working with OC clients is that they are experts at masking inner experience and inhibiting emotional expression, to such an extent that they may not even be aware when they are doing it. It's not that they don't recognize the utility of being more expressive, genuine, or self-revealing; it's that they don't know how to go about behaving differently (or fear being hurt or betrayed if they ever truly tried).

Plus, OC clients are highly motivated to appear in control, or competent, even when the house is burning down (the "don't ever let them see you sweat" phenomenon), and their superior capacities for self-control make this possible (at least most of the time). Yet, despite strong desires to be seen as competent, most OC clients, almost paradoxically, behave as if change is impossible or as if normal expectations of behavior should not apply, given their history or current toxic living conditions. Therapists can often unwittingly join with their OC clients' pessimistic point of view, forgetting that past trauma and current adversity do not necessarily equate to despair and defeat.

OC clients are also expert at blocking feedback they don't want to hear and disguising intentions (the art of disclosing without disclosing), without making it obvious that this is what they are doing (for example, pretending not to hear, ignoring, answering a question with a question, subtly changing the topic, turning the tables by asking an apparently innocent question). Complicating matters further (and exacerbating OC clients' self-hatred), they are usually highly aware of their compulsive needs to control, to win, or to dominate—desires they are likely to keep hidden from others and often privately use as "proof" of their nefarious and flawed personalities.

Indirect or disguised social signals are powerful because they allow the sender to influence (control) others or get what he wants without ever having to admit to it; for example, the silent treatment signals anger without saying a word and is easy to deny: "Who me? No, I'm not angry. I just don't feel like talking." Yet they arrive with a hidden cost for the sender. Indirect signaling often leads to misunderstanding or distrust between people because it is hard to know the true meanings or intentions of the sender (and for the therapist to know what to target for change). Regardless of the sender's actual intentions, indirect and ambiguous social signals (a flat facial expression, an expressionless tone of voice, a smirk, a yawn) are often interpreted by recipients to mean disapproval, dislike, or deception (even when never intended), which is precisely what makes them so interpersonally damaging.

Furthermore, deciding to ignore social signaling and to target internal processes instead (such as thoughts or internal emotional experience) only exacerbates the dilemma when working with OC clients, since internal experience is always the easiest to plausibly deny or obfuscate when the overt behavior or social signals on the outside are ambiguous. Targeting internal experience is much easier when working with individuals characterized by undercontrol (for example, people with borderline personality disorder) because it is harder for the client to appear credible that she is "perfectly fine" after throwing a chair through the therapist's window (see table 9.2).

Table 9.2. Social Signaling Differences Between Overcontrolled and Undercontrolled Personality Styles

	Overcontrolled (OC) Signaling	Undercontrolled (UC) Signaling
Expressivity	OC social signaling tends to be understated, controlled, predictable, and generally non-mood-dependent. There are two differing OC signaling styles: (1) inhibited, muted and flat expressions and (2) overly prosocial, insincere, and feigned expressions. Both styles rarely reveal or express vulnerable emotions, either publicly or privately.	UC social signaling tends to be dramatic, disinhibited, unpredictable, and mood-dependent. Flat facial expressions, when they occur, are temporary and almost always the consequence of dysregulated emotion (for example, overwhelming shame, extreme anger, dissociation, or panic). Vulnerable and extreme displays of emotion (such as anger and crying) are commonplace.
Control	OC individuals may have secret pride in their innate capacity for superior self-control and their ability to inhibit impulses, delay gratification, plan ahead, tolerate distress, and control expressions of emotion in any situation; for example, they can appear calm and disinterested on the outside despite feeling anxious on the inside.	UC individuals are painfully aware of (and may be embarrassed or ashamed about) their inability to control their expressions of emotion. They typically lack the inhibitory capacities needed to prevent an emotional outburst from occurring when under stress or conflicting demands.

Setting	OC individuals have been intermittently reinforced to inhibit or mask emotional expressions in public or around people who are not in the immediate family. They are highly self-conscious and dislike the limelight unless they have had time to prepare.	UC individuals have been intermittently reinforced to escalate expressions of emotion. Their low capacity for inhibitory control, combined with their high reward sensitivity, makes the factor of setting (that is, private or public) less salient or less noticeable to them; when highly excited, for example, they may be unaware that they are talking too much or too loudly. They are generally less self-conscious than most others in public, enjoy being the center of attention, and are less likely to spend their free time preparing, planning, or rehearsing prior to an upcoming social event.
Variability	OC individuals display little variability in how their emotions are expressed, either in valence or intensity. Their low reward sensitivity makes spontaneous displays of excitement or joy less likely.	The emotional expressions of UC individuals are diverse and labile, both in valence and intensity. Although in general they strive to inhibit or control extreme expressions of negative emotion (often without success), they rarely attempt to control or inhibit expressions of positive emotion.

Essentially, undercontrolled maladaptive social signaling is by definition *big* (that is, more expressive, more dramatic, more labile). Treatment targets stand out and shout their presence when working with UC clients; their bigness is what makes them hard to ignore (and hard to deny), whereas OC social signaling is almost always understated, controlled, and small (except for instances of emotional leakage), making it hard know what to target for change in therapy. Fortunately, there is a way to get around this dilemma. It begins by noticing that when it comes to social signaling, size doesn't matter; for example, silence can be just as powerful as nonstop talking. Plus, from an RO DBT perspective, when it comes to interpersonal connectedness, what we think or feel on the inside matters less than how we communicate or signal our inner intentions and experience on the outside.

Thus social signaling matters, but knowing what to target out of the literally thousands of microfacial expressions, body movements, gestures, and verbal statements occurring in just one one-hour therapy session, let alone all the multitudes that occur outside of session, seems like an impossible task. But don't despair—there is a way forward, one that begins with the recognition that our personal social signaling habits can bias what we see as a maladaptive social signal.

We Don't See the World as It Is, We See It as We Are

There is no right or optimal way to socially signal—each of us has our own distinctive style of expression. Thus learning how to target indirect and ambiguous social signals can be a challenge for therapists because each of us is unique. Moreover, a core RO DBT principle is that we bring perceptual and regulatory biases with us wherever we go, including into the work we do with our clients (that is, we don't see the world as it is, we see it as we are). This is one of the reasons RO DBT encourages therapists to seek outside supervision and practice radical openness themselves (ideally in an RO consultation team).

Additionally, the discrete nature of most OC behavior can result in therapist self-doubt as to the veracity of a problem behavior—that is, is it really problematic? For example, a case conceptualization problem can be seen whenever a therapist without awareness automatically accepts her client's worldview or explanation as reasonable, normal, or adaptive. Thus a client reports, "I can't go on a date, because I don't have any money," and instead of questioning this response, the therapist accepts it as plausible, forgetting that poor people date all the time. Or a client says, "I can't allow myself to reveal my inner feelings, because I'm depressed," and the therapist then drops the behavioral change expectation and focuses instead on trying to get rid of the depression first, forgetting that the depression stems from the social signaling deficit of masking inner feelings in the first place.

Likewise, fundamental differences in desired intimacy, cultural differences, and personality differences (such as the extent to which a therapist leans toward overcontrolled coping or undercontrolled coping) not only make us unique but also can influence how we perceive the world—and, as a consequence, our treatment targeting. For example, therapists who lean toward an overcontrolled coping style themselves (and our research suggests that most do) can often find it more difficult (not easier) to identify maladaptive OC social signaling deficits because they often exhibit the same behavior themselves (albeit usually less rigidly).[51] Plus, if a therapist who leans toward overcontrolled coping has primarily lived solely with people who have the same style, then he is naturally more likely to perceive his own social signaling style as normal or even preferred. Asking a therapist who leans toward an OC coping style whether a particular social signal is maladaptive or not is a bit like asking a fish whether it is swimming in saltwater or freshwater—it all feels the same when you have nothing to compare it to. As one research therapist put it, "I have learned to use self-enquiry whenever I find myself saying to myself that my client's behavior seems reasonable. Often I discover that I engage in the same behavior as my client."

Finally, targeting social signaling can be challenging to learn because it requires the therapist to let go (at least to some extent) of prior training or other theoretical models that emphasize different mechanisms of change, such as the importance of directly changing internal experience (for example, dysfunctional thoughts, dysregulated emotions, or the salience of traumatic memories) or changing how we respond to internal experience (for example, avoidance, nonacceptance, rumination, or thought suppression). Indeed, most of us revert to old habits or what we know best when feeling uncertain; thus, therapists should anticipate that they are likely to respond similarly when first learning RO DBT (so be kind to yourself).

The good news is that I have been fortunate to receive a great deal of feedback from my OC clients, friends, students, and colleagues over the years, not only about the basic principles underlying RO DBT but also about how I have tried to explain these principles to others (for example, in trainings or during supervision). The consequence has been the development of two (that's right—not just one) methods of targeting maladaptive social signaling, which can be used independently, interchangeably, or in combination. They differ primarily by how structured and planned versus unstructured and spontaneous they are when being implemented, yet both lead to similar targeting success.

Treatment Targeting: Best When It's Curious

We both know and don't know other people. Research shows that within just a few minutes of exposure to the nonverbal behavior of another person (even just a picture), we are able to form reliable and valid impressions of a stranger's personality traits, socioeconomic status, and moral attributes like trustworthiness and altruism (Ambady & Rosenthal, 1992; W. M. Brown et al., 2003; Kraus & Keltner, 2009). Yet anyone who has ever truly tried to know another person from the inside out is likely to quickly point out that it's harder than you might think (or than the data just cited might suggest). From my perspective, when it comes to treating problems of emotional loneliness (like OC), what matters most about our intuitions is not how accurate they are but how we viscerally feel about the other person—that is, the extent to which we desire to spend more or less time with him.

Thus, when it comes to targeting maladaptive social signaling, therapists often need to retrain themselves to consider any overt behavior displayed by the client in session as a social signal, regardless of the intentions of the sender. For example, when a client begins to bounce her leg up and down repeatedly in session, an RO DBT therapist is likely not to automatically assume that this behavior is simply a habit or a symptom of anxiety (and thus ignore it); instead, the therapist is likely to evaluate the shaking leg from a social signaling perspective but discuss it directly with the client as a potential target only if it occurs across multiple sessions, in multiple contexts (not just in therapy), and only if it is collaboratively determined to interfere with the client's social connectedness or her ability to live according to her values (such as being seen by others as competent). Assuming that these criteria are met, at some point during treatment the RO DBT therapist is likely to directly discuss the social signaling aspects of the behavior with the client, as an initial step in determining its relevance as a treatment target, and to ask, with a warm closed-mouth smile, "Have you ever noticed that whenever we talk about certain topics, but not others, your leg starts to go up and down really fast? What do you think that shaking leg is trying to say?"

In addition, rather than telling OC clients what is wrong with their social signaling, RO DBT therapists encourage clients to examine the utility of their social signaling for themselves via self-enquiry, a process that can be initiated by two broad questions:

1. To what extent did my social signaling reflect my core values?

2. To what extent did the consequences of my social signaling achieve my original intentions?

The answers that emerge from these questions should not be considered definitive (absolute truth); instead, they are working hypotheses that are collaboratively shared with the therapist (or recorded in the client's RO self-enquiry journal) and targeted for change only after the client and the therapist have agreed that these hypotheses are relevant. The best therapeutic questions are those we don't already believe we know the answers to (that is, questions reflecting genuine curiosity). Rather than asking questions in order to change a client's mind or coerce him to think the way we do, RO DBT therapists ask questions in order to learn who the client is and encourage him to discover for himself how he wants to live. The essential difference between this approach and other therapeutic methods using Socratic questioning (Padesky, 1993) is the emphasis that RO DBT places on social signaling.

Targeting In-Session Social Signaling: Basic Principles

Targeting social signaling in session is easy (oops...I just contradicted what I said earlier; okay, *easier*) once you grasp just how much social signaling is going on between people at any given moment. It is all about retraining what you prioritize as a problem, and where you focus your attention. As highlighted repeatedly throughout this book, RO DBT prioritizes nonverbal behavior over verbal descriptions or reports. Indeed, huge amounts of information are transmitted, received, interpreted, and responded to, often at the subliminal level of awareness, within seconds of first meeting someone. We are constantly scanning the facial expressions and vocalizations of other people for signs of disapproval—that is, information about our social status, the extent to which our behavior is socially desirable, or the degree to which another person appears to like us. Slow-motion film analysis has robustly revealed that we react to changes in body movement, posture, and facial expressions of others during interactions without ever knowing it. Plus, research shows that we need at least seventeen to twenty milliseconds to be consciously aware of an emotional face, and yet our brain-body is already physiologically reacting at durations as low as four milliseconds (L. M. Williams et al., 2004, 2006), and researchers estimate that language-based appraisals don't even start until two hundred milliseconds (for example, a facial expression is labeled a smile)—which, from the perspective of the evolutionarily older subcortical processing, seems really slow. Moreover, top-down reappraisals (such as cognitive restructuring) of bottom-up primary appraisals are even slower because the person first has to label the experience (as a frown, for example) and then access a wide range of memories, contextual information, and prior learning to decide whether top-down regulatory processes at the central cognitive level agree with bottom-up primary appraisals at the subcortical level. (*Phew!*) So suffice it to say, "There's a whole lot of feelin' goin' on," according to Granny Moses of the 1960s TV hit series *The Beverly Hillbillies.*[32] The question is, is it possible to train a person to become better aware of nonverbal behavior that is often happening in milliseconds?

Fortunately, there is a wide range of research suggesting that we are pretty good at doing this. That is, we use other people's social signals to judge whether or not we trust them or would like to spend more time with them. Most therapists viscerally know what it feels like to trust another person or desire to be attached to them. What's more, research shows that, broadly speaking, humans are expert social safety detectors. Our brains have evolved ways to reliably detect the extent to which another person is likely to engage in reciprocal cooperative behaviors. For example, we recognize another's prosocial intent through emotion-based touching, smiling, and overall level of emotional expressivity (Boone & Buck, 2003; W. M. Brown & Moore, 2002; W. M. Brown et al., 2003; Hertenstein, Verkamp, Kerestes, & Holmes, 2006; Schug, Matsumoto, Horita, Yamagishi, & Bonnet, 2010), and we are adept at knowing whether a smile is genuine or phony and can accurately detect tension in the voice of a person (for example, Pittam & Scherer, 1993; Ekman, 1992). Indeed, one of the most reliable first impressions we form about others is whether they are warm (kind, friendly) or cool (aloof, prickly). Yet, as noted earlier, therapists should avoid the temptation of assuming their visceral observations represent the truth about their clients. Plus, research conducted by Paul Ekman and his colleagues over the past forty years, primarily centered on detection of deception, suggests that it is possible to train people to become better detectors of subtle indicators or microexpressions of emotion. For example, individuals with higher accuracy rates in detecting lies have been shown to use different and more varied verbal and nonverbal cues, in particular focusing on nonverbal signals and microexpressions of emotion. The accurate lie detectors also practiced their skill and sought feedback about their performance to improve their abilities, with respect to eye contact, for example (Ekman & O'Sullivan, 1991; Ekman, O'Sullivan, & Frank, 1999; O'Sullivan & Ekman, 2004). Thus, with a little training and practice, therapists can learn to notice subtle expressions of emotion in session. The next step in this journey is how to translate this into a relevant treatment target.

Targeting Problematic Social Signaling in Session: A Step-by-Step Protocol

Broadly speaking, whether identified from in-session behavior or derived from clients' self-reports of behavior occurring outside of session, the most important question to keep in mind when targeting social signaling is *How might my client's social signaling impact social connectedness?* The core idea is for the therapist to use her personal success in establishing close social bonds as a template to evaluate the potential effectiveness of her client's social signaling (this presumes, of course, that the therapist has had some success herself in forming long-term intimate bonds). To put it another way, the essence of this evaluation boils down to the following question: *If this person were not my client, would I enjoy spending time with him?* Or, to be even more colloquial, *Is this the type of person I would like to go have a beer with?* If not, why not? Or, more specifically, *What is it about my client's social signaling that might make people less likely to desire to affiliate with him?* However, there are some unique features associated with in-session social signaling targeting that, once mastered, can be iteratively integrated into targeting social signals outside of session (that is, social signals that are never seen directly by a therapist but only heard about via clients' self-reports). Thus I chose to begin with in-session behaviors.

The entire protocol (which I affectionately call the "yawning protocol") is summarized in detail by the clinical example presented in appendix 5. It includes not only detailed descriptions of the client's nonverbal social signaling, which can be used to determine whether a client is engaged or nonengaged in treatment, but also detailed accounts of how the therapist uses his own social signaling behavior to influence the client, without ever saying a word.

It is important not to become demoralized by the amount of detail or the number of steps in the protocol (there are fifteen in all), because in many ways this one clinical example contains the entire essence of RO DBT when it comes to treatment targeting; indeed, it makes this chapter almost superfluous. Plus, to go even stronger (let's be bold), when the clinical example in appendix 5 is combined with a thorough knowledge of the skills training manual, the therapist is basically equipped with the core principles of what to target and how to target (these principles are found in appendix 5) as well as how to intervene (these principles are found in the skills training manual). Another advantage of appendix 5 is that it illustrates just how much social signaling is happening in session that oftentimes we don't notice, or ignore, or believe to be irrelevant, or have no idea what to do with.[53]

The clinical example in appendix 5 should not be mistaken as relevant only to clients who yawn. It is also intended to be used as a template for applying the targeting principles to other potential problematic social signals. To do so, simply replace the word "yawn" and its variants with a word or a phrase representing another target (such as "flat face," "eye roll," or "furrowed brow"). It can also be helpful to keep in mind that, in general, there are two common indirect social signaling styles seen among OC clients that therapists should be alert for: *excessive* prosocial signaling, and a conspicuous *lack of* prosocial signaling (see table 9.3 for a summary of each).

Table 9.3. Absent vs. Excessive Prosocial Signaling in Overcontrolled Clients

Absence of Prosocial Signaling	Excess of Prosocial Signaling
Flat, deadpan expression	Frequent frozen, polite smiles displaying the teeth
Lack of head nodding or smiling	Excessive head nodding
Lack of friendly and cooperative signals	Overly attentive, ingratiating, or flattering behavior that is unnecessary or inappropriate
Staring	Frequent displays of submission or appeasement

Note: Regardless of whether the behavior represents an absence or an excess of prosocial signaling, it is unresponsive, pervasive, and context-inappropriate.

What's important is that the social signal you target should be relevant—is it keeping the client out of the tribe? This sometimes could even include how the client dresses or the type of jewelry she wears, as these, too, are social signals. Plus, nonverbal components of speech—rate (how fast or slow a person talks), pitch (the relative sound frequency, high or low), intonation (emerging pitch movements during speech), rhythm (how speech is organized into regular time intervals), and loudness (voice volume)—can also be important to target. For example, a flat and monotonic or expressionless voice, long and unnecessary pauses before answering questions or when speaking, talking much more slowly than others, and exhibiting longer pauses during conversations are all patterns of speech commonly observed in OC clients. Depressed clients are also more likely to end a sentence with a downward rather than upward inflection, which can signify low mood, boredom, or disinterest. Any of these might function as relevant targets. Yet you can only target one at a time, and so what is important is to look for the one that is the most powerful—that is, most likely to be creating difficulties for the client in achieving social connectedness.

> The social signal you target should be relevant—is it keeping the client out of the tribe?

The silent treatment represents another good example of a powerful yet indirect social signal. It most often occurs following a disagreement with someone, or when a person fails to conform to expectations. It signals disagreement or anger without overtly disclosing it, involving a sudden reduction in verbal behavior, a flattened facial expression, and avoidance of eye contact. If asked by the recipient about the sudden change in social signaling, the sender will usually deny the change and, with a blank face and unemotional tone of voice, say, "No, I'm fine" or "Everything's okay." In addition, as noted previously, "pushback" and "don't hurt me" responses (described in chapter 10) are so common that they have complete protocols for targeting and intervention when they occur in session, and an entire RO skills training class is dedicated to them (see the skills training manual, chapter 5, lesson 16). Finally, although the clinical example in appendix 5 is self-explanatory, there is one particular step in the protocol that many therapists find difficult to perform, partly because it feels so different from how they have been previously trained. You may have already guessed what it is—I am referring to the sixth step (that is, demonstrating the potentially maladaptive social signal to the client). Some basic principles underlying this step are reviewed next.

Show, Don't Just Tell

Demonstrate the maladaptive social signal; don't just talk about it. This principle represents classic RO DBT. The fundamental principle is for the therapist to act out or model the social signaling deficits rather than intellectually describe what they look like. This allows OC clients to viscerally experience what it might feel like to be on the receiving end of their social signal. Therapists should avoid explaining, justifying, or preparing an OC client beforehand; this not only takes up valuable session time but is not necessary and can lead to clients' reluctance to engage in role playing because they feel self-conscious. Instead, as shown in appendix 5, rather than explaining, simply ask clients to show you what the social signal is in order to ascertain its seventy.

Plus, contrary to what many therapists might expect, it is important when demonstrating to exaggerate the social signal, not downplay it in order to protect the client or avoid personal embarrassment. When done well, exaggeration functions to ensure that the client notices the social signal during role playing and makes it clear that the therapist is not mocking or criticizing the client, whereas serious and realistic depictions of a client's social signal are more likely to be taken as criticism because the client can painfully see himself in the therapist's realistic depiction. Exaggerated depictions are like watching a pantomime or comedy show, thereby making it less personal while still getting across the main point—that is, how the social signal being depicted may function as maladaptive. Exaggerating a social signal also models that it's okay to be expressive (recall that OC clients will not believe it is socially acceptable for a person to play, relax, or openly express emotions unless they first see their therapists model such behavior). When we freely express ourselves, tease one another, or allow ourselves to be silly around others, we transmit a powerful prosocial signal of nondominance, equality, and friendship. An exaggerated, silly demonstration of an OC social signaling behavior not only makes obvious to the client any potential downsides of the signal but also provides an opportunity for the client to viscerally experience what it is like to be on the receiving end of the signal. Thus, rather than talking about the social signaling problem, the RO DBT therapist demonstrates it and then works collaboratively with the client to determine the extent to which the social signal negatively impacts the client's social connectedness or accurately reflects the client's valued goals.

Refrain from Soothing or Expressing Concern

It is also important for therapists not to react strongly or with overt concern or soothing when a client expresses embarrassment during role playing. Not only is this normal, but expressions of embarrassment are almost always prosocial and signal willingness for self-examination. People like and trust those who display embarrassment. We feel more connected with people who show embarrassment (by blushing, for example) because it signals that they care about social transgressions (such as stepping on someone's toe or being insensitive).

Keep It Short

Finally, a common mistake for a therapist when conducting a demonstration or role playing with an OC client is making it last too long (most often because it just doesn't seem right that a client could grasp the impact of the social signal quickly). However, as described earlier, the type of visceral learning we are hoping for often takes only milliseconds to occur. So keep the demonstrations short. If the performance is exaggerated sufficiently by the therapist, then the client's subcortical emotion-processing system gets the point. In other words, if a therapist finds himself trying to explain to a client what she "should have" experienced, then the therapist should consider three possible options:

1. The social signal demonstrated by the therapist was not exaggerated sufficiently for the client to experience its impact, in which case the therapist should simply try again and increase the intensity of the signal (this is almost always the best first thing to do).

2. The client is nonengaged and is communicating this indirectly by pretending not to have seen or experienced the problem with the social signal, thereby triggering the protocol for repairing an alliance rupture.

3. The social signal is not maladaptive or relevant, meaning that most people would not find it distressing or off-putting.

The third of these options is less likely to occur, albeit, as can be seen in the example shown in appendix 5, at least initially the yawning client would have been perfectly happy for the therapist to simply go with the original hypothesis: that the client was just tired. Thus it is important to be tenacious. And one last point before moving on—it is important to note that not once in the example shown in appendix 5 does the therapist make any attempt to fix, solve, or change the maladaptive social signal. Focusing on solutions or skills (that is, how to change the behavior) during treatment targeting sends the wrong message; not only does it imply that you already understand the behavior (that is, that it is maladaptive and thereby needs to be changed), it also reinforces OC clients' tendencies to compulsively fix. Remember, OC clients need to learn how to chill out.

Next, I outline how to incorporate the OC social signaling themes into treatment targeting. The themes are helpful because they ensure breadth of targeting (so that core issues are not overlooked), and they are helpful early in therapy when treatment targeting would be useful but in-session displays of maladaptive social signaling have yet to occur sufficiently or repetitively enough for the therapist to use the in-session targeting protocol (see appendix 5).

Using OC Social Signaling Themes to Enhance Targeting: Basic Principles

There are five OC social signaling themes. Ideally, by the fourth or fifth session, the therapist should have begun the process of identifying individualized targets (albeit, as noted earlier, informal targeting could theoretically begin as early as the first session). Targets should be modified and refined over the course of treatment, partly as a function of new ones emerging, older ones improving, or simply as a function of getting to know the client better. Thus the therapist should not make the mistake of thinking that once he has come up with a target linked to one of the five OC social signaling themes, his work is done—far from it. Treatment targeting is a continual process in RO DBT that ideally gets increasingly detailed and relevant to the specific problems the client is struggling with as the client becomes more adept at revealing rather than masking inner experience, and has had the experience of collaboratively repairing alliance ruptures with their therapist (recall that a strong working alliance in RO DBT is posited to have been established only after there have been multiple ruptures and repairs; see chapter 8).

The OC themes are not targets themselves; they are too broad and not specific enough to function as targets. Instead, they ensure that the major relevant problem areas most commonly seen in OC clients are covered during the course of treatment. Thus, although the protocol described later in this chapter may appear formal or structured (indeed, it is labeled as such), this does not mean it should be followed rigidly. As mentioned earlier, therapists should feel free to integrate both formal and informal targeting approaches (and this often proves the ideal approach). The majority of therapists report finding the more formal approach most helpful when initially learning RO DBT, as it ensures that they are not inadvertently overlooking potentially important targets. Yet, with increasing experience, most therapists naturally become more flexible and often end up integrating both formal and informal approaches to targeting, depending on what they observe in session and according to the needs of their clients. What's important is not the style of targeting (that is, formal or informal) but the outcome—was the therapist able to identify relevant social signaling targets that are specific to the client? Here are examples of some features and social signaling deficits linked to each OC theme:

- Inhibited emotional expression (saying, "I'm fine" when not; exhibiting blank facial expressions; smiling when angry; "never let them see you sweat"; low use of emotional words; low use of big gestures and cooperative signals, such as eyebrow wags, hand gestures when speaking, head nods, eye contact)

- Overly cautious and hypervigilant behavior (planning compulsively before every event; obsessively rehearsing what to say; avoiding novel situations; taking only calculated risks; obsessive checking behaviors)

- Rigid and rule-governed behavior (regardless of the context, acting in ways that are dominated by prior experience and by such rules as "always be polite," "always work hard," "always think before acting," "always persist," and "never complain")

- Aloof and distant relationships (secretly smiling when people find it hard to understand one; rarely revealing personal information or weakness to another person; abandoning a relationship rather than dealing directly with a conflict)

- Envy and bitterness (making frequent social comparisons; engaging in harsh gossip about a rival; pouting when angry; engaging in revengeful acts; secretly smiling when a rival suffers; refusing help from others, or refusing to give help to others)

Finally, how themes and targets manifest behaviorally varies considerably among individuals. Therapists should attempt to be as behaviorally specific as possible; that is, identify the form, frequency, intensity, and function of the behaviors associated with the theme. For example, under the theme of "aloof and distant relationships," one client's aloofness might be represented by his covertly changing the topic of conversation to avoid disclosing personal information; another client's aloofness is exacerbated by his stern glances of disapproval directed toward someone who is doing something he dislikes; and yet another client might maintain his aloofness by getting others to talk whenever the topic gets personal. In order to ensure that interventions are relevant, it is important to determine exactly how aloofness and distance are socially signaled (for example, a person who habitually changes the topic whenever the conversation gets personal requires an intervention that is different from the one needed for a person who walks away from conflict). But before I review the formal protocol—*formally!*—I will mention a number of common pitfalls that I have observed over the years. If these are avoided at the outset, the therapist can save time and prevent unnecessary confusion on everyone's part.

Treatment Targeting: Common Pitfalls

Information Overload

Avoid the temptation of introducing all five OC themes at the same time. Although orientation and commitment strategies are a core part of RO DBT, when it comes to treatment targeting, too much information delivered too soon and too fast usually creates more problems than it solves (and can be iatrogenic). For one thing, the therapist has now placed herself in the position of needing to explain, justify, or defend broad concepts about OC coping that were never designed to fully capture the complexity of every OC client. OC themes are broad descriptors that help improve therapists' treatment targeting, not statements of fact about all OC clients. Therefore, introduce only one OC theme at a time (that is, one per session).[54]

The Struggle to Identify a Target

Even though the learning curve is sometimes steep for therapists, most OC clients (when engaged) not only immediately grasp the significance of social signaling but can also, without much trouble, generate several examples linked to a particular OC theme during treatment targeting. When they struggle and yet appear engaged, reassess their understanding of what a social signal means to them, and clarify any misunderstandings. However, when a client struggles and appears less engaged (for example, averting his eyes, mumbling, repeatedly saying, "I don't know"), the therapist should not only reassess the client's understanding of a social signal but also consider the possibility of an alliance rupture; that is, this change in behavior is a social signal (to the therapist). The question is, what is the client trying to signal? This means dropping the treatment agenda (that is, the agenda of identifying a social signaling target) and instead instituting the protocol for repairing an alliance rupture (see chapter 8)—for example, by asking directly about the change in behavior: "I don't know about you, but I've noticed that your behavior seemed to change as soon as we started to talk about identifying a social signal linked to this theme. What's going on with you right now? What are you trying to tell me?" Once the alliance rupture is repaired, most often the struggle disappears.

The Need for More Insight

Encourage self-enquiry when a client reports as adaptive or normal a social signal that you consider maladaptive. Present the client with the following self-enquiry questions to help facilitate this process (but don't feel compelled to present all of them):

- To what extent am I proud of the way I am behaving? Would I encourage another person or a young child to behave similarly when they interact with me? What might this tell me about my values or how I feel about the way I am behaving or thinking? What is it that I might need to learn?

- If I am proud of how I am behaving or thinking, then what is preventing me from more directly signaling my true intentions or feelings to the other person or persons rather than being so indirect or ambiguous?

- Would I feel embarrassed, distressed, or annoyed if my true reasons for signaling this way were to be revealed to others or made public? What is it that I might need to learn?

The Tendency to Tell Rather Than Show

Get into the habit of demonstrating to the client what the social signaling deficit looks or sounds like rather than just talking about it. As noted earlier, this is an essential component of RO DBT therapy and a skill that most therapists need to learn and practice. It allows the client the opportunity to be on the receiving end of her social signal, rather than just talking about it, and then to decide for herself whether this is how she wants to behave. It can be a source of great fun and laughter, and it can be done with almost any type of social signal, from an eye roll to a scowl to a whisper or a long-winded rambling reply to a question that is never actually answered. It is essential that therapists let go of being overly concerned about how a client might react to a demonstration, mainly because the entire point of the demonstration is to provide feedback to the client. Recall that in RO DBT, whenever we feel invalidated we have an opportunity to practice self-enquiry by asking ourselves *What is it that I might need to learn?* rather than automatically expecting the world to validate us by changing. Without a robust demonstration of the maladaptive social signal, the therapist is left having to persuade the client that a social signal is a problem (through appeals to logic, for example, or by way of verbal descriptions or anecdotes). Not only is this a lot of work, it is rarely (if ever) as powerful as the visceral impact of a good demonstration.

The Desire for a Quick Fix

Block automatic desires on the part of the client (and yourself) to quickly fix problems. Broadly speaking, most OC clients are compulsive fixers, and it is easy for them to fall into the trap of trying to fix their compulsive overcontrol once they have recognized it as a problem. The therapist should feel free to slow the pace of the targeting process (but not too much) when a client appears to compulsively rush recovery. For example, one OC client arrived at her fifth session with a written list of eighteen treatment targets she had decided should be immediately addressed. The therapist validated the client's commitment to treatment (the list of targets) while asking whether the client's strong motivation to fix herself might actually represent more of the same (OC behavior in disguise). This smuggles the idea that most problems in life do not require immediate solutions—and, ideally, the pacing of the treatment targeting process throughout treatment reflects this.

Step-by-Step Formal Treatment Targeting with OC Social Signaling Themes

Step 1: Introduce the Theme for the Session

- At the start of the session, during agenda setting, introduce the OC theme you want to work on (for example, aloof and distant relationships), but remember to work on only one theme per week.

- If necessary, briefly remind the client of the purpose of OC themes in general; for example, "OC themes are guides to help us improve treatment targeting." Long explanations or detailed discussions about the themes are unnecessary and can often prove unhelpful.

- Remind the client about the importance of identifying social signaling treatment targets: "Problems of overcontrol are posited to most often pertain to feeling like an outsider, emotionally estranged from others, and lonely. How we socially signal strongly impacts social connectedness. Thus, rather than prioritize how you feel inside, or what you might be thinking, RO DBT prioritizes how you communicate your inner experience to others because how we socially signal impacts not only how we feel about ourselves but how others feel about us."

Step 2: Ask What Words Come to Mind in Connection with a Particular OC Theme

This helps build a shared language between you and the client and gives you a sense of how the client thinks about the concept itself. It also personalizes the targets (and the treatment) for the client. Make a note of the client's words as an aide-mémoire for future dialogues. However, it is important to not belabor this step; you only need a few words before moving on to the next step.

Step 3: Link the OC Theme to Valued Goals

Ask, for example, "How does the theme of envy and bitterness apply to your life, and with whom? What valued goals does it prevent you from achieving or living by?"

Step 4: Ask the Client How You Would Recognize His or Her OC-Themed Behavior

You might say, for example, "If I were a fly on the wall, how would I know you were behaving in an aloof and distant manner?" This question functions to help both the client and the therapist identify specifically what the maladaptive social signal looks like to an outside observer. Thus therapists should encourage their clients to imagine what others might see when they do this behavior—that is, to see it as would a fly on a wall watching them when the problem behavior emerges. Since the fly cannot read a client's mind, the metaphor helps both the therapist and the client remain focused on finding a social signaling target linked to the theme and then agree on the words that best describe it (that is, a label for the client's diary card). A fly would be unable to see thoughts or internal emotions.

Verify that the social signal identified is both relevant (as when it prevents the client from achieving her valued goals) and pervasive (as when it is habitual, frequent, or occurs across contexts). Thus a social signal that is highly predictable or infrequent (for example, it occurs only on Sundays at 9 a.m.) or that occurs with only one person (for example, a particular neighbor), though perhaps still being a problem, may not be relevant or pervasive enough to warrant targeting. Often the best way to accomplish this is to simply ask the client to "prove" why the social signal is really maladaptive—for example, by saying, "Yeah, but what's wrong with telling your husband he doesn't know how to stack the dishwasher properly? Maybe he doesn't" or "But maybe it's honest to yawn when you find your husband boring—what's wrong with that?" The major point is to not automatically assume that client self-reports of social signaling targets are necessarily valid or relevant. This approach has the added advantage of making the target more precise while simultaneously assessing the client's actual commitment to change (because the client must convince the therapist that the maladaptive social signal is a problem, not the other way around). Also—again—*demonstrate* to the client what the social signaling deficit looks or sounds like; don't just talk about it.

Step 5: Agree on a Behavioral Label That Describes the Social Signal

For example, the label "artificial concern" might be used for an insincere expression of sympathy or caring (behavior linked to the OC theme of inhibited emotional expression). The label "apparent engagement" might be used for answering a question with another question (behavior linked to the OC theme of aloof and distant relationships). The label "false humility" might be used for the client's criticizing of herself before others can (behavior linked to the OC theme of envy and bitterness). Or the label "walking away" might be used for her leaving abruptly when conflict occurs (behavior linked to the OC theme of aloof and distant relationships).

Step 6: Identify Thoughts and Emotions Linked to the Social Signaling Target

Most often this translates to identifying one thought and one emotion associated with the social signaling target that had just been identified. For example, one client, after agreeing to target a social signal collaboratively labeled "walking away" (abruptly ending conversations the client disliked by walking away, abandoning the relationship, or hanging up if talking over the telephone, all behaviors linked to the OC theme of aloof and distant relationships), was asked about what types of thoughts she noticed just before she walked away. The client reported that she was often thinking *I don't need this. Don't they realize how much I have done to help them, without ever asking for anything in return?* This behavior was labeled "being a martyr" (the client, by the way, both hated and loved this target). The client and the therapist then identified and labeled an emotion (resentment) that was linked to both walking away and being a martyr—and decided to track all three (that is, walking away, being a martyr, and resentment) at least initially and then refine or modify each over time as needed.

Step 7: Monitor New Targets and Block the Urge to Fix Deficits

Monitor new targets using the RO DBT diary card, and block automatic urges to fix the social signaling deficit immediately. Encourage the client to see himself as a scientist or independent observer who has been trained to observe the extent of a potential problem before attempting to change it. Thus, at least initially, any newly identified social signaling target should simply be monitored the first week after it has been identified (for frequency and intensity), along with the covariates (thoughts and emotions) associated with it, before trying to do anything about it. This also helps smuggle the idea that not every problem in life needs to be fixed immediately and helps ensure that the treatment target actually matters (is relevant). Thus, if after monitoring a newly identified social signal for a week and discovering that it never occurred once during the preceding week, rather than just automatically continuing to monitor the target, the therapist and the client might decide to explore how it suddenly became such a rare event, or to make adjustments in how the target is defined or monitored. As noted earlier, low-frequency and nonpervasive social signals, although perhaps disruptive when they do occur, may be less relevant to obtain a life worth sharing. The only exception to this is life-threatening behaviors; because of the serious consequences linked to these behaviors, they remain important to monitor (especially if a client has a history of suicidal behavior or self-injury), regardless of frequency, severity, or pervasiveness.

Step 8: Rank-Order Themes and Targets

OC themes and individualized targets should be rank-ordered (flexibly). Since there are five broad OC themes, therapists can expect that it will take up to five sessions to discuss all five themes and identify individualized targets for each theme. Theoretically (and numerically), this could result in the generation of fifteen or more individualized targets by the end of the ninth session for the highly diligent therapist and equally diligent OC client. So chill out! The aim is to have fun exploring social signaling, not to rigidly adhere to an arbitrary protocol. The good news is that secondary targets (emotions and thoughts) linked to primary social signaling targets almost always overlap—for example, anger might be the emotion related to the social signaling target known as "the silent treatment" as well as to the social signaling target labeled "walking away"—and in this way the number of items monitored on a diary card is naturally reduced. In addition, all targets do not have to be monitored immediately or at the same time. Instead, therapists should collaboratively decide with their clients which targets they believe most important to change first and then focus on them rather than trying to fix everything all at once (that is, being rigid about how they apply a protocol designed to change maladaptive rigidity). Quality is more important than quantity, and the best tests of the quality of treatment targeting are the client's improvement and change that is sustainable.

OC Theme-Based Targeting: A Clinical Example

In the following transcript of a session, a therapist uses the procedure just described and the client's self-report of perfectionism to individualize targets around the OC theme of rigid behavior:

Therapist: Okay, as we discussed earlier, one of my agenda items for today's session was to introduce a new OC theme, known as "rigid and rule-governed behavior," with the aim of identifying a new treatment target. Are you ready to move on to this?

(Client nods affirmation.)

Therapist: Okay. So when I say the words "rigid and rule-governed," what comes to mind? What words or images appear?

Client: The first thing that came into my mind was an image of myself as a little girl, getting furious at my sister when she rearranged my collection of china horses. I have always preferred structure and order. Other things that came to mind were the words "perfectionism" and "obsessive planning" as well as "being correct."

Therapist: So one of the things you are saying is that you noticed desires for order and structure from a young age, and words like "perfectionism," "planning," and "being correct."

(Client nods affirmation.)

Therapist: How do you think the theme of rigid and rule-governed behavior manifests in your life now? What valued goals does it prevent you from achieving or living by?

Client: Hmmm…I don't really know for sure. My sis always says I am a stickler for details, and it does seem to annoy her. *(Pauses.)* I know that I'm definitely considered a control freak at work, but I see this as a virtue.

Therapist: Okay, so something about being a control freak, controlling things, being highly organized, perhaps structured—something about this— and you think this type of rigid behavior may be upsetting to others? *(Links rigidity to negative social consequences.)*

Client: Not upsetting. They just don't seem to like it.

Therapist: So if I were a fly on the wall, watching you, what would I see you doing that other people would find annoying or unwelcome? How would our fly on the wall know you were doing something that they did not like? What actions would the fly see you do? *(Helps client refine the target.)*

Client: I don't know—maybe they're jealous. *(Smiles slightly, pauses, looks at therapist.)* I guess it is annoying to have someone telling you what to do. It is my job, but not really for my sister. I just think most people don't know how to keep things organized.

Therapist: So the fly on the wall would notice you telling others what to do or how to organize something? And I am aware of imagining that the telling is not about something the other person has asked you to help them out with or advise them about. Is that correct? *(Keeps focus on topic of perfectionism and rigid behavior by ignoring comment about jealousy; notes client's use of the word "jealous" for later discussions about the OC theme of envy and bitterness; suggests instead that telling others what to do is likely to be problematic to others because they have not requested client's help or advice.)*

Client: Yeah, that's it.

Therapist: So maybe we could start to monitor how often you tell others what to do or try to organize things. Shall we label this behavior of telling others what to do and use the diary card to see how often it shows up over the next couple of weeks?

(Client nods in agreement.)

Therapist: (*Smiles*) This should help us know better whether this behavior of telling others what to do is actually preventing you from reaching important goals like the one you mentioned about improving relationships. For example, you are aware of imagining that people find this annoying. What evidence do you have for this? (*Uses client's own words to describe the target to be monitored and asks for clarification regarding how client knows others are annoyed, to help verify the target's importance and its consequences.*)

Client: Hmmm…that's a good question. (*Pauses.*) My sis just tells me. She'll say things like "I already know what to do" or "All right, already—I see your point! Stop trying to fix me!" Things like that. (*Pauses.*) But at work it's more subtle. Sometimes people just walk away. They don't respond to my email even after I've sent it four times! It's really frustrating because my job is to make sure that the policy and procedures for quality control are followed. People just don't understand the importance of this.

Therapist: It sounds like you feel you're not appreciated for your work.

(*Client nods in agreement.*)

Therapist: Maybe we can look at how being appreciated is linked to all of this. When you don't feel appreciated, what emotion do you think you are experiencing? (*Looks for non–social signaling behaviors and targets linked to the overt problem behavior of telling others what to do.*)

Client: Hmmm…not sure. I feel frustrated and annoyed that I'm the one that always has to make sure everything works out. Yeah, now that you say it, I am definitely not appreciated!

Therapist: Okay, good. How about we just start out with these three behaviors? One is overtly telling others what to do. Another involves thoughts of not being appreciated and always needing to be responsible, or something along those lines. And the third is an emotion of anger or annoyance. Really, this should be interesting. The idea is for us start having you rate these three behaviors over the next couple of weeks, and then, when we find a day when you had high-intensity bossing or telling others what to do, we can do some analysis around telling others what to do and see if we can make sense of it, and change things if needed. Would you be willing to do this? (*Highlights two non–social signaling behaviors and targets that are linked to telling others what to do—one related to cognition, the other to emotion—and assesses client's willingness to target these behaviors in treatment.*)

Client: Yeah, that sounds good. I do feel it's my job to make things right, but I can be very bossy—not one of my most redeeming qualities. (*Smiles slightly.*)

255

Therapist: Okay, how about this? What if we put on the diary card, under social signaling behaviors, the behavior of telling others what to do, rated on a scale of 0 to 5, with 0 meaning that it didn't happen at all that day. Let's say a 3 means that you were telling people what to do fairly often that day, and a 5 means that you were really a control freak that day. *(Pauses.)*

(Client nods in agreement.)

Therapist: *(Shows client diary card)* Then, under non–social signaling or private behaviors and targets, we monitor anger or annoyance and rumination about not being appreciated, labeled something like "People are ungrateful," and see if our hypothesis that high-frequency brooding or thinking about how ungrateful people are, high annoyance or anger, and high bossiness (telling others what to do) occur on the same day and are linked to a particular interaction on that day. How does this sound to you? *(Uses words that are the same or similar to how client described her experiences when labeling the three targets linked to the OC-themed rigid behaviors; reviews how the targets will be rated, shows client where on the diary card they will be rated, and explains what the ratings might accomplish.)*

The therapist purposefully did not generate solution analyses for the targets and instead encouraged the client to practice enjoying self-enquiry by first observing rather than fixing a potential problem. Moreover, the therapist purposely did not pursue other potential targets (for example, jealousy and envy) unrelated to the goal of exploring the OC theme of rigid behavior. Instead, the therapist noted these privately, as possible targets that could be discussed in future sessions.

After reviewing all the OC themes and obtaining targets for each, the therapist and the client decided which targets were most problematic in preventing the client from achieving her valued goals. In this case, the client's feelings of ostracism, isolation, and loneliness were considered core factors underlying her refractory depression. The therapist and the client agreed that the most important target was related to the OC theme of aloof and distant relationships, with two social signaling targets—"walking away" from conflict and "silence around others," or going quiet when annoyed. Since suicidal behaviors were not present, the therapist and the client agreed that their first priority would be to monitor and conduct chain and solution analyses around these two social signaling targets (see "OC Behavioral Chain and Solution Analyses: Broad Principles" and "Conducting a Chain Analysis, Step-by-Step," chapter 10).

The theme of rigid and rule-governed behavior was ranked a very close second for this client because it was clearly associated with feelings of isolation. The social signaling target chosen for monitoring was "bossiness" (telling other people what to do), and it was linked to feelings of resentment and anger as well as to thoughts about being unappreciated. The third and fourth themes—inhibited emotional expression, and envy and bitterness—were considered equivalent in importance for this client, and both were linked to the client's primary OC theme of aloof and distant relationships. Individualized targets for these themes were pretending, the "I am fine" phenomenon, secret pride, and urges for revenge.

The final OC theme for this particular client—overly cautious behavior and hypervigilance—was evaluated as less relevant; nevertheless, this theme was targeted, albeit indirectly, via skills that emphasized activation of the client's social safety system (PNS-VVC) during social interactions, which helped her enter social situations with a less guarded or wary manner.

Monitoring Treatment Targets with Diary Cards

Diary cards are designed as a means for the client to record the presence, frequency, and intensity of targeted behaviors on a daily basis over the course of one week. The therapeutic rationale for a daily diary card should be explained to the client, usually during the fourth session (see "Introducing the RO DBT Diary Card," chapter 5). The diary card is reviewed each week at the beginning of the individual therapy session (including use of skills), and a new card is provided to the client (with any new targets or modifications in targets) at the end of each session. When introducing diary cards, it is important to emphasize that the information monitored on them will represent a core means for the therapist to find out about what has happened during the past week with a client, without the client's having to say a word (okay, maybe a *few* words).

However, when first learning RO DBT, many therapists wrongly assume that flexibility means complete lack of structure, or that having an easy manner means never having an opinion. This was never intended, nor do I consider it remotely close to competent RO DBT. Despite often being experts at hiding their suffering, the lives of OC clients are often miserable, even though it might not always be apparent. Like all of us, OC clients often need to be pushed to make major lifestyle changes. Changing old habits is hard, whereas staying the same often feels easier and safer. My point is this: effective therapy with an OC client requires the therapist to be highly committed, highly flexible, and highly structured in order to genuinely make a difference, and diary cards are an important structural component of this process.

Diary Cards: Three Things to Remember

1. Diary Cards Are Essential

Diary cards are essential, despite often being frustrating to complete. Diary cards are not the treatment, but they are one of the core components that enable the treatment to be delivered effectively. They mitigate storytelling and long explanations about events that happened during the past week, which otherwise must be heard (when there is no diary card) in order for the therapist to know how to structure the session and define the problematic behavior that will be the focus of the current session's behavioral chain analysis. Thus diary cards save valuable session time for work on solving problems, and research shows that they improve the accuracy of the information obtained. Indeed, if all is going to plan, only about six minutes are allocated for in-session review of a diary card. The major point is that without a diary card, therapy becomes a bit like finding a needle in a haystack when it comes to identifying the most maladaptive and relevant social signaling deficit that has occurred during the client's preceding week.

2. Noncompletion of a Diary Card Is a Powerful Social Signal

Most OC clients are treatment-compliant to a fault; they are likely to feel obligated and duty bound to thoroughly complete the diary card as requested and can sometimes provide so much detail that a therapist is hard pressed to complete the review of the diary card in the six minutes allocated. Thus an OC client who does not complete the diary card is sending a powerful social signal of nonengagement to the therapist. Rather than automatically assuming that the client should be more committed, should try harder, or should do better, the RO DBT therapist sees noncompletion of a diary card as indicating an alliance rupture.[55] Thus therapists who are struggling with obtaining diary cards, or who find themselves demoralized about getting them completed, should use this as an opportunity for self-enquiry and practice outing themselves to fellow RO practitioners, if possible (for example, the RO consultation team). Therapists should practice self-enquiry to determine how they might be contributing to the problem and then engage the protocol for repairing an alliance rupture, to address any potential rifts or stimulate self-enquiry on the client's part. The following questions can often facilitate this:

- What is it that might be leading me to desire to abandon diary cards? Is it possible that I am burned out or demoralized? If yes or maybe, have I shared this with anyone? What is it that I might need to learn?

- How committed am I to the concept or idea of diary cards in general? Is there a chance I was never fully committed to using them in the first place? If yes or possibly, what might this tell me?

- To what extent do I believe it important to follow protocols or a manualized treatment? What might this tell me about how I am implementing diary cards?

- Is it possible that my client is shaping my behavior? What is it that I might need to learn?

- In my professional practice, do I normally find it difficult to obtain diary cards or similar information from my clients? If no or rarely, then what might this tell me about my current client? If yes or frequently, then what might this tell me about myself?

- How much energy do I have in my body when I ask these questions? What might this tell me about my personal commitment to using diary cards? About myself? About my professional practice?

Thus, broadly speaking, noncompletion of diary cards by an OC client is considered evidence of an alliance rupture, thereby triggering the protocol for repairing an alliance rupture. It is a powerful social signal, especially when the client has agreed to complete them in prior sessions and, perhaps, even more so when the client has already been completing them but then suddenly stops or begins to be less thorough in how they are completed. Often noncompletion means lack of relevancy (for example, the client can't see how monitoring targets will help him). When the problem is unable to be repaired quickly, or when the client continues to have problems with diary cards (for example, he keeps forgetting to bring them to session), despite assurances by the client that there will no longer be difficulties, the therapist can provide a copy of the following questions to facilitate self-enquiry on the client's part (the client should also be advised to note any observations in his self-enquiry journal):

- What am I trying to communicate or socially signal to my therapist (or other people) by not completing my diary card? If I have completed diary cards before, what's changed? Have I told my therapist about this? What is preventing me from doing so? Is there something here for me to learn?

- To what extent am I proud of having not completed my diary card? Would I encourage another person to behave similarly? What might this tell me about my values? What does it tell me about my commitment to therapy or getting better?

- Do I find myself wanting to automatically explain, defend, or discount any questions about how I am completing my diary card (or not completing it)? If yes or maybe, then what might this mean?

- To what extent do I feel that I know the rationale behind using diary cards? If I am uncertain or disagree with the rationale, have I let my therapist know this? What might this tell me?

- Do I find myself disliking this self-enquiry practice about diary cards? What might this tell me about my commitment to therapy? About myself?

- Do I believe diary cards are relevant to my treatment? Have I let my therapist know about this? If not, what might this say about my commitment to treatment?

- Do I feel that the treatment targets that are being monitored on my diary card are important? If not or possibly not, have I told my therapist about this? If I have not told my therapist about my concerns, then what is preventing me from doing so?

- Am I using this experience as another opportunity to beat up on myself or to prove to myself or others that I am worthless or unworthy? What is it that I might need to learn?

- Is there any part of me that feels it is unfair for me to be expected to complete a diary card? What does this tell me about my willingness to make important changes?

- Do I believe—because of my exceptional suffering, traumatic history, or prior sacrifices—that it is unfair for me to be asked to complete a diary card? To what extent do I expect my therapist to treat me as special or different from other clients? What might this tell me? What is it that I need to learn?

- To what extent do I believe that others should know, without my having to tell them, what I am thinking, wanting, or expecting to happen, thus making diary cards unnecessary?

- Is there any part of me that is secretly hoping that the treatment will fail? Am I purposefully choosing to not complete diary cards in order to punish my therapist, myself, or someone else?

- Do I simply not believe in diary cards, no matter what my therapist says to try to convince me otherwise? What might this tell me about my commitment to therapy or, more broadly, my world view?

- Am I holding on to a grudge or resentment about my therapist or the treatment itself? If yes or maybe, is this interfering with my completion of diary cards? What is it that I might need to learn?

3. What Matters Is Social Signaling

Finally, it doesn't matter so much what the diary card actually looks like—handwritten, computerized, or smartphone text (with an app on the side). What matters most when treating OC clients is finding accurate means to record the presence of social signaling deficits on a daily basis; everything else is simply gravy. Thus maladaptive social signaling matters, since this is what is hypothesized to be keeping the client out of the tribe. Three or four social signaling targets, with nothing else filled out on the rest of the card, will be preferable by far to no card whatsoever or a phony card (one completed just prior to session in order to please the therapist).

The RO DBT Diary Card: Structural Features

The diary card templates shown in figure 9.1 and figure 9.2 can be photocopied. The therapist can modify the templates as necessary to suit the specific needs of a particular client or clinical population (for example, adolescents diagnosed with anorexia nervosa).

Many clients find that placing the diary card next to their beds functions as an aide-mémoire to complete the card for the day's events before falling asleep. Here are the two most common methods of rating:

1. Simple presence or absence of a particular behavior, usually signified by writing Y (yes) or N (no) in the relevant column, to indicate that on a particular day the behavior either did or did not occur

2. A dimensional rating of intensity that includes an overall assessment of frequency and comparison with other times the behavior occurred

The dimensional scale ranges from 0 to 5:

0 = the behavior was not present

1 = the behavior was slightly present (low frequency and low intensity)

2 = the behavior was definitely present, but at a low level

3 = the behavior was moderately present

4 = the behavior was severely or intensely present (frequency and/or intensity high)

5 = the behavior was the most intense ever experienced by the client and at extremely high frequency (frequency and intensity abnormally extreme or severe)

In general, changes in dimensional ratings that are 3 or more points higher than what is normally reported by a particular client should be highlighted and analyzed. This means that the therapist must be adept at orienting the client on how to use the dimensional rating scale accurately. For instance, it would be extremely rare for a client to consistently report a 5 for a particular behavior every single day of the week. Doing so suggests that the client is unable to notice differences in intensity and frequency or is attempting to signal something important to the therapist about the behavior (for example, the client may feel hopeless that she will ever fully change this behavior, or she may wish the therapist to pay more attention to this behavior). When this occurs, the therapist must be careful not to reinforce maladaptive responses that may function to keep the client stuck (for example, the client's belief that change is impossible). Most human behavior, emotions, and mood states vary over time (during sleep, for example, fear and depression dissipate). Furthermore, most humans can change how they behave, even under high duress (a depressed client can still be active enough to save a child from a burning building).

Radically Open RO DBT Diary Card	Initials/Name ID #	Major OC theme this week	**Filled out in session: Y/N** **Started Card:** Date ___/___/___	How often did you fill out this side? ____ Daily ____ 2–3x ____ 4–6x ____ Once

Cirlce Start Day Day of Week	Urge to Committ Suicide	Private Behaviors: Thoughts, Sensations, Emotions										Medications: Med as Prescribed	Medications: Other Drugs or Alcohol	Social Signaling or Other Overt Behaviors									
	0–5											Y/N	What										
MON																							
TUES																							
WED																							
THU																							
FRI																							
SAT																							
SUN																							

Notes/comments/chain analysis:	Valued goals sought this week:	New self-enquiry questions:

Figure 9.1. Front of Diary Card (Blank), Showing Treatment Targets

Radical Openness Skills (circle each day of the week you practed a particular skill)	Hand-out or Work-sheet	Week-day	Week-day	Week-day	Week-day	Week-day	Week-end	Week-end
Flexible Mind DEFinitely: Three Steps for Radically Open Living	1.B	Mon	Tue	Wed	Thu	Fri	Sat	Sun
The Big Three + 1: Activating Social Safety	3.A	Mon	Tue	Wed	Thu	Fri	Sat	Sun
Practiced Loving Kindness Meditation: Maximizing Social Safety	4.1	Mon	Tue	Wed	Thu	Fri	Sat	Sun
Flexible Mind VARIEs: Engaging in Novel Behavior	5.1	Mon	Tue	Wed	Thu	Fri	Sat	Sun
Flexible Mind SAGE Skills: Dealing with Shame, Embarrassment, and Feeling Rejected or Excluded	8.A	Mon	Tue	Wed	Thu	Fri	Sat	Sun
Flexible Mind Is DEEP: Using Values to Guide Social Signaling	10.2	Mon	Tue	Wed	Thu	Fri	Sat	Sun
Practiced Being Kind to Fixed Mind	11.2	Mon	Tue	Wed	Thu	Fri	Sat	Sun
Practiced Learning from Fatalistic Mind	11.3	Mon	Tue	Wed	Thu	Fri	Sat	Sun
Practiced Going Opposite to Fatalistic Mind	11.B	Mon	Tue	Wed	Thu	Fri	Sat	Sun
Practiced the Awareness Continuum	12.1	Mon	Tue	Wed	Thu	Fri	Sat	Sun
Mindfulness "What" Skills: Observe Openly	12.2	Mon	Tue	Wed	Thu	Fri	Sat	Sun
Mindfulness "What" Skills: Describe with Integrity	12.2	Mon	Tue	Wed	Thu	Fri	Sat	Sun
Mindfulness "What" Skills: Participate Without Planning	12.2	Mon	Tue	Wed	Thu	Fri	Sat	Sun
Mindfulness "How" Skill: With Self-Enquiry	13.1	Mon	Tue	Wed	Thu	Fri	Sat	Sun
Mindfulness "How" Skill: With Awareness of Harsh Judgments	14.1	Mon	Tue	Wed	Thu	Fri	Sat	Sun
Mindfulness "How" Skill: With One-Mindful Awareness	14.1	Mon	Tue	Wed	Thu	Fri	Sat	Sun
Mindfulness "How" Skill: Effectively and with Humility	14.1	Mon	Tue	Wed	Thu	Fri	Sat	Sun
Practiced Identifying "Pushback" and "Don't Hurt Me" Responses	16.1	Mon	Tue	Wed	Thu	Fri	Sat	Sun
Flexible Mind REVEALs: Responding with Interpersonal Integrity	16.2	Mon	Tue	Wed	Thu	Fri	Sat	Sun
Flexible Mind ROCKs ON: Enhancing Interpersonal Kindness	17.1	Mon	Tue	Wed	Thu	Fri	Sat	Sun
Practiced Kindness First and Foremost	17.B	Mon	Tue	Wed	Thu	Fri	Sat	Sun
Flexible Mind PROVEs: Being Assertive with an Open Mind	18.A	Mon	Tue	Wed	Thu	Fri	Sat	Sun
Flexible Mind Validated: Signaling Social Situation	19.A	Mon	Tue	Wed	Thu	Fri	Sat	Sun
Flexible Mind ALLOWs: Enhancing Social Connectedness	21.1	Mon	Tue	Wed	Thu	Fri	Sat	Sun
Practiced MATCH + 1: Establishing Intimate Relationships	21.3	Mon	Tue	Wed	Thu	Fri	Sat	Sun
Flexible Mind ADOPTs: Being Open to Feedback	22.1	Mon	Tue	Wed	Thu	Fri	Sat	Sun
Flexible Mind DARES (to Let Go): Managing Unhelpful Envy	27.A	Mon	Tue	Wed	Thu	Fri	Sat	Sun
Flexible Mind Is LIGHT: Changing Bitterness	28.A	Mon	Tue	Wed	Thu	Fri	Sat	Sun
Flexible Mind Has HEART: Learning How to Forgive	29.A	Mon	Tue	Wed	Thu	Fri	Sat	Sun

Figure 9.2. Back of Diary Card (Blank), Showing Client's Use of RO Skills

Preferably, cards are double-sided, with targets on one side and skills usage on the other. The day of the week a particular RO skill was used should be circled, thereby providing both the client and the therapist a sense of what skills the client is using the most, which ones she still needs to learn (and, if deemed essential for a particular client, which ones should be taught informally in individual therapy), and the client's overall commitment to skills usage. As can be seen in the diary card template, in the far left-hand column of the card (going down) are listed the days of the week, with each day having a corresponding row. Two broad sections of blank columns can be seen, one for recording secondary non–social signaling behaviors and targets (thoughts, sensations, emotions) and the other for recording primary social signaling behaviors or other overt behaviors. The columns are left blank so that the therapist and the client can individualize what is targeted, with the exception of the three columns that address the client's urges to commit suicide, the client's compliance with taking prescribed medications, and the client's use of nonprescription drugs and alcohol. However, all of this can be modified according to the needs of the client (or the program). Thus, for example, a program that targets eating disorders may wish to add several additional prelabeled columns for high-risk behaviors related to eating disorders. The therapist can keep a copy of each weekly diary card as part of the client's record and as a means of monitoring progress.

A Brief Overview of the RO DBT Diary Card Template

As mentioned earlier, the RO DBT diary card should be considered a working example or template; that is, it can be used as is or modified as needed. The general features of the card are as follows:

- Initials or ID number: Instead of the client's name, the client's initials can be used for confidentiality. The client may have an ID number assigned if he or she is part of a research study.

- Indication of whether the card was filled out during the session: If the client filled the card out during the session, circle Y. Otherwise, circle N.

- Indication of how often the card was filled out during the preceding week: The client should record how often he filled out the diary card during the past week (for example, every day, two to three times, four to six times, or just once).

- Starting date: The client should record the date that corresponds to the start of the week during which the card was completed.

- Major OC theme for the week: The client should record the major OC social signaling theme he is primarily focused on for the week.

- Urges to commit suicide (rated from 0 to 5): For any particular day, the client should rate urges to commit suicide, with the rating reflecting both the frequency of suicidal thoughts and the intensity of suicidal urges. Blank columns can be individualized to include tracking of other suicidal behaviors that may be relevant to different clients (for example, urges to self-harm, overt actions of self-harm, suicidal ideation, and so forth).

- Client's compliance with prescribed medication instructions: This portion of the diary card is relevant to any current prescribed medications that a client is taking and that may be important to monitor (for example, antidepressants). The client should write Y (yes) or N (no) to indicate whether medications were taken as prescribed.

- Client's use of nonprescription drugs or alcohol: For alcohol, clients should specify the type of drink (beer, cocktails or other mixed drinks, whiskey, wine, and so forth) and the amount (number of glasses). For illicit drugs, the client should specify the type of drug used (marijuana, heroin, speed, cocaine, and so forth). In general, most OC clients do not abuse illicit drugs, because they tend to be rule-governed and are motivated to appear proper and socially desirable.

- Client's notes, comments, and chain analysis: This section is designed to allow clients a place to record any additional comments or observations that might be relevant.

- Valued goals sought during the week: This optional section is designed to help remind clients to focus on seeking valued goals. Therapists should feel free to modify this section or even eliminate it entirely if it is discovered not to be particularly useful.

- New self-enquiry questions: This is a very important section on the diary card. It helps the client remember to practice self-enquiry and simultaneously provides a structured means for the client to practice outing herself. When this section is left blank, the therapist should consider the client's lack of completion to be a social signal that may reflect the presence of an alliance rupture or confusion about self-enquiry. Regardless, when this section is left blank, the therapist should not ignore it.

Protocol for In-Session RO DBT Diary Card Review

In the following transcript of a client's twelfth session, a therapist reviews the diary card of an OC client with a history of suicidal ideation and chronic depression; the client's valued goals are to have improved relationships with her family (her sister and her daughter), to find a healthy romantic relationship, and to learn how to relax more and work less. The client and the therapist had previously identified several social signaling targets: the silent treatment (not talking to someone in order to punish him, but without admitting that this is what is being done), pretending (the client saying that she is feeling fine when she is not), walking away (abandoning a conversation without warning because it is getting too uncomfortable), and emotional leakage. They had also identified two habitual thoughts: *People are users* and *Why do I have to do everything?* The emotions and thoughts represent non–social signaling behavioral targets.

Therapist:	*(Looks at card)* Okay, let's take a look at the rest of the card. *(Pauses.)* Hmmm…no suicidal thoughts or urges. Well done! *(Smiles warmly, reinforcing lack of life-threatening behavior.)* Hmmm…let's see. *(Pauses; reads aloud the scored numbers reporting the intensity of the behavior that was recorded.)* On Tuesday, you rated anger as high—it was a 4. And envy/resentment was even higher—it was a 5. Plus, you rated blaming others high, too—it was a 5. But on Wednesday you had some high shame—this was a 4. When you look back on it, which day last week do you think was your worst—your most problematic? *(Works to identify which day and specific behavior to discuss in more detail, and to conduct a chain analysis.)*
Client:	On Tuesday, my sister and her husband came over for a visit. Sometimes I just think they like to make me feel bad—they always act like they're so happy.
Therapist:	Hmmm…yeah, we have noticed this type of thinking before, especially when it comes to your sister and her husband. I see, too, that on Tuesday you checked off the silent treatment and walking away. Well done on noticing all these behaviors! *(Reinforces self-enquiry, smiles briefly, pauses.)* What happened that made Tuesday so difficult?
Client:	Well, I decided that I would work on improving my relationship with my sister by asking her and her husband over for dinner. I spent all day making her favorite foods. It was maddening. All her sycophantic husband could do was nod and agree with everything she said. She didn't once comment on the food. Instead, all she talked about was how great her new job was. It was just too much, so I decided to leave.
Therapist:	Even though it was your house? *(Clarifies context.)*
Client:	I just couldn't stand to be there any longer. I pretended that I wanted to take a walk. But I was so worked up, I left without a coat. Even though I was freezing, I just kept saying to myself, *I'll be damned if I go back.*
Therapist:	Hmmm…wow, that seems like a really difficult time. And a perfect opportunity for us to use our newly developed chain analysis skills. *(Pauses momentarily.)* Should we target walking away as the problem behavior?

Client: Yeah, I guess so. I think I am still down on myself about what happened.

Therapist: Hmmm…yeah, maybe feeling down is the natural consequence of things like this, especially since one of your valued goals is to reconnect with your sister. *(Links targeted problem behaviors with valued goals.)* Perhaps our chain analysis can help make sense of this. *(Pauses momentarily.)* Before we go there, let's take a quick look at the rest of the card.

The therapist then quickly looked over the remainder of the card to ensure that there were no other major problems to address, and to gain a sense of how well the client had been using RO skills (diary card reviews should be done quickly—within five to seven minutes). Once this was completed, the agenda was set for the session, and a chain analysis was begun to examine the social signaling behavioral problem of walking away as well as how it was linked to the non–social signaling targets of envy and resentment and blaming others, and to examine how these functioned as obstacles to the client's achieving her goal of an improved relationship with her sister.

Valued Goals, Themes, and Targets

Together, table 9.4, table 9.5, and table 9.6 provide an overview of how valued goals, themes, and targets can be integrated in order to formulate a case conceptualization. The client was a forty-five-year-old female with a twenty-five-year history of chronic depression and comorbid obsessive-compulsive personality disorder. She was married (to an engineer), had no children, and was not working. With respect to the themes targeted for this client, the highest priority was her aloof, distant relationships with others; additional major themes were envy and bitterness, inhibited emotional expression, and rigid, rule-governed behavior. Table 9.4 shows the client's values and goals; table 9.5 and table 9.6 show, respectively, her non–social signaling targets and her social signaling behavior, along with the particular feelings, actions, and outcomes to which the targets and the behavior were linked.

Table 9.4. Client's Values and Goals

Client's Values	Client's Goals
Close social and familial bonds	Having closer relationships with her husband and other family members, especially her sister
Self-sufficiency Competence Achievement Productive work	Finding a job or volunteer work that will use her skills and contribute to her family's income
Fairness Kindness Respect and caring for others	Being kinder to others Offering help without expecting anything in return Accepting help from others

Table 9.5. Client's Non–Social Signaling Targets

Non–Social Signaling Target	OC Theme/Behavior
Emotions	
Anger, resentment	Envy, bitterness Aloof, distant relationships
Loneliness	Aloof, distant relationships
Sensation	
Exhaustion	Rigid, rule-governed behavior Aloof, distant relationships Compulsive cleaning, taking care of others
Thoughts	
My little schemer…[a]	Envy, bitterness Fantasies of revenge Resentment Exhaustion Aloof, distant relationships

I'm not being appreciated.	Rule-governed behavior
	Envy, bitterness
	Exhaustion
Why don't they know better?	Aloof, distant relationships

ᵃ This is the label used on the client's diary card in connection with certain behaviors.

Table 9.6. Client's Social Signaling Behavior

Social Signaling Target	OC Theme/Behavior
Giving others the silent treatment	Aloof, distant relationships
	Resentment
	Thoughts of not being appreciated
Walking away (most often from a conflict with her husband)	Aloof, distant relationships
Smiling when angry	Inhibited emotional expression
	Resentment
	Envy, bitterness
	Rigid, rule-governed behavior (for example, following the "always be polite" rule)
Turning down help	Bitterness
	Resentment
	Exhaustion
	Sadness
Overapologizing	Rigid, rule-governed behavior (following the "always be polite" rule)
	Resentment
	Exhaustion
Giving an honest opinion	Improved social connectedness (through increased honesty in sharing opinions rather than masking true feelings)

From Targeting to Intervention: An Overview of Treatment Strategies

After identifying the problem behavior that is preventing the client from achieving valued goals, the next step is to determine what to do about it. Most often, in most psychotherapeutic approaches, this translates into helping the client either change or accept the problem behavior (or some combination of the two). However, RO DBT adds an additional step between the identification of a problem and what someone does about it—that is, a practice of self-enquiry. Thus, before rushing in with change or acceptance strategies, don't forget to encourage your clients to practice self-enquiry. Furthermore, the interventions outlined in the sections that follow are only part of the intervention picture. Therapists should be highly familiar with and, ideally, practicing the RO skills themselves (see the skills training manual) and weaving them into their individual therapy as needed (that is, either formally or informally). Finally, the solutions described in the following sections are intended to augment the skills taught in RO skills training classes, not replace them.

RO DBT Treatment Strategies Addressing OC Themes

Inhibited Emotional Expression

As outlined in other chapters of this book, RO DBT links the communicative functions of emotional expression to core OC deficits in forming and maintaining close social bonds. This theme is divided into two subthemes:

1. Inhibited or disingenuous expression (for example, frozen, blank, flat, or feigned and insincere expressions not genuinely representing inner experience): Pervasive attempts to conceal, disguise, or suppress emotional expressions, or to simulate or pretend to be exhibiting genuine emotional expressions, are core problems for OC. They have a massive negative impact on interpersonal relationships. Therefore, targeting inhibited or disingenuous expressions is considered an essential component of treatment success.

2. Diminished emotional experience and low emotional awareness: OC clients frequently report diminished emotional experience and awareness in situations that most others would report as highly emotionally charged (for example, a funeral, a birthday party, a retirement celebration, or a disagreement with a spouse). Emotional attenuation is diminished or undifferentiated experience of emotions, which may be a consequence of low awareness of emotional sensations, thoughts, or images; little experience in labeling emotions; motivational factors (for example, not labeling or discussing emotions) that may lessen heated conflict or reduce possible social disapproval;

biotemperamental differences in emotional reactivity; and mood states common among OC clients (such as dysphoria, bitterness, anxiety, and irritability) that may make it difficult for OC clients to detect when a new emotion has appeared (that is, in OC there may be a lack of contrast effects; sadness is easier to notice if one was experiencing joy a few minutes earlier). Therapists should remember that emotional attenuation does not mean that clients are unemotional, despite the fact that they may genuinely be unable to detect emotions or to label their experiences as emotions. For example, without fear-based responses, an OC client would have long ago been run over by a bus, since emotions allow quick reactions to relevant stimuli prior to conscious awareness. Therapists should retain an open-minded, inquisitive stance when clients report emotional attenuation, a stance that communicates belief in clients' self-reports and yet challenges them to go deeper.

Treatment Strategies for Subtheme 1: Inhibited or Disingenuous Expression

Provide Didactics on the Benefits of the Free Expression of Emotion

Therapists must repeatedly orient, teach, and model to clients the benefits of free expression of emotion. For example, free expression of emotion can enhance creativity, validate one's inner experience, and signal openness and lack of deception to others. It is the essential glue needed in order to develop genuine intimacy with others. Free expression of emotion enhances intimacy because it signals to others that you trust them (because you are revealing your inner self) and that you are trustworthy because you are not hiding anything. Despite the majority of people considering blushing a highly undesirable response, resulting in attempts to control or suppress it (Nicolaou, Paes, & Wakelin, 2006), research shows that individuals who blush and openly display embarrassment are more likely to be trusted by others and judged more positively, and observers report greater desires to affiliate with them, compared to a nonblushing individual in a similar context (Feinberg et al., 2012; Dijk, Koenig, Ketelaar, & de Jong, 2011). Therapists must also describe how micromimicry works in provoking empathy; that is, one way we understand others' emotions is to experience those emotions ourselves via facial micromimicry. For example, if a person observes someone grimacing in pain, the observer immediately microgrimaces. This sends signals to the observer's brain, and by experiencing the emotion, the observer is now able to understand how the other person is feeling. Explain that consciously masking facial expressions still communicates a message (Adler & Proctor, 2007). An observer is likely to recognize that an emotion is happening within the other person, even if it is denied or masked (J. J. Gross & John, 2003). Explore with clients the pros and cons of expressing emotions, and remind them that expression of emotions is context-dependent (for example, when playing poker, a blank face is useful for placing a bet). Ask for a commitment to work on learning how to express emotions freely.

Change Physiological Arousal Prior to Social Interactions

Therapists should review handout 3.1 ("Changing Social Behavior by Changing Physiology") in the skills training manual.[56] See also the skills training manual, chapter 5, lesson 3, for the "Hunting Dogs, Shields, and Swords" teaching point, and recount "The Story of the Disliked Friend." Explore in a collaborative manner with the OC client how bringing particular mood states or behaviors (hunting dogs, shields, and swords) into social situations can make the situation worse. Review the rationale for changing physiology and getting into one's social safety system prior to social interactions; when we viscerally feel safe, we are able to naturally and freely express our emotions. Therapists should look for opportunities to practice changing physiological arousal in session and assign homework designed to enhance this skill. Lastly, therapists should encourage the use of RO DBT loving kindness meditation (LKM) as a social safety mood induction that naturally facilitates free and open expression.

Break Down Overlearned Inhibitory Barriers

OC individuals have developed inhibitory barriers that make free expression difficult. To break these overlearned barriers down, therapists must be careful not to confirm clients' beliefs that emotions should always be regulated or controlled. Therapists need to model this understanding by throwing themselves wholeheartedly into exercises designed to enhance spontaneity, playfulness, and uninhibited emotional expression; in the skills training manual, chapter 5, lesson 5, see "The Extremely Fun Extreme Expression Workshop" and the mindfulness practice called "The Oompa-Loompa" or, in lesson 30, "The Mimicry Game." Therapists should teach how specific body postures, facial expressions, and gestures influence physiological arousal and communicate important nonverbal information to others; in the skills training manual, chapter 5, lesson 3, see the exercise called "The Big Three + 1." Creativity and playfulness can be important (for example, viewing in-session pictures or video clips showing facial expressions of differing emotions while mimicking them together). The importance of therapist modeling cannot be overemphasized; free expression by a therapist signals that it is a socially appropriate behavior. Homework assignments can further enhance this (for example, practice making different emotional expressions in a mirror or experimenting with big gestures that signal cooperation, such as eyebrow wags combined with expansive, out-turned hand gestures). The overall goal is to shape increased emotional expression via graduated exposure to increasingly challenging but not overwhelming expressive opportunities.

Use Contingencies to Shape the "I Am Fine" Phenomenon

As described earlier, the "I am fine" phenomenon refers to the tendency of many OC clients to verbally underreport or misreport their genuine emotional states. Frequently a functional analysis of the "I am fine" phenomenon reveals that the behavior is negatively reinforced; for example, by denying feeling upset, a client is able to avoid discussion of a potential conflict. Therapists can influence this by changing the consequences or reinforcers. For example, a therapist can inform clients that whenever they say they are fine, it will be taken to mean that they are actually *not* fine. Here, the therapist stops and has the client redescribe vague emotional wording or apparent underreporting by momentarily stopping the in-session conversation, highlighting the language used by the client ("I'm fine"), and then asking the client to describe his experience in more detail, using emotional words. This playfully irreverent strategy, or therapeutic tease, provides a mild aversive contingency for undifferentiated labeling, all the while shaping the client to be more descriptive of what he may actually be experiencing. Frequency counts by the client of how many times "I am fine" is said throughout the day can serve similar functions.

Treatment Strategies for Subtheme 2: Diminished Emotional Experience and Low Emotional Awareness

Use Behavioral Exposure

For some individuals, emotional attenuation, numbing, feelings of detachment, or shutdown may be classically conditioned responses. The neuroregulatory model underlying RO DBT posits that classically conditioned shutdown responses are mediated by activation of the dorsal vagal complex (DVC) in the parasympathetic nervous system (PNS; see chapter 2). The PNS-DVC is triggered by overwhelming threat leading to a physiological state associated with numbing, lowered pain sensitivity, and flattened affect (Porges, 2003a). The therapist must be alert for signs of this type of response in session (for example, the client's facial expression goes blank, or the client finds it difficult to speak, understand, or hear what the therapist is saying). When this appears to be occurring, the therapist should drop her agenda and enquire about the change or shift in the client's behavior. The goal of this exploration is to identify the cue that triggered the shutdown or numbing response and determine the function of the response (that is, whether it is respondent, operant, or some combination of both; see chapter 10 for a discussion of respondent and operant behaviors). Thus the assessment of a shutdown response, at least initially, is the same or similar to how a therapist might assess an alliance rupture—that is, the agenda is dropped, and enquiry regarding the sudden change in behavior occurs. The differences between the two rest in how they are treated.

Classically conditioned shutdown responses are best treated using exposure techniques. Behavioral exposure involves exposure to the cue that elicits the conditioned response while avoidance or escape behaviors are blocked (Foa & Kozak, 1986; Barlow, 1988). Exposure is hypothesized to involve the acquisition of new learning, usually safety signals (T. R. Lynch, Chapman, Rosenthal, Kuo, & Linehan, 2006; Bouton, 2002). However, exposure treatment for emotional attenuation, to our knowledge, has yet to receive much attention in the research literature on behavioral exposure. Traditional exposure therapy targets sympathetic nervous system (SNS) arousal involving automatic fight-or-flight responses; for example, arachnophobia (extreme fear of spiders) involves SNS-mediated fear and avoidance.

For OC clients, the cue or conditioned stimulus for a shutdown response might be as simple as a request for personal information, being asked for an opinion, or being praised. Neutral stimuli of this nature become classically conditioned because requests for information or praise in the past preceded harsh punishments (for example, if the client's answer was incorrect, or if she displayed too much pleasure). A shutdown response is protective because it blocks awareness and sensitivity to incoming stimuli, yet it also prevents new learning from occurring. Thus a client who automatically numbs out or shuts down whenever she is praised or given a compliment will be less likely to learn that compliments are not dangerous.

Exposure therapy for emotional attenuation involves first orienting the client to the principles just described and obtaining commitment prior to proceeding. Secondly, exposure therapy for emotional attenuation involves preventing PNS-DVC-mediated responses by coactivating an antagonistic autonomic nervous system (ANS) response (for example, SNS appetitive arousal). Essentially, therapists should combine exposure principles with antagonistic ANS arousal procedures (for example, repeatedly complimenting a client while she jumps up and down and smiles broadly or waves her arms while eyebrow wagging). To my knowledge, Martin Bohus and his colleagues in Germany are the only research team to have studied this type of exposure intervention. In their procedure to prevent dissociation in BPD clients, a client rides a stationary bicycle while listening to an audiorecording with cues from a past trauma (personal correspondence). For some clients, activation of the sympathetic nervous system may not be necessary because their shutdown response still allows them to attend to incoming stimuli; in this case, simple presentation of the cue (that is, praise) while blocking avoidance will likely be sufficient to achieve similar effects. That said, research on this proposed mechanism of action is sorely needed, and clinicians should take this into account when applying these principles to emotional attenuation.

Monitor Numbness and Body Sensations

Raising awareness of changes in body sensations (or sudden lack of sensation) can help improve emotional awareness (for example, heart rate going up, feeling flushed or hot, sweating, tremors, feeling numb or flat, urges to urinate). For precision, it is usually best to monitor lack of sensation (numbness) separately from change in sensation (feeling hot), and the specifics of what is monitored on the diary card will vary from client to client. These emotional signs can then be incorporated into chain analyses.

Use Overt Actions to Facilitate Labeling of Emotions

Raising awareness of emotion can be enhanced by using the overt behaviors linked to emotional experience as a means to facilitate labeling. For example, a personal attack of someone (such as harsh criticism) suggests that the client is feeling anger (action urge of anger is to attack). Bowing one's head or covering one's face suggests shame (action urge of shame is to hide). By knowing which actions are linked to which emotions, a client can learn to label inner experience in a manner similar to others. Labeling emotions makes it easier to identify likely thoughts, sensations, and action tendencies linked to emotions and predict one's future behaviors. Plus, using the same words that others use to describe emotional experience enhances social connectedness because it signals a shared or common bond. When first starting this practice, clients may lack an emotional vocabulary. For example, one OC client was only able to use words like "plastic," "raw," "fresh," "dry," "polished," and "tidy" when first describing what were posited to be inner emotional experiences. Other OC clients dislike basic emotion labels (anger, fear, disgust) because to them they are too extreme. They may be willing to admit that they are frustrated but may find it hard to say they are angry because to them anger equates to yelling and screaming. In the skills training manual, chapter 5, lesson 7, therapists can read about how to teach the way in which emotions are linked to the five neural substrates; lessons 6 and 22 show how to teach more broadly on emotions. Therapists should look for opportunities for the client to practice labeling emotions in session; for example, the therapist can check in with a client periodically during session by asking, "How are you feeling now?"

Help Clients Learn How to Grieve

OC clients can find it difficult to experience and label vulnerable emotions; for example, when sad, they may label their sadness as fatigue. During the orientation and commitment stages of therapy, it is important for therapists to assess the presence of trauma, long-held grudges, and other losses that may be important obstacles preventing client growth. Grief work can become an important means to help a client let go of these painful experiences. Successful grieving requires the brain to learn that what was before is no longer. Grief work means feeling the loss and then letting it go (practicing regulation). Over time, the brain adjusts to the changing circumstance; that is, we give up searching for the lost object and begin to build a new life (see the skills training manual, chapter 5, lesson 29).

Encourage Self-Enquiry

It is important for therapists not to focus solely on changing aversive emotions. RO DBT emphasizes the importance of self-enquiry—that is, pausing to question one's reactions, in order to learn, before applying a regulation strategy (such as accepting, distracting, or reappraising). Rather than redirecting attention away from aversive emotions (for example, by attending to neutral, non-emotion-based body sensations), RO DBT encourages clients to redirect attention *toward* aversive emotions (even when they are of low intensity) and use self-enquiry first. For example, sadness may signal that something important in one's life has changed or that one needs to do something different. Self-enquiry of emotion means pausing to ask oneself *What might this emotion be telling me? How open am I to feeling this emotion? Do I desire to get rid of the emotion, deny it, or regulate it immediately?* If yes or maybe, then *What am I avoiding? Is there something here to learn?* Self-enquiry is nonruminative because it is not looking to solve the problem or to regulate or avoid the discomfort. Indeed, quick answers are considered to most often reflect old learning and desires to avoid genuine contact with the pain associated with not having a solution. Thus self-enquiry can be differentiated from other mindfulness approaches because it actively seeks discomfort to learn and blocks immediate answers rather than prioritizing dispassionate observing, metacognitively distancing from thoughts, and waiting for the experience to fade away. This is why most self-enquiry practices are encouraged to last over days or weeks. Clients are encouraged to keep a weekly journal, a small book in which they can record self-enquiry questions and what arises during self-enquiry practices.

Foster Nonjudgmental Awareness

Mindfulness training can also influence the appraisals or thoughts we have about emotions. We sometimes refer to this skill as "having but not holding" an emotion— that is, allowing oneself to fully experience, without judgment, the sensations, images, and thoughts involved in an emotion and then to let it go (for example, by using a change strategy) while maintaining a willingness for the emotion to return. In addition, clients can be reminded that their thoughts or appraisals can influence emotional experience. What we think about during an emotional experience can prolong the emotion or trigger another one (for example, the thought *I hate being angry* can be a bit like putting gasoline on a fire and can refire the same emotion). Mindfulness teaches a person to observe the response tendencies of an emotional event (for example, when fearful, observe without judgment the urge to escape). T. R. Lynch and colleagues (2006) have posited that this approach automatically alters the meaning or appraisal associated with an emotion (for example, from something bad to something that just *is*) without the need to use executive control to reappraise or modify one's original emotional perception. By allowing emotions to be experienced (exposure) without judgment, new associations are acquired (the emotion just *is*, the thought just *is*, and the memory just *is*). With repeated practice, associations between emotionally evocative stimuli and new ways of behaving or thinking become increasingly dominant, thus making it less likely, for example, that fear will be refired by appraisals that it is bad or dangerous (see T. R. Lynch et al., 2006). This approach— that is, observing emotional sensations, urges, thoughts, and memories dispassionately—is the core of most traditional mindfulness awareness treatments (J. M. G. Williams, 2010; Segal, Williams, & Teasdale, 2002). RO DBT values both dispassionate awareness and passionate participation.

Assign Homework Practices Aimed at Developing Mindfulness of Emotion

Homework assignments should be assigned to help clients improve mindful awareness and labeling of inner experiences (for example, mindfully taking a hot bath while practicing "observe openly" and "describe with integrity" skills to label sensations, thoughts, and, ideally, any emotions associated with the experience; see also the Awareness Continuum in the skills training manual, chapter 5, lesson 12). However, many OC clients have purposefully arranged their environments and activities such that they rarely encounter strong emotions (for example, by going to work the same way every day, eating the same food every day, and planning carefully before going to the store). Thus therapists must encourage clients to engage in behaviors that evoke emotions (for example, behaving more prosocially, smiling more, sharing vulnerable or personal experiences with others, walking home using a different route, joining in with singing at church, or participating in a dance activity) while nonjudgmentally observing their old response tendencies (such as being silent, looking away, or leaving early). With repeated practice, the client develops new (neutral, more positive) associations about previously avoided situations and internal emotional experiences.

Overly Cautious and Hypervigilant Behavior

Overly cautious and hypervigilant behavior in OC is posited to stem from biotemperamental predispositions for heightened threat sensitivity and diminished reward sensitivity. Consequently, when contemplating a valued activity (for example, attending a daughter's wedding), OC clients may not experience anticipatory pleasure, and when actually engaged in the activity they may experience lower excitement or pleasure than others. Approach motivations and cautiousness can also be influenced by family and environmental factors; for example, fears of making a mistake or being the center of attention may stem from early childhood experiences punishing difference or lack of precision. Despite this, a number of OC clients may appear, at least on the surface, to not be afraid of social or novel situations. Rather than avoiding such situations, they may dutifully attend church, school, work, or scheduled social events on time and make important contributions to community events (for example, by speaking out against injustice, organizing future meetings, or recording meeting minutes). However, when queried, their prosocial contributions may stem from a sense of obligation rather than anticipated pleasure or social connectedness. Indeed, they may consider the pursuit of pleasure or enjoyment decadent, perverse, or self-indulgent. As a consequence, when treating OC overly cautious and hypervigilant behavior, it is important for therapists to account for the factors just cited and to adjust their interventions accordingly. In addition, the biotemperamental basis of this theme implicates the importance of RO DBT strategies designed to activate differing neural substrates, most notably the social safety system (PNS-VVC; see chapter 2).

Treatment Strategies for Overly Cautious and Hypervigilant Behavior

Activate the Social Safety System (PNS-VVC) Prior to Engaging in Novel Behavior

Biotemperamental biases for heightened threat sensitivity make it more likely for OC clients to perceive new or uncertain situations as threatening (that is, defensively arousing). Therefore, it is essential for therapists to teach OC clients how to activate the social safety system prior to assigning behavioral activation tasks as homework. Individual therapists should not assume that skills training classes will be sufficient in helping OC clients learn these skills. Didactic instruction in social safety activation and troubleshooting commitment are essential parts of individual therapy, ideally occurring by the sixth session and using the same handouts as skills classes. This ensures that social safety skills are taught early in treatment and at least twice (that is, once in individual therapy and once in skills class). Therapists should also not assume OC clients to be competent in social safety activation simply because they have been instructed in skills usage or have rehearsed these skills in a therapy session. Many OC clients fail to appreciate the significance of these skills (at least initially), often because they assume they should be easy, secretly regard the skills as "woo-woo" or silly (for example, loving kindness meditation, eyebrow wags), or may not fully grasp the science behind them. Thus therapists must assess not only commitment to practice social safety activation skills but also competency in their performance. Without this, clients may dutifully comply with social signaling assignments yet fail to benefit from them because they are unable to downregulate biotemperamental predispositions for defensive arousal. The problem is not lack of willingness on the client's part to behave differently; the problem is that the client has insufficient experience in activating social safety to be able to viscerally link it to positive outcomes.

Teach Flexible Mind VARIEs

Flexible Mind VARIEs skills (see the skills training manual, chapter 5, lesson 5) are designed to facilitate success in trying out new things and going opposite to avoidance. Although these skills are formally taught in skills class, individual therapists should informally teach them and reinforce their use via individualized homework practices. Practices can start out with something as simple as the client's rearranging the furniture at home, wearing different clothes (for example, brighter colors), taking a new route when driving to the store, or trying a new type of food. Contrast is introduced as making life interesting. Flexible Mind VARIEs skills should not be taught or assigned for practice before an OC client has become adept at activating the social safety system. Over time, with increasing successful practice, the therapist can increase the intensity of exposure to previously avoided situations, places, or people.

Rigid and Rule-Governed Behavior

Inflexible and rigidly held beliefs are prototypical of OC, although OC clients' natural tendency to not reveal inner thoughts and experiences will not always make this immediately apparent. Rigidity is defined as resistance to changing beliefs, attitudes, or personal habits, whereas rule-governed behavior refers to learned behavior that is language-based. Verbal rules describe relationships between a behavior (such as openly revealing vulnerable emotions) and a potential consequence (for example, people who are open and vulnerable are more likely to be hurt). Problems arise whenever rule governance becomes so dominant that the majority of the person's responses become determined by past learning, not by the present moment's experience. The majority of OC clients are both rigid and rule-governed, most often manifested by compulsive needs for order and structure, strong desires to be correct, hyperperfectionism, compulsive problem fixing, maladaptive hoarding, hyperplanning, excessive rehearsal, and insistence on sameness.

Problems with rigid and rule-governed behavior most often become apparent whenever the client encounters environmental feedback that disconfirms a self-construct or worldview or does not match expectations for what should be occurring. Often, rigid beliefs have a history of intermittent reinforcement (that is the observation, rule, thought, or belief was effective in solving a problem in the past). Treatment strategies targeting rigid and rule-governed behavior can be distilled down to the following basic approaches:

- RO DBT radical openness and self-enquiry practices designed to question one's perception of reality and encourage openness to disconfirming feedback (see the skills training manual, chapter 5, lessons 1, 11, and 13)

- RO DBT neuroregulatory skills designed to activate differing neural substrates, in particular the neural substrate associated with the ventral vagal complex and social safety (see the skills training manual, chapter 5, lesson 2)

Treatment Strategies for Rigid and Rule-Governed Behavior

Ask, Don't Tell

OC clients are hypersensitive to criticism, fear making a mistake, and often have a long history of intermittent reinforcement associated with rigid beliefs, which makes them less amenable to normal persuasion or logic. A type of calcified thinking can emerge that grows stronger when challenged or exposed; like the hard external skeleton of the marine organisms that form coral reefs, direct disturbance makes the hard deposits grow thicker.

RO DBT works with rigid beliefs and behavior by first assuming that the therapist may be mistaken or incorrect in how she understands the problem. This provides breathing room for the client and an opportunity for learning on both the client's and the therapist's part. Thus, instead of telling an OC client that his rigid behavior or belief is invalid, distorted, or ineffective, the therapist should ask the client, with an open mind, how his belief or why his behavior is beneficial to him. This models radical openness on the therapist's part while encouraging the client to practice self-enquiry and self-disclosure. For example, a therapist noted that his OC client described waking up in the middle of the night in order to get some pain medication for her ailing husband as "selfish" and "controlling" rather than as an act of kindness. In this situation, asking rather than telling might involve a question like "Can you help me understand how helping your husband in this manner was a selfish act?" A query of this type helps the client practice revealing inner feelings and avoids providing leading information that could influence how the client responds.

Since a strong working alliance may not emerge until midtreatment (around the fourteenth session), prior to this OC clients may tend to report what they think the therapist wants to hear. When an OC client appears to be struggling with describing something, quickly moving in to provide helpful suggestions (therapeutic mind reading) or therapeutic interpretations will not give the client the space and time to describe her experience (or her struggle to do so) in her own words. For example, much more is likely to be learned through open-ended questions ("What prevents you from labeling your actions as kind?") or questions with no clearly correct or socially appropriate answer ("When you help your husband out in the middle of the night, does this behavior make it more likely or less likely for you to achieve what is important for you in life?") than through interpretations ("Maybe you can't allow yourself to feel kindness because you are so self-critical"). The therapist must not overcorrect and assume that competent RO DBT involves asking questions only. On the contrary; didactic teaching, therapeutic mind reading, case formulation reviews, and explicit demands for change are also necessary components.

Allow Natural Change, and Slow the Client's Compulsive Fixing

Individual therapists should look for opportunities to help their OC clients let go of rigid desires to immediately fix or solve problems when they arise. For example, one OC client arrived at her third RO DBT session with a list of 117 new things she had tried out the previous week, a task that was not requested by her therapist. This behavior, though representing a strong attempt to correct her avoidance of novelty, also represented a core issue in being able to tolerate uncertainty. The client was applying maladaptive control efforts to correct another maladaptive OC problem. In general, therapists should adopt a stance of nonurgency when working with OC clients rather than somber problem solving, particularly when it comes to rigidity. Therapists should encourage OC clients (as well as themselves) to practice allowing problems to just be, without assuming that every apparent problem requires immediate resolution. This functions as informal behavioral exposure to uncertainty and ambiguity. Compulsive fixing can be monitored on diary cards, and therapists should use this to help clients realize that sometimes apparent fixing makes matters worse. One OC client recalled how she had immediately ordered a brand-new dishwasher after discovering that her old one was full of dirty water. It was only the next morning, when the new one arrived, that she discovered the actual problem—a blocked drainage pipe that was not even part of the machine. Her desire for quick control resulted not only in lost time and money but also in the aggravation of knowing that her solution had been inappropriate. If she had allowed herself the grace of not trying to immediately solve the problem, she might have discovered the next morning that the problem was a drainage issue, not a mechanical one. Awareness of this pattern became an important turning point for this client in being able to allow natural change to occur and to let go of compulsive fixing.

Encourage the Art of Nonproductivity

Therapists should look for opportunities for OC clients to practice not working all of the time. OC clients have forgotten the importance of play and laughter in healthy living. Therapists can remind clients that as children (at the age of three, for example) they were able to play without self-consciousness. Doing something new or different every day helps break down old habits and encourages spontaneity naturally. Therapists should look for ways for their clients to practice being less work-focused, without giving themselves a hard time about it. For example, instead of reading another self-improvement book, OC clients should be encouraged to read magazines or books that are fantasy-oriented, recreational, nonserious, or fictional. Homework assignments might include practices such as leaving work early once per week, going out for a beer with work colleagues, taking naps, daydreaming, watching comedies, taking long baths, or spending only a set amount of time to complete a task.

Use Playful Irreverence to Challenge Rigid Beliefs and Block Compulsive Rule-Governed Behavior

Playful irreverence combined with stories and metaphors can smuggle important information about problems or treatment strategies that otherwise might have been dismissed if presented more formally. For example, therapists can playfully take advantage of OC tendencies to comply with rules to block compulsive fixing by creating a new rule that must be followed—specifically, the new rule is "You are not allowed to attempt to solve or fix a problem until twenty-four hours after it first occurs." Delaying compulsive fixing behaviors over a twenty-four-hour period has several benefits for an OC individual:

- It provides time for new information about the problem to emerge naturally and blocks rash decision making that only later is discovered to have been in error or unneeded.

- Compulsive fixing is driven by fear and avoidance of uncertainty or ambiguity, but delaying a decision or solution by twenty-four hours ensures that the person has slept on it (during sleep, cue-driven emotional responses fade, and so it is more likely for a new perspective on the problem to emerge in the morning).

- It provides the client an opportunity to not work so hard and practice developing a nonjudgmental sense of humor about himself and his personal foibles (see the skills training manual, chapter 5, lesson 5, for teaching about the art of nonproductivity).

The strategy should be delivered using playful irreverence (that is, a slightly tongue-in-cheek manner). Playfully insisting it is imperative to adhere to the new twenty-four-hour rule on delay of fixing, while nonverbally communicating affection, encourages the client to join with the therapist in experimenting with novel ways to change old habits.

The following examples from therapists' transcripts demonstrate the use of irreverence to challenge literal belief in thoughts and help loosen rule-governed thinking (see chapter 10 for a more detailed discussion of playful irreverence):

Therapist: Last night I made this delicious cheesy pizza with fresh mozzarella cheese, roasted tomatoes and garlic, a bit of fresh pepper and parsley sprinkled on top, and a crunchy crust drizzled with olive oil. I just can't wait to get home tonight and warm it up in the oven! (*Pauses, looks at client.*) But why am I telling you this?

(*Client shrugs.*)

Therapist: The truth is that I lied. I never made that pizza! The point is that if you, like me, are salivating now, then we can know for a fact that thoughts don't have to be true to influence us. So just because you think it, that doesn't mean it's true. (*Uses this experience to help client understand that thoughts, even when untrue, exert a powerful influence, both physiologically and emotionally.*)

Therapist: (*Wears glasses*) I don't wear glasses.

(*Client freezes.*)

Therapist: No—I mean it. I don't wear glasses! (*Touches the glasses he is wearing, pauses, looks at client.*) Do you believe me?

(*Client shakes head no.*)

Therapist: My statements about glasses are just like the thoughts in your head—they sound convincing, but they're not necessarily true. (*Uses this experience to irreverently challenge client's literal belief in thoughts, and uses the story to facilitate teaching.*) Perhaps because thoughts are inside of us, we tend to believe them, even though we can easily discount thoughts about things outside our heads. For example, we easily discount the words coming from a radio insisting, "Send me your money, or the world will end." Or when a child proclaims, "I am a seven-foot-tall giant," we know these words are fantasy. But we don't easily discount our own internal verbal behavior—our own words and thoughts. (*Weaves in other examples demonstrating the importance of seeing thoughts as thoughts, not as literal truth.*) So my suggestion is for us to start practicing the skill of observing our thoughts and not seeing them as literally true. The goal is to be able to watch them like a movie playing. As you get better at this, you might find that some of your negative beliefs about yourself or others will start to have less power over you. How does this sound to you? (*Checks in with client to confirm agreement.*)

Highlight Rigidity's Negative Impact on Relationships

Rigid rule-governed behaviors, perfectionism, and compulsive desires for structure and control can negatively impact relationships. For example, one OC client reported that she felt compelled to redo other people's work if she believed that they might not have done it properly, a behavior that the therapist and the client decided was most likely reinforced by the client's pride or sense of accomplishment after having done a job well. However, her behavior of compulsive redoing negatively impacted her relationships; that is, her family and coworkers experienced her redoing as demoralizing, since their efforts rarely appeared to meet her perfectionistic standards. Moreover, the consequences for the client were often exhaustion (redoing other people's work required additional effort) and an increasing sense of resentment and bitterness because she felt that she was the only one ever doing any work (her family had essentially abandoned helping out with most domestic chores). For other clients, rigid behaviors may have more to do with rules pertaining to social etiquette ("always behave politely" or "always send Christmas cards") or dutifulness ("always reply promptly to all emails"). Mindfulness practices can focus on the importance of nonjudgmental participation in relationships while letting go of unhelpful rumination about what should have happened or how the other person should have behaved.

Urge-Surf Compulsive Desires for Structure and Control

RO DBT conceptualizes compulsive desires for structure and control as inner experiences with predictable action tendencies (action tendencies or urges that are transitory in nature). Clients can be taught how to mindfully urge-surf compulsive desires to control, fix, or correct without getting caught up in the thoughts associated with the urge or mindlessly giving in to the action tendencies associated with it (for example, ruminating about a solution or rushing to fix an apparent problem). With repeated practice, the client is able to learn that the urge, like a wave, crests and then passes (Marlatt & Gordon, 1985). See the skills training manual, chapter 5, lesson 12, for an urge-surfing mindfulness script.

Learn to Love Perfectionistic Tendencies

Therapists should avoid the trap of trying to change perfectionism. RO DBT encourages OC clients to practice embracing fallibility rather than always trying to improve themselves. Treatment of maladaptive perfectionism must start, therefore, with loving one's shortcomings. One RO DBT therapist, when asked by an OC client to target perfectionism, replied in a playfully irreverent way: "I'm sorry. I can't ethically treat your perfectionism. If I do so, I buy into your belief that you are never good enough. That is, if I try to help you get rid of your perfectionism, I am essentially agreeing with you that you are flawed, and I think that would be morally wrong. There is an alternative way out of this, though, assuming you might be interested. The path is a difficult one. Instead of changing your perfectionistic tendencies, it requires you to first fully love or appreciate them. Interestingly, once you have genuinely achieved this, you are by definition, in that moment, no longer a perfectionist, because you have stopped trying to improve yourself."

Aloof and Distant Relationships

Since OC is considered fundamentally a problem of social isolation and loneliness, the overarching goal of treatment is to help the OC client establish or enhance one or two long-term and highly intimate relationships (for example, a romantic partnership or marriage). Most OC clients desire a healthy long-term romantic relationship, despite the fact that many may have become bitter, cynical, or resigned about ever achieving this. An in-depth intimacy assessment of existing long-term relationships (or lack thereof) should be undertaken, and commitment to change obtained. It should be explained that genuine progress in this area is essential if the client is to truly obtain a life worth sharing and to experience long-term benefits from treatment (for example, no longer being chronically depressed). Genuine progress, in RO DBT, is more than planning or talking about relationships; it is defined as engaging in new behaviors (for example, progress may be defined in terms of the client's having started dating by the eighteenth session). The importance of this goal should be briefly introduced during the first four orientation and commitment sessions and then revisited frequently. Therapists should be careful not to join with the OC client's worldview about interpersonal relationships (for example, that long-term romantic relationships are either impossible or undesired, or that what the client currently has is fine). The client's resistance to this topic should be anticipated (see information on "pushback" and "don't hurt me" responses in chapter 10) but not taken to mean that work on this theme should be dropped.

Treatment Strategies for Aloof and Distant Relationships
Link Repair of Alliance Ruptures to Relationship-Enhancement Skills

Since OC clients are risk-averse, they tend to be wary, cautious, and less trusting when entering into new relationships, thereby making the establishment of a therapeutic alliance more difficult (see chapter 5). Fortunately, the problems associated with establishing a strong therapeutic alliance with OC clients are the same as or similar to those experienced by the client with others in the real world. For example, OC clients consider abandonment the solution to interpersonal conflict. However, conflict is inevitable in all intimate relationships. Clients should be encouraged to view individual therapy as the ideal (and safe) place to practice conflict-resolution skills instead of walking away, and it can be explained (using playful irreverence) that because part of good therapy will be to provide corrective feedback (invalidating maladaptive behavior), there should be plenty of opportunities for practice. This is why alliance ruptures are prioritized over other behavioral targets in RO DBT for OC (second only to life-threatening behaviors) and not considered problems per se but opportunities for skills practice. Details for managing alliance ruptures and repairs are provided in chapter 8.

Reinforce Disagreement

For many OC clients, aloofness manifests as overly agreeable behavior that may on the surface appear intimacy-enhancing. For example, a client may dutifully comply with homework assignments (spending hours on detailed completion of diary cards, for instance) and may never or only rarely disagree overtly with the therapist, and yet inwardly the client may not understand the importance of completing a diary card, despite its having been explained, or may believe diary cards are a waste of time or irrelevant to her problems. Despite this, she may never reveal these concerns, while inwardly remaining disillusioned about therapy or angry at the therapist. Consequently, therapists should consider expressions of compliance, agreement, or commitment (particularly in the early stages of treatment) as information that may or may not reflect a client's true inner experience. Instead, therapists should encourage disclosures of dissension, discomfort, ambivalence, or disagreement by redefining them as representing therapeutic progress, not problems, and as essential steps for enhancing intimacy.

Thus, if a client discloses to the therapist that he doesn't agree with something that the therapist just said, the therapist should take the following three steps:

1. Thank the client for being honest about his feelings, and point out that doing so goes opposite to the natural OC tendency to mask inner feelings

2. Seriously consider the feedback as possibly accurate, and practice self-enquiry (that is, look for ways in which the therapist may have contributed to the issue) without automatically assuming that the criticism reflects the client's pathology

3. Work with the client on deciding what to do about the feedback (for example, continue to observe the issue, make a change in how things are done, or stay the same), and use this as an opportunity to teach principles associated with Flexible Mind (see the skills training manual, chapter 5)

Enhance Relationships by Increasing Openness to Critical Feedback

For some OC clients, an aloof and distant interpersonal style has been intermittently reinforced because it functions to help them avoid painful interpersonal feedback. Appearing cold or unapproachable can create an impression that interpersonal feedback does not matter or is unimportant. Over time, others may stop providing feedback. Radical openness means giving up being right, without losing your point of view. This requires a willingness to be flexible and fallible. Therapists should encourage OC clients to use Flexible Mind ADOPTS skills as a means for encouraging interpersonal feedback from others (see the skills training manual, chapter 5, lesson 22).

Teach Validation Skills to Signal Social Inclusion

A major skill deficit for many OC clients is that of being able to communicate understanding and acceptance—that is, validation—of another person's feelings, thoughts, desires, actions, and experience. Validation enhances intimate relationships because it communicates to others that their responses are acceptable and valued, and that they themselves matter. Individual therapists should explicitly teach validation skills to OC clients and look for opportunities for in-session rehearsal (see the skills training manual, chapter 5, lesson 19).

Teach Match + 1 Skills to Enhance Personal Self-Disclosure

Most OC clients avoid revealing vulnerability or disclosing personal information to others, making the formation of intimate relationships more difficult. Close interpersonal relationships involve reciprocal disclosures of potentially damaging, embarrassing, or socially inappropriate feelings, thoughts, or experiences, not just prosocial or positive experiences. Therapists should help their OC clients recognize that sharing vulnerability or past mistakes with others communicates to receivers that the sender considers them trustworthy. This makes it more likely for receivers to respond similarly. Individual therapists should teach Match + 1 skills (see the skills training manual, chapter 5, lesson 21) to facilitate this. Match + 1 skills are based on a simple relationship principle: revealing personal information allows us to get closer to another, and this reciprocal process provides the basis for all close interpersonal relationships. Match + 1 skills can be practiced in session (for example, via role playing) and with homework assignments that start by practicing the same skills with individuals whom the client does not have strong feelings toward (for example, grocery clerks, postal workers, or neighbors) and observing their impact. However, it is important for therapists to remember that the primary goal of Match + 1 skills is to establish or enhance long-term and highly intimate relationships (that is, a romantic partnership or marriage).

High Social Comparisons with Envy or Bitterness

OC clients are achievement- and performance-focused; appearing competent is not optional but imperative. Thus they must engage in frequent social comparisons in order to verify that their performance is superior or at least adequate relative to others. The search for evidence that they are better, faster, smarter, or fitter than others can become a compulsive means of regulating negative affect and enhancing self-esteem. Although social comparisons can verify personal success, they carry with them a hidden cost when unfavorable. Unhelpful envy arises when a person compares herself disapprovingly to others and believes that others' advantages are unjust. It is an important emotion to understand because it can prompt passive-aggressive and sometimes overtly aggressive behavior.

Within one month of a romantic betrayal, individuals with a high capacity for inhibitory control reported greater symptoms of trauma, depression, stress, embarrassment, and less forgiveness compared to those low in inhibition (Couch & Sandfoss, 2009). Research shows that interpersonal transgressions (that is, perceptions that another person has harmed the subject in a painful or morally wrong way; see M. E. McCullough, Root, & Cohen, 2006) can have negative effects on mental health. For example, an experience of humiliation has been found to be associated with a 70 percent increase in the risk of major depressive disorder (Kendler, Hettema, Butera, Gardner, & Prescott, 2003). As previously noted, our research suggests that approximately half of all OC clients can be expected to have a past trauma or that they have reported holding on to a grudge toward another person. High social comparisons are common among OC individuals and function as a precursor to envy and bitterness. Though it is normal to feel less positive toward someone who harms us, individuals who are able to let go of grudges or transgressions and forgive have been shown to become less avoidant, less vengeful, and more benevolent toward the people who have hurt them (see M. E. McCullough et al., 2006). The following transcript conveys an OC client's experience linked to bitterness and revenge:

> I had to fill my car up on Friday morning, which is annoying in itself because it seems like a waste of time. When I got there, there was a line, and I remember thinking Why are these stupid people taking so long? Finally my turn came, and I realized that I had to stretch the hose across my car because the gas cap was on the opposite side of the pump. This took time, and the people in the car behind kept staring. I felt humiliated. So I said to myself, Let them wait. With that, I went through my usual routine, found my rubber gloves in the trunk, wiped the hose and nozzle with a cloth, double-checked the receipt, and, all in all, just made sure that I took care of things properly. The fact that this took time just didn't matter. I simply ignored the honking, and in the end I felt vindicated because I had stood my ground.

Following this incident, the client's back pain intensified, he ruminated about the event, and he fumed about the stupidity of people. He also thought of ways he might get back at the owners of the gas station. The individual therapist worked with the client on finding the dysfunctional links in the situation, via chain analysis, and generating more effective ways of responding. This included labeling the emotion he experienced and examining the consequences of his behavior, such as increased back pain. The therapist used this experience to work on the client's commitment to learn skills to let go of unhelpful anger and resentment. This included forgiving himself for parking on the wrong side of the pump and empathy for the frustration expressed by others at the station.

Unhelpful envy involves a painful blend of shame and resentment, which we describe as secret anger. In addition, repeated failures to achieve what one believes one is entitled to, or repeated conclusions that others have been unfairly advantaged, can lead to the mood state known as bitterness. Bitterness is characterized by an overarching sense of pessimism, cynicism, and ungratefulness. Both bitterness and envy negatively impact interpersonal relationships and make it less likely for others to desire affiliation. As one OC client described her untreated OC mother, "It's difficult to be around her—she is always raining on someone's parade."

Treatment Strategies for Envy and Bitterness

Teach Opposite-Action Skills for Envy and Bitterness

Therapists should teach opposite-action skills for envy and bitterness during individual therapy, despite the fact that these skills will also be covered in training classes. Opposite action for envy requires acting opposite to two differing urges—the urge to hide and the urge to attack—whereas opposite action to bitterness involves helping others and allowing others to help, reflecting on commonalities among people, and practicing gratitude.

Model Kindness First and Foremost

Kindness is a core way of behaving in RO DBT. It encourages others to join with us rather than go against us or move away from us. Kindness means practicing genuine humility by acknowledging our place in the world and appreciating how all things are connected. Kindness means giving another person the benefit of the doubt until we have more information, and even then practicing a willingness to be wrong. Crucially, it does not mean just being "nice" to others. In fact, sometimes the kindest thing a person might do for another is to say no or be tough. Therapists should model kindness with their clients and encourage homework practices that will help strengthen kindness (see the skills training manual, chapter 5, lesson 17).

Teach Loving Kindness Meditation

It should be explained to clients that the goal of LKM practices, when used to help treat envy and bitterness, is different from how LKM is normally practiced in RO DBT. The primary aim of LKM is activation of the PNS-VVC-mediated social safety system. When LKM is used to help clients with high envy or bitterness, the primary goal shifts from activating social safety to enhancing compassion and connection with community. When used in this manner, LKM practices can be extended to having clients direct affection, warmth, and goodwill not only toward people they already care for and neutral others but also toward people they are struggling with (feeling envy toward, for example), toward themselves, and toward the world. Short four-minute LKM practices have been shown to bring significant increases in positivity and feelings of social connectedness toward strangers as compared to a closely matched control (Hutcherson, Seppala, & Gross, 2008). Therapists can use the LKM script provided in the skills training manual (chapter 5, lesson 4) as a basis of practices for targeting envy and bitterness, ideally audiorecording the practice during individual therapy (the audiorecording can be given to the client to use at home).

Finally, therapists are reminded that LKM practices for envy and bitterness are optional and used only on an as-needed basis, whereas LKM practices aimed at activating the PNS-VVC-mediated social safety system are required (that is, part of the standard RO DBT protocol).

Offer Forgiveness Training

Most OC clients find it difficult to forgive themselves and other people for transgressions, mistakes, or past harms. What is important to realize is that we all struggle with forgiveness, no matter who we are. Forgiveness is a process, and it involves a decision to let go of pain, a commitment to change our habitual ways of responding, and a willingness to practice skills shown to help us be more compassionate and forgiving. It is not a promise that if we forgive, the pain will go away. Forgiveness training is one of the most powerful clinical tools in RO DBT. It provides an essential means of rejoining the tribe and regaining compassion for oneself and others. Although forgiveness training is formally taught in skills training classes (see the skills training manual, chapter 5, lesson 29), individual therapists should also teach forgiveness principles as part of individual therapy (normally after the fourteenth session). Therapists should remind clients that forgiveness is not approval or denial of the past but instead means taking care of ourselves. Forgiveness is a choice; it requires an ongoing commitment to let go of past hurts in order to grow and be mentally healthy. Finally, forgiveness is liberating because it means letting go of past grievances, grudges, or desires for revenge in order to care for ourselves and live according to our values; yet, as a process, it takes time and requires ongoing practice.

Using Social Signaling Subtypes to Improve Treatment Targeting

As mentioned in chapter 3, there are two social signaling OC subtypes—the *overly agreeable* subtype and the *overly disagreeable* subtype—and they differ primarily in how the person described by the features of each subtype desires to be perceived by others in his or her social environment (that is, the subtypes have to do with the OC individual's public persona). The core social signaling deficit characterizing OC pertains to pervasive masking of inner feelings from others—that is, what is expressed on the outside (publicly revealed) often does not accurately reflect what is felt on the inside (privately experienced). Thus treatment targeting can be improved simply by knowing the client's public persona (that is, OC subtype) because the very opposite of this persona often represents the core issue the client needs to address in order to rejoin the tribe and reduce emotional loneliness.

Both subtypes are motivated to appear competent; however, the overly disagreeable subtype is less concerned about social approval or politeness. The words "agreeable" and "disagreeable" refer to the outer mask or persona most commonly exhibited by the person when challenged, not to his or her inner emotional state per se. Both subtypes experience the full range of human emotions and mood states internally (such as anger, hostility, anxiety, fear, shame, and guilt), yet how they express their internal emotional experience depends on their self-control tendencies (see chapter 2 for information about RO DBT's neuroregulatory model). Thus the persona or outer expressive style of the overly disagreeable individual may appear strong-willed, dogmatic, aloof, disdainful, or skeptical when under stress or confronted with disconfirming feedback and unexpected events. In contrast, the persona of the overly agreeable individual is more likely to appear deferential, compliant, intimate, or people-pleasing.

The Overly Disagreeable Subtype

Individuals falling within this subtype are motivated to be seen as competent but not compliant, obsequious, or submissive. Their manner of speech may be business-like, and their facial expressions tend to be serious, concerned, or flat, particularly when under stress. They tend to value having a strong will and may be able to recall vividly times they have stood up against injustice or resisted social pressures to conform in ways they believed immoral. They tend to strongly dislike enthusiastic or expressive individuals and people whom they consider to be weak, whiny, phony, or incompetent. Interestingly, although they are willing to confront others about moral wrongdoing or strongly proclaim the importance of doing the right thing, when it comes to more intimate interpersonal conflict they usually prefer to walk away or abandon the relationship rather than deal with the problem directly.[57] However, they are willing to appear unfriendly or bad-tempered in order to achieve an objective, even if it harms an important relationship. For example, the overly disagreeable subtype is more likely to engage in "pushback" responses (such as answering a question with a question) rather than "don't hurt me" responses (such as acting weak or fragile) when confronted with unwanted feedback. Despite this, these individuals are most often highly prosocial and friendly, especially when around people they do not know well. Thus therapists should anticipate a polite and prosocial manner from overly disagreeable clients during the early stages of therapy, until the first alliance rupture.

Despite an apparently tough or confident exterior, inwardly the overly disagreeable subtype feels insecure, apprehensive, uncertain, and vulnerable, experiences that these individuals are unlikely to reveal to others. They may secretly believe that their hard outer exterior covers a fundamentally flawed and weak inner self. Indeed, they are likely to believe that it is imperative to hide this vulnerability from others and may assume that any person revealing personal vulnerability is either a fool or a manipulator. This often results in an inability to allow themselves pleasure, rest, or self-soothing, since this could imply they need it, a stance that leads to burnout and cynical bitterness.

Thus treatment targeting for the overly disagreeable subtype emphasizes the importance of revealing vulnerability, rather than hiding vulnerability, in order to establish and improve close social bonds with others. Individual therapists should focus on RO DBT skills emphasizing validation (see the skills training manual, chapter 5, lesson 19) and helping these clients learn to do the following things:

- Be more playful, spontaneous, and less obsessive about being productive (lesson 5)

- Be assertive with an open mind (lesson 18)

- Reveal vulnerability to others (lesson 21)

- Deal with conflict openly rather than abandoning relationships (lesson 21)

- Repair a damaged relationship (lesson 21)

- Apologize after a transgression (lesson 21)

- Be open to critical feedback (lesson 22)

- Let go of envy and bitterness (lesson 28)

- Forgive themselves and others (lesson 29)

Here are some examples of individualized homework tasks that I have found useful when working with someone who may be more overly disagreeable:

- Complete a task without looking back over the details or double-checking your work.

- Practice being lazy, or decrease excessive work behaviors; for example, leave work at the same time as others, take a nap on Saturday afternoon, or read an entertaining magazine or book that is not designed to improve who you are or make you a better person.

- Practice playing and developing hobbies or leisure activities that are not designed to improve you.

- Spend only a set amount of time to complete a task, and if you're unable to complete the task during this time period, practice accepting that the task can always be completed later; allow yourself to go back to work on the task only the following day.

- Develop a sense of pride in being capable of letting go of rigid desires to work and in not always having to be right.

- Practice the art of resting; for example, take a twenty-minute power nap every day.

- Practice being loose and relaxed, and find ways to be less serious; reward yourself for letting go of rigid desires to always fix or solve problems.

- Practice making minor mistakes and watching the outcome, and notice that a mistake does not always mean that something bad will happen; at times, new learning or unexpected and beneficial outcomes can emerge from apparent mistakes.

- Practice interacting with individuals who are different, less serious, or less work-focused; for example, go to a fair where hippies hang out.

- Let go of hoarding behavior; for example, throw a newspaper away daily.

- Reinforce yourself for a job well done rather than automatically moving on to the next task; for example, after cleaning the garage, take time out to read a fun novel or sunbathe for an hour.

- When in situations that are uncertain or ambiguous, practice revealing your uncertainty rather than always pretending to be in control.

- Practice letting go of urges to tell another person what to do or how to manage a problem.

- Practice confiding in others.

- Increase prosocial behaviors; for example, engage in three practices of chit-chat per week, say thank you to praise, and practice apologizing after making a mistake.

- Decrease avoidance of situations where positive emotion could occur; for example, buy a puppy.

- Decrease expectations that all grievances should be repaired or wrongs righted; for example, notice times when you are not able to fix or repair a situation, despite your best intentions.

The Overly Agreeable Subtype

Individuals falling within this subtype are motivated to be seen as competent and socially desirable. The words "overly agreeable" refer to their public persona or overt style of interaction as well as to a common mood state. Individuals who are overly agreeable fear social disapproval or going against the tide. They have a strong desire to avoid conflict and to appear normal or proper when in public. They maintain a mask of social politeness that is removed only in private (for example, around family members or when they are alone). They tend to obsessively rehearse or plan what they will say or do during social interactions and may practice behaviors that are designed to appear spontaneous or fun. Maintaining this prosocial persona is exhausting because they are always performing rather than being. Consequently, they may report higher rates of sick leave, migraine headaches, and other somatic problems, which may often follow periods when they have felt greater social pressure to perform (for example, at a wedding or at an off-site all-day retreat for work).

Despite the apparent cooperative and prosocial nature of their overt behavior, overly agreeable individuals experience high rates of anger, resentment, and envy, emotions they may deny or work hard to cover up. They tend to obsess about their social status or standing among their peers and will secretly scan their social environment for signs of disrespect, disapproval, or lack of appreciation. They are more likely to believe their interpretations of others' behavior or expressions as accurate, despite no evidence or evidence to the contrary. They can ruminate for days or weeks (sometimes years) about perceived slights or betrayals without ever checking out the accuracy of their perceptions with the other person. Often only their immediate family members may know the extent of their anger, which can be expressed vehemently within the privacy of the home (in temper tantrums, for instance, or sarcastic belittling). Individuals outside the home may describe the overly agreeable client as a wonderful person who is always polite and caring. However, beneath the mask of social desirability, overly agreeable clients feel socially inadequate, inferior, and inauthentic. They may feel like frauds because their outward expressions of caring and concern often don't match their inner state. For example, they may frequently have negative thoughts about others, may secretly enjoy seeing misfortune befall another, may actively seek ways to undermine a person by whom they feel slighted, or may revel in harsh gossip. Similarly, they may tend to downplay or minimize personal accomplishments while at the same time secretly yearning for praise or recognition for a given talent. In addition, they may insist on taking the blame or may behave in a self-deprecatory manner when conflict arises yet may inwardly be blaming others or be seething inside with righteous indignation. Because they are adept at hiding their anger, resentment, or envy from others, they tend to believe that others behave similarly. Thus they are likely to distrust others and may consider others' candor or expressions of emotion to be manipulative or deceptive. This perception usually extends to their therapists and skills instructors, particularly during the early stages of treatment.

The facial affect and the manner of speech most frequently associated with individuals of this subtype involve prosocial displays that may often appear out of place or exaggerated, considering the circumstances or the situation (for example, excessive politeness, caring, or sympathy directed toward someone they hardly know or may never see again), or expressions of emotion that do not match inner feelings and thoughts (smiling when distressed, for example). They may have developed strategies to lessen their social awkwardness (sitting rather than standing during interactions, smoking cigarettes because it gives them an excuse to be away from the group, asking questions about the other person's life in order to avoid having to talk about themselves, feigning interest in or excitement about something in order to change the topic). They may appear to be listening attentively during a conversation yet inwardly be shut down, berating themselves, rehearsing a response, or judging the other person (see also the material on the "deer in the headlights" response, chapter 6). They may work hard to appear friendly and may report having a number of friends or may describe a talent for being able to get others to confide in them. Yet, when examined

293

in greater depth, very few people actually know who they are (for example, few are aware of these individuals' inner doubts or fears, few are knowledgeable about their angry outbursts, and few feel a sense of intimacy or social safety around them).

Individuals of the overly agreeable subtype are more likely to engage in "don't hurt me" responses when confronted with unwanted feedback (see chapter 10), and they may be more difficult to treat than clients of the overly disagreeable subtype precisely because their strong desire for social approval may make it more difficult for them to reveal their true feelings or thoughts. Furthermore, once they have determined that flexibility may be socially desirable, overly agreeable clients may quickly become adept at convincing their therapists that they are indeed flexibly controlled. This may involve admitting to the right number of problems needed to convince a therapist that they are not in denial, or steering the conversation away from hot topics, or subtly punishing feedback or questions they do not want to hear. Therapists should refer to the RO DBT assumptions about OC clients (see chapter 4) to help retain phenomenological empathy when working with overly agreeable individuals (recalling, for example, that, despite tendencies to avoid revealing vulnerability, these clients are inwardly suffering, are exhausted by their self-control efforts, and most often are keen to learn how to establish a genuinely intimate bond with another person).

In general, when working with overly agreeable individuals, therapists should target genuine self-disclosure of critical thoughts, distress, and behaviors that are not prosocial as an important step toward authenticity. Treatment targets, skills training, and homework assignments for individuals who fit the overly agreeable subtype focus on helping them learn to do the following things:

- Genuinely play without pretending (see the skills training manual, chapter 5, lesson 5)

- Reveal critical or judgmental thoughts or emotions (lessons 19 and 21)

- Be open to critical feedback without falling apart (lesson 22)

- Let go of needless social comparisons (lesson 28)

- Forgive themselves or others (lesson 29)

Individualized homework tasks that I have found useful when working with someone who may be overly agreeable include those that follow:

- At least once a day, practice talking without rehearsing beforehand what you are going to say.

- Three times per week, practice revealing to others your honest opinion about something, and let go of sugarcoating your opinion or trying to make it sound cooperative.

- Practice being bold and confrontational; during individual therapy, say aloud to your therapist three judgmental thoughts you have about others, and block your attempts to minimize any judgments or shame you may have about being or feeling judgmental (in other words, don't judge your judging).

- Twice per day, practice being more self-interested and doing things that might only benefit yourself rather than other people; for example, watch the television program you like, turn off your telephone for the evening, go to the restaurant you desire in order to eat the food you want, or make sure your boss is aware of a recent accomplishment.

- Practice appreciating and valuing your desire to behave in a socially acceptable manner (societies need individuals to behave cooperatively in order to survive); at the same time, practice the art of noncooperation, saying no, and standing up for yourself rather than automatically agreeing or complying with others in order to avoid conflict (for instance, three times per week, practice disagreeing without apologizing).

- Practice listening to another person with full attention rather than rehearsing what you will say next, and trust that you will know what to say when the time comes.

- Develop your rebel spirit; practice revealing dissent when you experience it, communicate your concerns directly, and then be open to feedback.

- Block harsh gossip about others, and use opposite-action skills for envy.

- Practice revealing distress or negative emotions when you experience them, and let go of pretending to be happy or caring when you are not.

- Practice trusting what others say and giving them the benefit of the doubt; practice trusting rather than distrusting, and allow yourself the luxury of distrust only after three or more interactions have provided evidence that distrust is warranted.

- Practice directly expressing justified anger, annoyance, or frustration in a manner that communicates a willingness to understand the other person's perspective.

- Let go of distrustful thoughts and of the assumption that others are out to get you.

- Remind yourself that others don't always see the world the way you do or cope in the same manner when it comes to how they express themselves (many people freely express emotions or inner experience without giving it much thought; for example, an undercontrolled individual is less likely to inhibit emotional expression).

Now You Know...

▶ The key to effective treatment with problems of overcontrol is to target indirect, masked, and constrained social signaling as the primary source of OC clients' emotional loneliness, isolation, and misery.

▶ The individual RO DBT therapist continually asks how the client's social signaling may be impacting his or her social connectedness.

▶ RO DBT posits that therapists and clients alike bring perceptual and regulatory biases into the treatment environment, and that these biases influence both the therapeutic relationship and treatment outcomes.

▶ The most effective therapists are both humble and open, which means that, with the exception of imminent life-threatening behavior, they let the client ultimately be the judge of what is, for him, maladaptive.

CHAPTER 10

Dialectical and Behavioral Strategies

Treatment strategies in RO DBT are principle-based. They are informed not only by neurobiological and evolutionary theory (see chapter 2) but also by core philosophical principles or ideas in RO DBT—dialectics, behaviorism, radical openness, and self-enquiry—that strongly impact the manner in which a therapist delivers the treatment. Radical openness and self-enquiry were addressed in earlier chapters; the primary aim of this chapter is to review the remaining two philosophical principles—dialectics and behaviorism—with an emphasis on strategies designed to maximize flexible responding, improve social signaling, and maximize social connectedness.

Why Dialectics?

Dialectical strategies in RO DBT share roots with the existential and dialectical philosophies found not only in Gestalt therapy (Perls, 1969) but also and most prominently in the dialectical principles guiding interventions in standard DBT (Linehan, 1993a). Dialectical thinking involves three developmental stages: a *thesis* (for example, "inhibition is useful") that gives rise to a reaction, its *antithesis* ("disinhibition is useful"), which in turn contradicts and seems to negate the thesis, whereas the tension between these two opposite perspectives is resolved by way of a *synthesis* of the two opposite perspectives, which ideally results in higher-order functioning, not simply in a compromise (a synthesis between the polarized statements concerning the value of inhibition versus disinhibition might involve a willingness to flexibly relinquish self-control when the situation calls for it).

Hegelian dialectics includes five key concepts or assumptions:

1. Everything is transient and finite.

2. Everything important in life is composed of contradictions (that is, opposing forces).

3. Gradual changes lead to crises or turning points, when one force overcomes its opponent force.

4. The world is holistic, and everything is connected and in relationship.

5. Change is continual and transactional (that is, opposing perspectives influence each other and evolve over time).

In RO DBT, the therapist uses dialectical principles to encourage cognitively rigid OC clients to think with more complexity as well as with more flexibility.

An example of dialectical thinking can be seen in the RO mindfulness skill of self-enquiry. As described in detail in chapter 7, self-enquiry requires a willingness to question one's beliefs, perceptions, action urges, and behaviors without falling apart or simply giving in. The dialectical tension involves balancing *trusting* versus *distrusting* oneself. Essentially, the question is *To what extent can I trust my personal perceptions at any given moment to accurately reflect reality?* Perhaps never, at least in absolute terms. The synthesis in RO DBT involves being able to listen openly to criticism or feedback, without immediate denial (or agreement), and a willingness to experience new things with an open heart, without losing track of one's values.

Dialectical thinking is also highly useful in loosening OC clients' tendencies toward inflexible rule-governed behavior, rigid Fixed Mind beliefs, and high moral certitude ("There is only one right way to do or think about something"), which can interfere with the ability to flexibly adapt to change and the ability to form close social bonds. For example, many OC clients consider "dependence" a dirty word (as reported by one OC client, "Dependence makes you weak and vulnerable to abuse"). Yet, regardless of our personal preferences, all humans are dependent on something or someone, at least some of the time; for example, we depend on our grocer to provide us with fresh milk, on our friends to tell us the truth, on our rock-climbing instructor to show us how to tie a knot properly, and on our parents' affection as infants. Moreover, our dependence on others does not negate the value of independent living, as in standing up against moral wrongs, striving to go where no one else has gone, saving for retirement to avoid burdening others, or voicing an unpopular opinion. Thus dialectical thinking is an important therapeutic tool in RO DBT. It allows a therapist to genuinely validate a client's perspective ("Being independent keeps you from being hurt") while maintaining its opposite ("Being dependent is essential for survival"), thereby creating the possibility for the emergence of a new way of thinking and behaving (a new synthesis). Finally, dialectical thinking also informs therapists' behavior during interactions with their clients.

In my work with OC clients, I have found that two dialectical polarities are most likely to arise:

1. Nonmoving centeredness versus acquiescent letting go

2. Playful irreverence versus compassionate gravity (see figure 10.1)

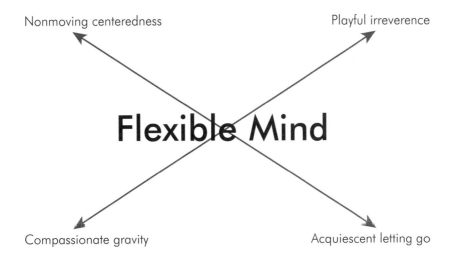

Figure 10.1. Dialectical Thinking in RO DBT

The next two sections of the chapter describe how these two polarities are used in RO DBT to enhance treatment.

Nonmoving Centeredness vs. Acquiescent Letting Go

The phrase *nonmoving centeredness versus acquiescent letting go* refers to the therapist's dialectical dilemma of knowing when to hold on to (rather than let go of) a case formulation, a theoretical insight, or a personal conviction when working with an OC client, in order to model core RO principles, maintain client engagement, repair an alliance rupture, or spur new growth. It is informed by an overarching RO DBT principle positing that therapists and clients alike bring perceptual and regulatory biases into the treatment environment, and that these biases influence both the therapeutic relationship and treatment outcomes. Therefore, being able to recognize and know when to let go of a bias represents an essential dialectical dilemma for the therapist in terms of the following therapeutic tasks:

- Maximizing the likelihood of forming a strong therapeutic alliance (RO DBT posits that a strong working alliance with an OC client is unlikely until multiple alliance ruptures have been successfully repaired over multiple sessions)

- Effectively modeling radical openness for the OC client

- Providing alternatives for the client's habitual ways of behaving and thinking

No small tasks, these! However, mindful awareness of the dilemma does not necessarily lead to synthesis, nor will it necessarily mitigate the emotional distress that can accompany the therapist's attempts to grapple with it (that is, both letting go of firmly held convictions and standing up for one's convictions can be painful therapeutic choices). Plus, to make matters more complicated, therapists *need* to be biased, at least to some extent; that is, the role of a health care provider necessitates professional opinions about a client's presenting problems and about the best course of treatment (such opinions are also known as a case conceptualization). Indeed, case conceptualization has been described as "the heart of evidence-based practice" (Bieling & Kuyken, 2003, p. 53). Therapists are usually trained to see their case conceptualizations as reliable and generally accurate descriptions of clients' behavior, despite research showing that therapists often formulate widely divergent case conceptualizations for the same client (Kuyken, Fothergill, Musa, & Chadwick, 2005). Yet, despite these difficulties, RO DBT posits that there is a way forward. It involves the therapist's creation of a temporary state of self-doubt whenever feedback from the environment or the client suggests that the case conceptualization may be in error.

Healthy self-doubt is a core construct in RO DBT (see chapter 7). It provides therapists with a coherent means of relinquishing control without abdicating their professional responsibilities, and without having to abandon earlier perspectives. To cite one example of the advantages of acquiescent letting go, a therapist in one of our research trials reported to his consultation team that he was struggling with knowing how to resolve a potential alliance rupture with his OC client. The client had been repeatedly dismissing any suggestion by the therapist that she was a decent human being or had prosocial intentions by saying, "You just don't know me. I am an evil person. I have a lot of resistance to joining the human race. I'm essentially not a very nice person, and my past, although I have shared little of it with you, is my proof." The therapist had attempted to point out factors that discounted or disproved the client's conviction, and yet each attempt appeared only to increase the client's insistence that she was inherently evil. Moreover, the therapist reported feeling increasing angst, since in his worldview it was impossible for humans to be inherently evil. The team encouraged the therapist to practice self-enquiry (that is, to create a state of temporary self-doubt), which eventually led the therapist to the discovery that it had been arrogant of him to assume that no one in the world could ever be inherently evil, an insight that enabled him to be radically open to his client's perspective, despite the pain it generated. In the next session, the therapist revealed his insight to the client—that he had been behaving arrogantly in prior sessions by assuming his worldview regarding evil to be the only correct one. His personal work on himself and his willingness to out himself immediately changed the dynamics of the therapeutic relationship and, to the surprise of the therapist, resulted several sessions later in the client independently revealing, "I've been thinking lately that maybe I'm not so evil after all." This clinical example demonstrates the therapeutic value of being able to radically give in, or let go of strongly held convictions, no matter how logical or viscerally right they may seem. The creation of a state of *temporary* self-doubt (via self-enquiry) does not mean approval, nor does it require a therapist to permanently let go of prior convictions; instead, it recognizes the therapeutic utility of closed-mindedness as one possible outcome (that is, nonmoving centeredness).

Consequently, nonmoving centeredness is the dialectical twin of acquiescent letting go. It refers to the importance of an RO DBT therapist holding on to a personal conviction or belief about a client, despite strong opposition from the client or the environment. The rationale for this stance may be best represented by the RO principle of kindness first and foremost, whereby, as discussed in previous chapters, kindness may sometimes mean telling someone a hard truth (in a way that acknowledges one's own fallibility) for the sake of helping her achieve a valued goal. Thus RO DBT therapists recognize that they may need to disagree with their OC clients to facilitate growth, albeit the vast majority of RO DBT confrontations involve asking (not telling) clients about their apparent problems, combined with offering nonverbal, nondominant social signals (a slight bowing of the head and a shoulder shrug along with openhanded gestures, warm smiles, eyebrow wags, and direct eye contact to communicate equity and openness to critical feedback). Nondominance signals are especially important when one person is in a power-up position yet desires a close relationship (as in the therapist-client relationship). This dialectical dilemma also allows for the possibility of less open-minded signaling (or urgency) and the use of dominant assertions of confidence in order to block imminent life-threatening behavior.

Playful Irreverence vs. Compassionate Gravity

Playful irreverence versus compassionate gravity is the core dialectic in RO DBT. It represents the fundamental dialectical dilemma therapists face when working with emotionally lonely and socially isolated OC clients: to welcome them back home and yet challenge them at the same time. The playful, irreverent part of this dialectic is the therapeutic cousin of a good tease between friends. Friends playfully and affectionately tease each other all the time. Teasing and joking are how friends informally point out flaws in each other, without being too heavy-handed about it. For example, research shows that teasing is how families and tribes provide informal feedback to individual members about minor violations of social norms ("Oops…did you just fart?"), selfish behavior ("Somebody made popcorn but forgot to clean up—I wonder who that could have been?"), and misjudgments about social status ("Of course, Your Majesty, we would be delighted to serve you").

As described in chapter 6, a good tease is always kind and is generally followed by a smile and other signals of friendliness, appeasement, and nondominance. A therapist who adopts a playful, irreverent style is challenging the client with humility, in a manner that is reserved for our most intimate relationships. Thus therapeutic teasing sends a strong, powerful message of social safety to emotionally lonely and socially isolated OC clients, one that essentially and wordlessly says, "You are part of my tribe."

Yet humans are not always nice, and teases are not always kind. As a species, we can be ruthlessly callous and deceptive to those we dislike, or to rival members of another tribe. Unkind teasing can be recognized most frequently by its lack of response to feedback, meaning that the tease just keeps on going, even when the recipient of the tease makes it clear (either verbally or nonverbally) that the tease has gone on too long, that she is not enjoying it, that she doesn't find it particularly amusing, and that she would like it to stop. Thus, when a smile or other appeasement signals arrive too late, a tease suddenly feels more like a put-down. Unkind teasing is similar to bullying but much scarier because it has plausible deniability: "Don't worry—I like you. The reason I never laugh at your jokes is simply because I don't find them funny." In RO DBT, I refer to unkind teasing as *niggling*, a way of getting back at people, punishing someone, or undermining the efforts of a rival without ever having to admit or take responsibility for one's nefarious intentions: "Who, me? No, I'm not trying to give you a hard time. Can't you take a joke?" (Niggling is also related to "pushback" responses, as we'll see later in this chapter.) It is the essence of dirty fighting and a source of secret pleasure (akin to envious schadenfreude, or experiencing pleasure when a rival is in pain or suffers a loss). Niggling and niggles are powerful because their function is to secretly control others, and yet the indirect manner in which they are expressed makes it plausible for the sender to deny doing so: "I really don't know what you're getting all upset about. It was only a joke." In fact, the more upset the recipient of a niggle becomes, the more powerful the niggler is likely to feel. Yet we hide our niggling from others (and often ourselves) because inwardly we know that niggling is an indirect way of communicating disapproval or dislike and represents a form of deception; the seemingly innocent joke or comment is intended to wound rather than help the other person, nor would we like to be treated by others in a similar fashion.

The good news is that therapeutic teasing is not niggling, so therapists can relax. Yet I am aware of imagining that all humans (assuming they have ever interacted with another person) have at least occasionally mistaken a kindhearted tease as a dig or a purposeful put-down, when none was intended, and so therapists might worry that their attempts to tease, joke, or be playfully irreverent with their clients might be taken the wrong way. My comment about this concern, using my best approximation of a Bronx accent, is "Fuhgeddaboudit." (That was a tease; you just couldn't see the smile and eyebrow wag that accompanied it). But, seriously now, why do you think I just said that? The reasons underlie much of what might be considered the essence of the RO DBT therapeutic style. But before we go there, I would like to introduce what I mean by the term *compassionate gravity* because doing so will help make sense of the why.

Niggling and Self-Enquiry

When niggling appears to be a significant pattern of behavior exhibited by an OC client, the therapist should encourage the client to practice self-enquiry. The following sets of questions can facilitate this process and help a client determine the extent to which this type of indirect social signaling reflects his core values:

- Do I ever secretly enjoy niggling others? Have I ever been secretly proud that I can appear nonjudgmental when in fact I am highly judgmental? Do I ever purposefully use a niggle to control or dominate others, block unwanted feedback, or achieve a goal?

- Am I secretly proud of my ability to niggle someone? What might this say about how I see the world and other people?

- Would I encourage a young child to niggle others when things don't go her way or she dislikes someone? If not, then what might this tell me about my values?

- Do I enjoy being niggled? If not, then what might this tell me about my own niggling behavior?

- How would I feel if I were to suddenly discover that others actually knew my true intentions or secret thoughts when I niggle them? What might my response to this question tell me about my core values, or about how I truly feel about the way I behave toward others? What is it that I might need to learn?

Compassionate gravity represents the dialectical opposite of the stance of playful irreverence. Rather than aiming to tease and challenge, it seeks to understand and signal sobriety (that is, it signals that the therapist is taking the client's concerns or reported experience seriously). It also functions as a way of taking the heat off a client, whereas playful irreverence puts the heat on (see also "Heat-On Strategies" and "Heat-Off Strategies," chapter 6). A stance of compassionate gravity is designed to slow the pace of the interaction and communicate social safety to the client. Here are the most common nonverbal behaviors that accompany a stance of compassionate gravity:

- Slowing down the pace of speaking

- Speaking with a softer voice tone

- Slightly pausing after each client utterance in order to allow the client time to say more (if so desired)

- Warm eye contact (not staring)

- A warm closed-mouth smile

- A therapeutic sigh of contentment

The therapeutic use of these nonverbal signals mimics how we speak to those we love in our most intimate moments. They function as powerful social safety signals and reinforce client engagement without ever having to say a word. Here are some additional nonverbal signals that commonly accompany a stance of compassionate gravity:

- Leaning back in one's chair

- Raising one's eyebrows when listening to the client (or speaking)

- Signaling nondominance and a willingness to be wrong, especially during an alliance rupture repair, via a slight bowing of the head, a slight shoulder shrug, and openhanded gestures combined with a closed-mouth smile

A stance of compassionate gravity also signals openness and humility. For example, a therapist who is able to admit that he is fallible, or that his personal worldview may have interfered with his understanding of the client's perspective, is practicing compassionate gravity. Indeed, compassionate gravity is invariably an essential part of a successful alliance rupture repair, or it can help balance a playfully irreverent comment in order to ensure that a therapeutic tease is not taken the wrong way. The overall aim is to communicate a genuine desire to know the client, from the client's perspective.

Both compassionate gravity and playful irreverence are powerful social safety signals; a good tease can make a person feel at home as much as a compassionate comment. Nevertheless, of the two dialectical poles, compassionate gravity is the easier one for most therapists to operate from, and it is often their default set point when in doubt (that is, most therapists, when in doubt about what to do, seek to validate, soothe, or empathize), whereas playful irreverence can make therapists feel that they are doing something wrong. Often this feeling of wrongdoing is a function of therapists' prior clinical training, or of common beliefs—myths, in my opinion—about how therapists should behave ("always assume the client is right" or "always be compassionate"). RO DBT obviously has similar values; otherwise, why would I use the word "compassionate" in the first place? The difference is that, broadly speaking, RO DBT prioritizes kindness over compassion when it comes to helping emotionally ostracized OC clients learn how to rejoin the tribe (refer to table 9.1).

What's important for therapists to remember, regardless of their personal experience or past history of teasing or being teased, is that the research shows that teasing is how friends, family, and tribes give each other feedback all the time, and it doesn't lead to major meltdowns or personal crises. Playful teasing between people is a statement of intimacy and trust, not of nefarious intent or malicious deception (that is, playful teasing is not niggling). It occurs only among friends and always ends with a nondominant or friendly signal, such as a smile, a head bow, or an appeasement gesture. Such signals of nondominance and friendliness are universally displayed across cultures, from the taunting laughter that ends with food giving of the forest Pygmies of the Congo (Turnbull, 1962) to the playful trickery and celebratory smirk of the Yanomamö tribe in South America (Chagnon, 1974) to the feigned aggressive giggle followed by gaze aversion and a smile common among the Japanese to the flat-faced barb that ends with a smile and an affirmative head nod seen in the British culture (see also Mizushima & Stapleton, 2006; Keltner, Capps, Kring, Young, & Heerey, 2001). That said, within a single culture there is a wide range of individual differences regarding the types of teasing that are deemed acceptable (such as a satirical comment or a cold bucket of water poured over someone else's head), the types of occasions deemed suitable for teasing (at funerals, some families celebrate the life of the deceased by teasing and joking, whereas other families would see this kind of behavior as disrespectful or uncouth), and who is allowed to be teased by whom (in some families or cultures, for instance, a child teasing an adult is considered inappropriate). Teasing is also moderated by individual differences in biotemperament, social status, and personality or coping style.

Therapists are not immune to any of these influences. Plus, how therapists have been trained, and the beliefs they hold about what is appropriate or inappropriate professional behavior (based on prior professional training), can also influence the ease with which they feel comfortable being playfully irreverent with their clients. Thus, when first learning RO DBT, therapists may find therapeutic teasing and playful irreverence anxiety-producing or uncomfortable. However, most often, upon reflection (self-enquiry), their discomfort with teasing is discovered to reflect personal preferences, personal beliefs, and past training, not the notion that teasing is terrible or damaging in itself; otherwise, why would friends affectionately tease each other and still remain friends, why would teasing occur across all cultures and in similar ways, why would so many people genuinely find kindhearted teasing amusing or fun, and why would teasing be a core part of flirting?

Nevertheless, most therapists find therapeutic teasing difficult because their OC clients are expert at subtly punishing any form of feedback, regardless of how it is expressed. For example, any attempt to tease, joke, or play in session may be met with an immediate flat face. Recall that the powerful impact that flat facial expressions exert on others is not solely a function of the absence of expression. Instead, the power of the flat face is derived from the conspicuous absence or low frequency of expected or customary prosocial signals (smiling, affirmative head nods) in contexts (such as a therapy session) that call for free expression of emotion. Another common reaction can be a "don't hurt me" response, characterized by gaze aversion and postural shrinkage, which implies that the therapist's playful irreverence is hurting the client and should stop immediately. The problem is that if the therapist immediately stops the playful irreverence, the therapist reinforces the very behavior for which she is attempting to provide corrective feedback via use of a therapeutic tease. Indeed, anthropological research examining the use of teasing within tribes shows that a tease is not removed until the errant member of the tribe admits to his wrongdoing and signals his willingness to repair the damage he has done (see the story of Pepei in Turnbull, 1962). Thus tribes are both tough and kind because their survival depends on every member contributing. Similarly, as tribal ambassadors,

RO DBT therapists are willing to personally suffer the pain of seeing a fellow tribal member (the client) struggle, in order to facilitate growth, without removing the cue or opportunity for learning at the first sign of discomfort on the client's part. That said, as we'll see later in this chapter, the reason for the dialectic is that both polarities matter.

Essentially, not only do OC clients take themselves very seriously, they also subtly reinforce everyone around them to behave seriously as well. Most often these sentiments are conditioned to appear whenever anyone (including a therapist) dares to behave in a manner that the OC individual disapproves of, dislikes, finds challenging, or considers inappropriate, and the punishment is usually delivered indirectly or nonverbally (for example, a flat face, a slight scowl, an unexpected awkward silence, averting or rolling of the eyes, or a sudden bowing of the head). This is not meant to imply that OC clients necessarily engage in this type of behavior with conscious intent; on the contrary, they suffer greatly and are unsure of how to change (which is why they are seeking treatment). Yet, like most of us, OC clients know more about themselves than they might care to admit, and genuine change is painful.

Thus, rather than immediately removing the therapeutic tease and behaving seriously, the kindest act for therapists working with OC clients is, in my opinion, to allow themselves and their clients the gift of friendship. That is, therapists should drop their guard in the same manner they do when among their friends. Translated into the context of therapy, this means dropping their professional role (at least to some extent) in the interest of helping their emotionally lonely and socially isolated OC clients learn what it viscerally feels like to have a good friend, to playfully engage in dialogue, to experience the self-confidence of belonging to the in-group, and to have the sense of security that emerges from belonging to a tribe.

> The kindest act for therapists working with OC clients is to allow themselves and their clients the gift of friendship.

Before we move on, let's return to my earlier comment, where I suggested that therapists need not be concerned that their attempts to tease, joke, or be playfully irreverent with their clients might be taken the wrong way (see my earlier "fuhgeddaboudit" tease). The question I left us to ponder is "Why do you think I just said that?" Essentially, was my joke more than a joke? The short answer is yes, it was. My teasing was purposeful and meant to facilitate learning. It was intended to model a therapeutic tease and simultaneously highlight how a playful, irreverent stance can function to capture attention by not always revealing everything all at once. Hopefully, it functioned as intended (and, assuming you have not yet drifted off to sleep, thanks for waiting). Next I describe some of the more practical features associated with this dialectic.

How Does the Therapist Know When to Be Playfully Irreverent and When to Exhibit Compassionate Gravity?

Here is the quick answer: the more a client's social signaling appears to represent hidden intentions or disguised demands, the more playfully irreverent (or teasing) the therapist, whereas the more genuinely engaged, candid, and open a client is, the more compassionate gravity the therapist is likely to exhibit. The reason therapists need to be adept at knowing when to move from playful irreverence to compassionate gravity, and vice versa, is twofold. First, this type of back-and forth interchange (from play to seriousness, then back to play again) reflects the type of ebb and flow that characterizes normal, healthy social discourse, thereby allowing an OC client an important avenue for practicing skills. Second, it helps prevent unnecessary therapeutic alliance ruptures. Recall that, although RO DBT values alliance ruptures as opportunities for growth, they are not purposefully created, since that would be phony. Conflict is inevitable in all close relationships; as such, therapists should not try to make ruptures happen; instead, they should just be themselves, and *voilà*—ruptures suddenly appear, like magic! Plus, especially during the earlier phases of treatment, OC clients are less likely to reveal negative reactions. Most maladaptive social signals are indirectly expressed and implied; they are disguised demands that function to block unwanted feedback or secretly influence the behavior of others, and the person making the demand never has to admit it (see "Indirect Social Signals and Disguised Demands," later in this chapter). Therefore, being able to move from playful irreverence to compassionate gravity (for example, from teasing to validating) is a very useful skill to possess, both in real life and in work with OC clients.

However, unlike in real life, therapists have a job to do, one that requires not only that they understand their clients as best they can but also that they be willing to provide their clients with corrective feedback (that is, point out painful truths that may be preventing clients from achieving their valued goals). Thus the utility of a therapeutic tease is that it provides corrective feedback (for example, by expressing incredulity and amused bewilderment when a client uses speech to tell you that he is unable to speak, or reports a complete lack of animosity toward a coworker he admits having lied about in order to get her fired). An example of this is the "Oh really...?" response, a classic RO DBT therapeutic tease. This is a form of social teasing or questioning that most people automatically use whenever a friend suddenly reports engaging in a behavior or a way of thinking that is opposite to or different from what the friend has previously reported, but without acknowledging the sudden change (for example, a friend who has always reported feeling criticized by his parents suddenly describes them as warm and caring). The "Oh really...?" response is designed to highlight social signaling discrepancies. It is most effective when accompanied by a signal implying disbelief (an expression of astonishment or surprise, or a lip curl combined with a tilt of the head), which is followed almost immediately by a signal of nondominance (a slight shoulder shrug and a warm closed-mouth smile). It implies friendly disbelief and allows an opportunity for the client to better explain his sudden change in position, without the therapist being overly officious, serious, or presumptuous. The therapist can use the client's response to "Oh really…?" to explore the discrepancy further:

Therapist: Just last week you were telling me that you hated your parents and blamed them for everything. Now, this week, you are telling me that you have never blamed them. Isn't that amazing? What do you think this might tell us, and how did you ever get to this place? *(Offers eyebrow wag and warm closed-mouth smile.)*

As another example of RO DBT playful irreverence, a therapist may respond to a client's report of feeling anxious (for example, about attending skills training class) or finding it hard to change her habits by saying, with a calm smile, "Isn't that wonderful." It is irreverent because the therapist's statement is unlikely to be what the client expected, and it is playful because the smile and the warmth in the therapist's tone of voice signal friendliness while simultaneously smuggling core RO DBT principles, without making a big deal of it (for example, one can follow through with prior commitments and feel anxious at the same time, and finding new lifestyle changes difficult should be celebrated as evidence of new growth and commitment).

Thus playful irreverence is challenging and confrontational, both verbally (via an unexpected question or comment that highlights a discrepancy in a client's behavior) and nonverbally (via an expression of surprise, a questioning tone of voice, or a curled lip), and it is followed almost immediately (in milliseconds) by nondominant body postures and friendly facial expressions (a warm closed-mouth smile and a slight shoulder shrug), which universally signal to the client that the therapist actually likes him and considers him part of the tribe. Playful irreverence can also be used as a minor aversive contingency that functions to punish (reduce) passive and indirect social signaling by an OC client (through the therapist's behaving as if the indirect or disguised demand has not been seen) until the client more directly reveals what her intentions or wishes are. For example, rather than automatically soothing or validating an OC client who turns away, frowns, or bows her head whenever she is asked something she would prefer not to hear, playful irreverence continues the conversation as if all is well. This forces the OC client to escalate the expression of the passive social signal, thereby making the maladaptive behavior more obvious and treatment targeting easier (extreme pouting is harder to deny); or, ideally, the client decides to explicitly communicate (via words) what she dislikes or is unhappy about (representing therapeutic progress and also perhaps an opportunity for an alliance rupture repair).

To summarize, the rule of thumb [(I know—we aren't supposed to be rule-governed in RO DBT, so for my sake just keep this to yourself) Editor's note: I'm listening] to guide the use of compassionate gravity versus playful irreverence in session is essentially this: the more maladaptive the OC client's social signaling becomes, the more playfully irreverent the therapist becomes, and the more engaged an OC client is in session, the more compassionate and reciprocal the therapist is likely to be (the therapist doesn't need to provide corrective feedback, because the client is working hard on his own). From a behavioral perspective, playful irreverence functions in the following ways:

- It places a maladaptive social signal on an extinction schedule when the therapist behaves as if the indirect signal was never observed.

- It helps determine whether the behavior is operant or respondent (see "Discriminating Between Operant and Respondent Behaviors," later in this chapter); if it is operant, the therapist can expect the maladaptive social signal to initially increase in intensity after the application of an extinction schedule.

- It makes candid expression of inner experience and emotion the most effective means of getting one's point across without the therapist making a big deal about it.

Whereas compassionate gravity functions to validate the client and communicate a nonpretentious sense of warmth and caring, in order to enhance client engagement and reinforce therapeutic change, playful irreverence is an essential part of welcoming the socially isolated and lonely client to rejoin the tribe.

When a Therapeutic Tease Falls Flat, Move to Compassionate Gravity

Therapists should anticipate signs of distress, confusion, uncertainty, and resistance whenever therapeutic teases are employed, because playful irreverence is not about soothing, placating, or regulating a client. Indeed, therapeutic teases are intended to playfully provide corrective feedback in order to help a client learn. Plus, there are lots of reasons why an OC client might not respond favorably to a therapeutic tease. Perhaps the first question is "How do you know that a client is responding favorably?" The best way to tell whether a client is responding favorably to feedback (such as a therapeutic tease) is to examine the extent to which the client remains engaged during the tease and immediately after the tease. Negative answers to the following questions suggest nonengagement:

- Does the client stay on topic?

- Does the client answer the question that you asked?

- Does the client maintain eye contact?

- Does the client laugh, smile, or chuckle when you do?

- Does the client use full sentences when speaking, not one-word answers?

- Does the client spontaneously bring up new information that is relevant or personally revealing, without your having to ask for it?

No matter how competent therapists may be in establishing connections with their clients or providing helpful corrective feedback, they should always expect therapeutic teases to fail. (Okay—not *always*.) Sometimes therapeutic teases fall flat because they are expressed too weakly, whereas other times they fall flat because they are expressed too strongly. Regardless of what happened, or why, whenever you sense that your tease was somehow not received as intended, or that it created more confusion, simply drop the tease—that is, let go of playful irreverence, and move toward a stance of compassionate gravity that encourages the client to join you in self-discovery.

"Why Do You Think I Just Said That?"

The good news is that therapists can relax when being playfully irreverent because, regardless of a client's response, it's always possible to repair any confusion or misunderstanding after an unsuccessful tease by using the following nifty three-step process:

1. Take the heat off the client (for example, by briefly disengaging eye contact for one or two seconds) and nonverbally signal compassionate gravity (for example, by leaning back while offering a closed-mouth smile and therapeutic sigh; see "Heat-On Strategies" and "Heat-Off Strategies," chapter 6).

2. Encourage the client to explore for herself the rationale behind the therapeutic tease by asking, "Why do you think I just said that?" while using nondominance (for example, slight bowing of the head, a slight shoulder shrug, and openhanded gestures) and cooperative-friendly signals (such as a warm smile, eyebrow wags, eye contact, slowed pace of speech, and a soft tone of voice) in order to encourage candid disclosure (see "Signaling Openness and an Easy Manner," chapter 6).

3. If the client continues to signal nonengagement, use the alliance rupture repair protocol (see "Repairing Alliance Ruptures," chapter 4).

Step 1

Step 1 of the protocol moves toward compassionate gravity by taking the heat off the client, without making a big deal of it. What is important to remember is that heat-off signals work as intended because you are not doing them all the time. Thus, despite the constant reminders throughout this book to adopt an easy manner when working with OC clients, this does not mean that you should always look chilled out, always lean back in your chair, always smile, always have your eyebrows raised, and so forth. That would be pretending, and both your body-brain and the client would know it, even though nobody would talk about it. (You wouldn't, because you would think this was what you were supposed to be doing, and your client wouldn't, either, because he would assume that you knew what you were doing. Isn't life fun?) Behaving with an easy manner is also context-dependent. Smiling, teasing, and lightheartedness are not always appropriate, and many situations in life call for solemnity and expressions of concern. If you constantly appear chilled out, you will not only seem a little strange (phony), you will also lose important opportunities for connecting with your client. Moreover, you will no longer be able to take advantage of a core RO strategy: leaning back in your chair works to signal social safety only if you were leaning forward in the first instance; briefly removing eye contact works to take the heat off only if you've had eye contact beforehand.

In addition, don't forget to move—avoid sitting in the same position for too long, whether leaning back or sitting forward. In real life, we shift our position, scratch, adjust our posture, wiggle our fingers, tap our feet, wave our arms, and change our expressions, depending on what's happening in the moment (and those who sit in a frozen position or rarely adjust their posture are read by others as a bit strange or odd, unless everyone is meditating in a Zen monastery). So sit forward, sit back, gesture expansively when making a point, smile, frown, look concerned, take a sip of water— it's what real people do in real-life interactions, and I am aware of imagining it is exactly what you do when you are among friends. Sitting still is what therapists do (we are often trained to sit still so as not to influence the client or appear professional), and who wants to act like a therapist?[58] Sitting still is similar to the feeling we get when we are asked to smile for the camera but the picture is delayed by a fumbling cameraperson; our candid smile of genuine pleasure quickly fades into a frozen, polite smile that feels increasingly phony the longer we hold it. It sends a message to your brain that danger may be present, not safety (when a rabbit sees a fox, the first thing it does is freeze all body movement). Real people in real-life friendly exchanges do not sit still or appear frozen—unless they are doing some major drugs! Plus, in RO DBT, we don't think it is possible to convince or talk our socially ostracized and lonely OC clients into coming back to the tribe; our job as therapists is to show them how to rejoin the tribe by behaving in the same manner with them as we would with our friends (the only exception to this is when imminent life-threatening behavior is present). My main point is this: when your client is engaged, it doesn't matter how you social signal. Leaning forward, expressions of concern, eye contact, and serious voice tones don't matter, because your client is engaged! Therapeutic social signaling matters primarily when your client is nonengaged, or when you are directly challenging your client (using the RO strategy of asking rather than telling). So relax or be tense, frown or smile, but whatever you do, make it real.

Step 2

Step 2 of the protocol places the heat back on the client, with a sense of open curiosity. Rather than immediately soothing, justifying, or apologizing after an apparently unsuccessful tease, ask: "Why do you think I just said that?" Combine that question with nonverbal signals of nondominance and friendliness to encourage candid disclosure and reduce the possibility of inadvertently reinforcing maladaptive indirect OC signaling and disguised demands (see "'Pushback' Responses" and "'Don't Hurt Me' Responses," later in this chapter). You can deepen compassionate gravity by explicitly explaining your therapeutic rationale for the tease—but, ideally, only after the client has attempted to explore the possible reasons on his own. Interestingly, even though one of the most common answers to this question from OC clients is "I don't know," OC clients often know more than they care to admit. Thus, despite often claiming ignorance, they often have some idea about what is going on (why you are teasing them), but they just don't want *you* to know that *they* know (not until they know you better). That said, often they have no idea of what is happening. What's important is that the client's awareness of what is happening when therapeutic teasing is going wrong doesn't really matter; what matters is whether the tease actually functions to help the client move closer to his valued goals.

Step 3

Step 3 of the protocol is designed to ensure client engagement and mutual understanding when prolonged verbal and nonverbal indicators of nonengagement (such as gaze aversion, continued indirect and vague answers, or lack of reciprocal laughing or smiling) suggest the existence of a possible alliance rupture. When this occurs, therapists should use the following questions to encourage candid disclosure and initiate the alliance rupture repair protocol (see chapter 4):

- What is it that you are trying to say to me right now?

- Would you mind saying that again? I'm not sure I really understood.

- I don't know about you, but it seems to me that something has changed. When you look down at the floor the way you're doing now, what are you trying to tell me?

The good news is that no matter how the client responds to these types of questions, you are in a win-win situation. By asking, not telling, you avoid making assumptions and at the same time provide an opportunity for the client to practice revealing her inner experience more directly (a core aim of treatment). Therapists should get in the habit of reinforcing the candid and open self-disclosures of their OC clients, especially self-disclosures that involve critical feedback, because this is how they will get to know their clients. I sometimes playfully refer to a client's candid self-disclosure (as opposed to masking) as the "gift of truth," a process of open, honest, direct communication that is encouraged between therapist and client. Most OC clients like having their self-disclosures named in this way, since this is linked to valued goals for honesty and integrity. Plus, the gift of truth can be used as a therapeutic tease (with therapists seeking permission from their clients to return the favor by providing the gift of truth to their clients as well as receiving it) and as a metaphor to encourage further candid disclosure from the client as well as candid feedback from the therapist. Finally, it is important to identify candid self-disclosure as a sign of therapeutic progress and an essential part of healthy intimate relationships.

OC clients are experts at masking inner feelings. Therefore, don't automatically assume that your tease or playful irreverence is not working, or that it's not being received as intended, just because you fail to get any feedback, or because the feedback appears negative. For example, the staring, flat-faced client—the one you are starting to believe may deeply hate you—may actually be working hard not to smile or crack up and may be inwardly feeling delighted, challenged, and amazed by your antics, and yet he dares not let you know that you are getting to him, because he has spent a lifetime convincing himself and others that he is incapable of feeling joy or pleasure (this is a fairly common response). If he allows himself to laugh or smile, even once, then this will prove to him that his life has been an entire sham, because happiness and positive social connections might have been possible. When the dilemma is expressed by a client overtly, reinforce the self-disclosure (thank him, point out how it makes you feel closer to him, and link it to his valued goals for closer relationships), and then, rather than trying to solve the dilemma or make it go away, encourage the client to use his conundrum ("This just proves I'm a failure") as the target for his self-enquiry practice of the week. This functions to smuggle two critical RO principles:

1. The client, like all of us, is responsible for how he chooses to perceive the world and himself (at least to a large extent).

2. Not every problem needs to be fixed immediately.

Plus, what is perhaps most important is that playful irreverence, when balanced by compassionate gravity, allows a client to experience firsthand what it feels like to be on the inside of a healthy interpersonal relationship, and it reflects the type of natural give-and-take and reciprocal sharing that occur among close friends. As such, therapists should not despair when a therapeutic tease fails to elicit a reciprocal smile or chuckle of engagement; the client may be much closer to signaling engagement than the therapist knows. In general, since a therapeutic tease is a form of contingency management, it theoretically should stop only after the client stops engaging in the maladaptive social signal and engages instead in a more prosocial or socially competent behavior (which could include an explicit request to stop teasing—a good friend stops teasing when asked explicitly). It is also important to keep in mind that therapeutic teasing is intended for maladaptive operant behavior, not respondent behavior (see "Discriminating Between Operant and Respondent Behaviors," later in this chapter). And, finally, it is important for therapists to remember that not every atypical or off-putting social signal is maladaptive or necessarily operant; a PNS-DVC shutdown response and the "deer in the headlights" response are two examples of common OC client behaviors that are respondent.

Dialectical Thinking Helps Loosen Rigid Thinking

Dialectical thinking allows for the existence of two seemingly opposite points of view at the same time (for example, "both independence and dependence have merit"), which can often prove immensely helpful when working with OC clients, who often tend to think more in terms of absolutes ("there is only one right way to do or think about anything"). Thus it is particularly useful when working on issues pertaining to the OC social signaling theme of rigid and rule-governed behavior. Both hold utility. Dialectical thinking allows therapists to acknowledge the truth within the client's perspective ("independence is essential") while simultaneously proposing its opposite ("dependence is a fact of life"), without assuming that one is better than the other, thereby allowing space for the client to find her own personal synthesis. The following clinical example shows an OC client early in treatment; the therapist has just begun working on gaining commitment from the client to target rumination and brooding as a possible treatment target linked to the OC social signaling theme of high social comparisons with envy or bitterness (see "RO DBT Treatment Strategies Addressing OC Themes," chapter 9):

Client: I don't really see this as a problem for me. My brooding reflects deep thinking. Careless thinking is what is making our world fall apart.

Therapist: I see your point. Thinking things through carefully is really important, and we certainly don't want to change that about you. (*Validates the importance of reflection while reassuring the client that changing this important part of him will not be the focus of treatment.*) In fact, if anything, we probably need to get you to think even more. I mean, after all, what is the essence of deep thought? (*Pauses.*) Perhaps it's the ability to question things, or oneself. Not taking things for granted—a form of self-enquiry. What do you think? (*Adopts a playful irreverent stance to link deep thinking with self-enquiry and challenge the client by suggesting that deep thinking is so important that the client needs to do it even more—a perspective that the client is unlikely to have anticipated; checks out client's perception prior to moving on.*)

Client: Yeah, that makes sense. Most people don't think enough—I see idiots everywhere.

Therapist: Yeah. So, on the one hand, we need to get you to increase your self-enquiry—your ability to think deeply. (*Ignores judgmental comment by client in order to stay focused on the dialectic.*) On the other hand, we want to honor the fact that thinking deeply, at its core, means questioning everything. Right? (*Looks at client; offers a closed-mouth smile.*) Meaning, not taking things for granted.

            (*Client gives slight affirmative nod.*)

Therapist: So if we are really going to be expert at not taking things for granted, it would seem that we would need to practice questioning our own beliefs—perhaps even our personal convictions about deep thinking. *(Reframes brooding and rumination as a conviction or belief while maintaining a collaborative "we" stance by implying that both therapist and client need to practice this type of questioning.)* That is, if we think deeply about deep thinking, who knows what we might discover? At the very least, we could feel proud for practicing what we preach…*(Pauses; offers closed-mouth smile and eyebrow wag)*…by not even taking our own convictions about deep thinking for granted. Sounds kinda fun. *(Offers closed-mouth smile, eyebrow wag; uses playful irreverence and logic to challenge client's resistance to examining habitual use of brooding.)* So, on the one hand, we need to value brooding, thinking deeply, and rumination. I mean, after all, they can lead to great things. On the other hand, we need to be better thinkers by using the essence of deep thought to challenge even our most basic convictions—perhaps even our beliefs about the value of deep thinking itself. *(Proposes a synthesis for the dialectical poles "brooding is always good" and "brooding is always bad.")* When I say this to you, what kind of thoughts or feelings come into your mind? *(Offers closed-mouth smile and eyebrow wag; checks in with client to determine the extent to which he is engaged and willing to pursue this way of thinking.)*

Despite reporting some trepidation, the client agreed that it might prove useful to learn how to question his personal convictions about deep thinking and brooding. When asked about his trepidation, he revealed that his reluctance to target rumination reflected a fear of failure (in prior treatments for his depression, he had been unable to stop or control his rumination successfully). The therapist thanked the client for his candor and then obtained the client's agreement to explain how RO DBT treats unhelpful rumination. The therapist explained that, for one thing, rather than focusing on reducing ruminative thinking or regulating emotion (that is, targeting internal experience), RO DBT is informed by a collectivist (rather than individualistic) model of emotion and emotional health, positing that individual well-being is inseparable from the feelings and responses of the larger group or community. Thus, in RO DBT, what a person feels or thinks inside, or privately (as in rumination), is less likely to be targeted for change, whereas how a person communicates or socially signals his inner experience, and how that impacts his social connectedness, are given higher priority. The idea is that when we feel part of a tribe, we feel safe, and as a consequence we naturally tend to worry less. Plus, since OC is primarily a problem of emotional loneliness, the emphasis is on helping the client learn how to rejoin the tribe. The therapist explained that from an RO DBT perspective, feeling happy is great, but when you are lonely it's hard to feel happy no matter how much you might try to accept, reappraise, or change your circumstances, or how much you might try to keep busy, exercise, practice yoga, or distract yourself.

This became an important therapeutic turning point for the client. Over the next couple of sessions, the client and the therapist worked together to identify how the client's brooding might manifest as a social signal. It soon became clear to the client that he frequently brooded around others, and he began to notice a common trigger—that is, his brooding behavior most often appeared to be triggered by perceived slights and feelings of being unappreciated or unrecognized, whereupon he would indirectly signal his dislike to others by furrowing his brow, frowning, and looking away or down. Other brooding-related social signals included purposely not laughing when a transgressor told a joke (or yawning when the transgressor talked), answering a question with a question, dropping the names of famous people he had met, reciting lines from a poem or a book, and delivering long-winded lectures or monologues. These social signals were monitored as a collective on the diary card under the label "My Little Professor." (RO DBT prioritizes labeling treatment targets colloquially—and, ideally, with humor—in order to smuggle the idea to overly serious OC clients that it is healthy to laugh at personal foibles.)

Other Common OC Dialectical Dilemmas

A common dialectical dilemma seen in work with OC clients revolves around issues of emotional experience and self-validation. As a group, OC clients tend to deny the experience of emotions (such as sadness, shame, anger, fear, and anxiety). They may hold beliefs that emotions are unsafe, destructive, intolerable, or a sign of weakness. As such, they will frequently invalidate or criticize their personal experience of emotions, particularly those emotions they consider socially unacceptable. Furthermore, when OC clients experience emotional leakage by inadvertently expressing an emotion at a higher intensity than they would have preferred, they are likely to judge themselves harshly for lack of self-control. Indeed, OC clients tend to discount and invalidate emotional experience globally, regardless of its valence (for example, discounting the utility of both positive and negative emotions), and to overvalue strategic or logical means of solving problems.

Almost paradoxically, OC clients can also appear to relish, romanticize, or become enveloped in certain mood states or emotions. When acting from this extreme, OC clients may experience secret enjoyment in feeling sad or melancholic, may appear to wallow in self-pity, or may appear to relish despair. This can manifest in a number of ways. For example, they may write tragic stories and poems, describe despair or melancholy as intellectually pure or noble, and relish a sense of nostalgic longing by listening to sad songs of unrequited love. They may delight in nihilistic thinking or cynicism, enjoy reading obituaries, and romanticize suicide or death. They may enjoy isolating or being estranged because it reinforces beliefs that no one cares, understands, or appreciates them. It is important for therapists to be aware that suicide risk may be higher when a client is operating from this state of emotional envelopment, necessitating a careful assessment of suicide risk. Similarly, melancholy, misery, and despair often signal that OC clients experience themselves as the victims, scapegoats, or martyrs of an unfair or unjust world (or of an unjust family). Clients' reasonable desire for recognition for their self-sacrifices—they often work long hours, forgo short-term pleasures, and follow rules when others do not—can lead to a sense of bitter longing. This longing for appreciation, which is in many ways justified, can lead to pervasive resentment that exacerbates feelings of isolation and distance from others. The problem for OC clients is that they have not allowed themselves periods of rest and relaxation, which are core antidotes to the burnout that stems from compulsive and obsessive self-control.

Therapists working with OC clients on this dialectical dilemma need to be aware of two issues that may make finding a synthesis difficult. First, when working with OC tendencies to invalidate emotional experience, therapists must remember that many OC clients do not experience emotional sensations in the same way others do and may lack the ability to label emotions. In addition, static mood states common among OC clients (such as constant feelings of tension, anxiety, and irritability) may make it difficult for them to notice emotions because they lack a contrast effect (sadness is easy to notice if one has just been experiencing joy). Thus therapists should be mindful to let go of hidden judgments or beliefs that a client may be purposely misrepresenting or lying about emotional experience. This allows an OC client the space she may need to explore the sensations that may be linked to emotions, without feeling pressured. Second, when OC clients appear to be operating from a stance of emotional envelopment, therapists should recall that feeling unappreciated is a natural consequence of striving hard to be the best, of always behaving properly, of forgoing pleasure, and of always following the rules. Furthermore, keeping tight control over one's desires, impulses, and emotions is hard work and frequently exhausting; yet, because OC clients tend to dislike making a big deal of their accomplishments, their self-sacrifices often go unnoticed. RO DBT addresses this dilemma with self-enquiry, in order for clients to explore what motivates them to help others and the extent to which their self-sacrifices fit with their core values. The dialectical synthesis most hoped for, from an RO DBT point of view, is for the client to recognize that she alone is responsible for deciding whether to help or not help another person. Her self-sacrifices are freely chosen, and consequently those people she decides to help don't owe her anything in return. At the same time, however, the client is able to recognize that self-sacrifice and reciprocity are equally essential for long-term healthy relationships. One OC client, via self-enquiry practices, began to recognize that what she described as her "saintly" self-sacrifices most often carried with them strong expectations that others should similarly reciprocate, and she would become quietly enraged when others failed to respond accordingly. Moreover, her self-enquiry led her to the realization that she had not made her desires for appreciation or help known to others (because doing so would be "selfish"). Together with her therapist, she was able to recognize that her fear of being dependent on others prevented her from asking for help. This self-discovery became an important step toward her repairing damaged relationships (by practicing being vulnerable and dependent on others) and simultaneously helped her reduce her overall sense of fatigue (because she could now allow others to help her rather than doing everything herself).

The Enigma Predicament

OC clients have been shaped to believe that self-control is imperative, and that it is intolerable to make a mistake. One way to avoid being criticized is to adopt the position "My problems are fundamentally different from others' problems," or to imply "My problems are so complex that no one could ever possibly understand them—I am not like other people" (which is true, by the way, but it's true of all humans, not just of OC clients). I refer to this as the enigma predicament, and it is a problem because it functions to subtly maintain OC social isolation, aloofness, and distance from others and can negatively impact the therapeutic relationship or demoralize the therapist; as one OC client divulged, "No therapist has ever truly understood me." Four stances associated with the enigma predicament (see figure 10.2) are considered most relevant because of how they negatively impact OC clients' social signaling and exacerbate an aloof and distant interpersonal style:

1. "I am not like other people."

2. "No one is capable of understanding me."

3. "Always have an answer, even if it's a question."

4. "Don't label me."

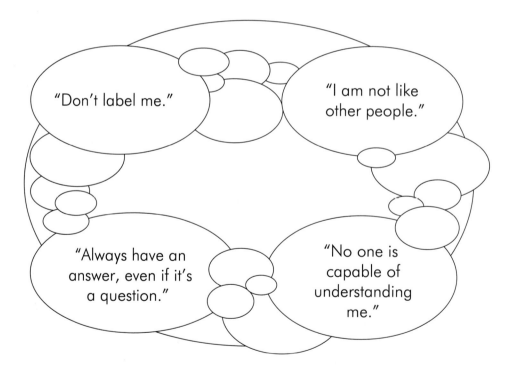

Figure 10.2. The Enigma Predicament

"I Am Not Like Other People"

The essence of this stance is that the OC client is fundamentally different or special. It implies that avoidance of social situations and of critical feedback is an appropriate response. As one client stated, "I'm not like most people. They seem to yearn to have others around. I learned long ago that most of that crap is phony." Another client revealed, "The reason I have never had a successful close relationship with anyone is because I am both discriminating and demanding. Most people settle for less." It is also one of the reasons why OC clients are sometimes misdiagnosed as having narcissistic personality disorder, since most people immediately respond to statements like these as being highly arrogant (and off-putting).

Therapists working with the "I am not like other people" component of the enigma predicament should look for opportunities to provide miniexercises in exposure to those interpersonal stimuli that OC clients tend to automatically avoid or discount as irrelevant (such as compliments, praise, offers of help, and normalization of their behavior). Doing so not only blocks maladaptive avoidance, which functions to maintain aloofness and distance, but also provides important corrective feedback, new learning, and opportunities to practice attachment and engagement behaviors with others. For example, often when OC clients are told that their behavior is normal, common, or understandable (since anyone in similar circumstances would have behaved the way they did), the result is a "pushback" response or an alliance rupture. However, the therapist should not take OC clients' frequent dislike of such comments to mean that he should stop sharing his observations of normality with his OC clients, since avoidance of this type of feedback maintains aloofness and distance. The following transcript illustrates some of these principles:

Therapist: I am aware of imagining that you are feeling misunderstood right now. Is that correct? (*Notices potential alliance rupture and asks about it.*)

Client: (*Shifts in chair*) No, not really.

Therapist: Hmmm. Are you feeling misunderstood about feeling misunderstood? (*Offers closed-mouth smile and eyebrow wag; uses a therapeutic tease to lighten the mood and encourage candid disclosure.*)

Client: Yeah, I guess I am. (*Chuckles, signaling engagement.*) It's hard for me to admit that I'm feeling misunderstood…(*Pauses*)…or feeling anything.

Therapist: Yeah, I can see this. (*Pauses slightly; moves toward a stance of compassionate gravity to reinforce candid disclosure.*) And at the same time, it makes sense to have a tear in your eye when you talk about your mom being in a wheelchair. Being sad about something like that is a normal reaction. (*Validates client's difficulty in talking about emotions and uses dialectics to guide the conversation back to what may have felt invalidating to the client.*)

Client: (*Looks directly at therapist*) I am *not* normal.

Therapist: *(Notices potential alliance rupture)* Well, you don't have a third eye, from what I can tell. *(Offers warm closed-mouth smile and eyebrow wag, signaling openness and playful irreverence to maintain the heat on the client and gently challenge the client's stance that she is different from others; pauses in order to allow the client time to respond.)*

(Client remains silent.)

Therapist: *(Leans back in chair; briefly disengages eye contact, and takes a slow, deep breath)* I guess what I am trying to say is that, whether you like it or not, you *are* normal, or at least similar to other people in some ways. *(Moves from playful irreverence to compassionate gravity by explaining the reasoning behind his teasing while retaining the perspective that client experiences normal human reactions.)* As we agreed earlier, part of our work is to get you to rejoin the human race. Every time you block a comment on my part that suggests you are part of a community, it seems to me that this only serves to make you feel *less* like you are part of something, not more. If anything, maybe we need to work together on getting you better at accepting that some of your responses, like your sadness about your mom, are the very things that tell us you are capable of joining the human race—because your reactions are normal! At least from my perspective. I suppose my question is this: What's wrong with being normal or like other people *(Pauses slightly)* at least some of the time? *(Offers closed-mouth smile, eyebrow wag; reminds client of prior commitment to work on improving relationships; uses "our work" and "we" to signal collaboration; uses strategies of asking rather than telling to signal humility and encourage self-enquiry.)*

Following this interaction, the therapist and the client agreed to target the client's avoidance of normality as maladaptive because it functioned to maintain her aloofness and distance from others. It was agreed that they would use behavioral principles of exposure to facilitate change in this area. The therapist obtained consent from the client to point out times in session when her responses appeared normal. It was explained that these moments would then be used as opportunities for the client to practice responding differently. Plus, informal exposure to even the word "normal" was introduced to the client as a playful way for her to overcome her aversion to the idea of being similar to other people. For example, it was explained that during discussion of an unrelated topic, the therapist might suddenly stop and, using a silly voice, playfully say aloud the word "normal" and then repeat it twice more (only louder). At other times, the therapist would ask the client to join him in repeating the word "normal," up to twenty times (this version soon evolved into a chant and, on one occasion, a song—much to the delight of both participants). These brief exposures laid down new associations to the word "normal" and helped the client learn how to laugh at some of her personal foibles and develop a sense of humor about her desires to "be an alien" (her words). Through self-enquiry practices, she was able to recognize that being part of a community, being similar to others, or being normal did not mean that she was doing something wrong, that she was boring, or that she had to give up her entire sense of self. For instance, the client considered idle talk to be a waste of time and stupid, and yet she did agree that social niceties or banter might be necessary early in a relationship, until the people involved got to know one another better. As such, one of her homework assignments included practicing chit-chat three times per week with someone she didn't know very well. Moreover, the client was encouraged to look for opportunities outside of session to go with the crowd or behave like others and then examine how this change in her social signaling impacted her relationships. The new social signaling insights that emerged from these exercises were then augmented by related RO skills, such as Match + 1 skills (see the material on Flexible Mind ALLOWs in the skills training manual, chapter 5, lesson 21).

This aspect of the enigma predicament can also manifest as secret pride in self-control. As mentioned repeatedly throughout this book, OC individuals are expert at inhibiting moaning, complaining, and crying when distressed; at planning ahead; at persisting in an uncomfortable task; and at ignoring short-term pleasurable rewards to achieve long-term goals. The value placed on self-control by most societies may function to reinforce these clients' beliefs that they are special or superior; indeed, oftentimes their pride is justified. At the same time, most OC clients have been socially anxious from a young age and have experienced themselves as socially awkward, odd, or inauthentic, compared to their peers (Eisenberg, Guthrie, et al., 2000; J. J. Gross & John, 2003). Thus, on the one hand, OC clients experience pride in their self-control, but on the other hand, deep down they feel inferior, socially excluded, or unsuccessful.

Yet sometimes discussing pride with OC clients can be difficult—they may consider pride morally wrong or inappropriate to acknowledge, since it implies that one is superior to others or may be seen as a form of boasting—and so secret pride is the most likely consequence. For example, as one OC client said, "This is really hard to admit, but deep down I feel that I'm better than most others at controlling myself, and this helps me maintain a belief that my standoffishness is not a problem." Some OC clients may push back when secret pride is discussed; as one client put it, "If I think so highly of myself, why am I so depressed?" The RO DBT therapist, using the moment to explore the extent to which the client was asking out of genuine curiosity rather than attempting to send the therapist a hidden message, said, "Hmmm." The therapist then paused, leaned back in his chair, offered an eyebrow wag, and said, "Interesting question. Do you believe you think highly of yourself?" This signaled to the client that the therapist had heard the question, and it also used the RO DBT strategy of asking rather than telling in order to assess the extent to which the client was genuinely engaged in seeing secret pride as a potential problem, as opposed to engaging in "pushback" behavior or signaling a potential alliance rupture (see "'Pushback' Responses" and "Indirect Social Signals and Disguised Demands," later in this chapter).

"No One Is Capable of Understanding Me"

This component of the enigma predicament makes it more difficult for others to desire to affiliate with OC clients or get to know them because it implies that there is no one with the intellectual or empathic capacity to truly comprehend their inner struggles, pain, or motivations. On the one hand, it is true that no one can truly understand the inner experience of another. On the other hand, people experience the feeling of being understood by others all the time, and this experience is an essential part of feeling socially connected. Persistently acting from a stance of being mysterious or incomprehensible is likely to punish attempts to understand. Eventually, people may simply give up trying to understand, which only confirms OC clients' original premise (that no one is capable of understanding them).

The stance just described not only exacerbates social isolation but can also block opportunities for growth. For example, whenever a topic is being discussed that the client dislikes, he or she may imply that the therapist is incapable of understanding. The therapist may then tend to avoid discussion of certain topics or inhibit certain responses in order to avoid upsetting the client. One client, asked about his emotional responses following a discussion in which he appeared to be upset, stated, "This sounds more about you than me," implying that the therapist's desire to understand the client's emotional experience more deeply was abnormal or reflected inappropriate needs. The therapist nondefensively and openly answered the client's disguised question and then used the RO DBT treatment strategy of asking rather than telling. "Hmmm," she said. "Actually, I was aware of imagining that you might have found our prior discussion somewhat distressing and wanted to make sure I gave you a chance to let me know what you were feeling…if you wanted to. Are you telling me that you don't want to talk about this right now?" The question was carefully worded in order to signal to the client that he could control the direction of the conversation if so desired, and, ideally, to help the client recognize that he is responsible for the decisions he makes in his life. This also provided an opportunity for the client to practice improving his social signaling by revealing his needs, wants, and inner experience directly rather than indirectly signaling them and either assuming that others understood him or blaming them when they appeared not to understand him.

When assessing this pattern, it is important for therapists to discriminate between "No one is capable of understanding me" and "You don't understand me." Unlike the distress most people experience when feeling misunderstood, an OC client whose behavior is being influenced by the enigma predicament may not be particularly distressed if misunderstood. In fact, being understood might actually be more distressing because it proves that being understood is possible and challenges a core premise needed to maintain an enigmatic persona. For instance, one OC client exhibited a slight burglar smile while stating, "I've seen over ten therapists, none of whom has ever been able to help me" (see "Burglar Smiles," chapter 6); the burglar smile leaked by this client suggested that he was secretly proud of his difficult-to-treat status, and so it also suggested the enigma predicament. To manage this, therapists must take the factors involved in treatment sequencing into account. For example, if this client's statement and burglar smile had occurred in the orientation and commitment stage of therapy, the therapist would have silently noted the behavior but ignored it for the time being (see appendix 5); the therapist's primary goal early in treatment is to establish a good working alliance with the client, not to address every potential maladaptive behavior. If it had been determined that this client's in-session reaction was secondary to feeling misunderstood or invalidated by the therapist (that is, secondary to something the therapist had done), then the protocol would have been to consider the statement and the burglar smile as indicating a possible alliance rupture and to work on repairing the rupture. If the same behavior had occurred after the alliance was well established, and if it had been determined that the function of the behavior was to allow the client to avoid participating, joining in, or connecting with others, then the therapist would either have ignored the behavior (in order not to reinforce it) or directly challenged the behavior (using strategies of asking rather than telling). For example, the therapist might have explicitly defined how and when the client's burglar smiles most often appeared and then conducted a brief chain analysis in order to determine the function of this social signaling behavior and the extent to which it impacted the client's social connectedness.

"Always Have an Answer, Even If It's a Question"

By always having some sort of response or answer for nearly everything, an OC client hopes to maintain an external persona or self-image of being knowledgeable, socially engaged, and competent. This component of the enigma predicament can manifest in a wide range of subtle behaviors. For instance, one OC client reported that she had become highly adept at steering any conversation away from herself by focusing on the other person, most often by asking what she referred to as "compassionate" questions about the other person's life. This helped her avoid discussing her own personal issues, revealing her true opinions, and appearing vulnerable or in the one-down position while also maintaining an outward appearance or persona of intimacy. On those rare occasions when someone would comment on her lack of personal self-disclosure, she would deny having any major issues needing disclosure, laugh it off, and change the topic, or she might turn the tables by suggesting that the other person seemed to worry too much or suddenly noticing that she was late for an appointment.

The "always have an answer" part of the enigma predicament often manifests in pretending: feigning interest (asking questions without real interest in the answers), signaling artificial concern (phony sympathy), pretending to be engaged (answering a question with a question in order to throw the other person off track), or falsely signaling openness (criticizing oneself before others can; as one client put it, "I'm happy to disclose a weakness as long as I identify it first"). The social signaling behaviors that accompany this component of the enigma predicament are often carefully rehearsed beforehand. In general, the aim is to create an outward persona or appearance of openness, connection, and humility while often secretly remaining closed, disengaged, or superior.

"Don't Label Me"

By shunning labels or categories and sidestepping public commitment, OC clients can avoid taking responsibility for their actions and can blame negative outcomes on others. If it is unclear what a person believes or feels, then it is very difficult to criticize or hold that person accountable. There is a wide range of ways in which this stance can be manifested. For example, one client indicated that, if pressed for an opinion about some problem, he would generally say, "I'll need to get back to you on that," with full knowledge that he would avoid ever doing so, and with the hope that the problem would go away. Some clients, despite explicitly admitting to characteristics of overcontrol, resist the "overcontrolled" label because acknowledging it might mean they would have to do something different. Other clients may resist diagnostic labels in general (such as "depression" or "personality disorder"), the conventional use of certain terms (for example, the word "normal" as a label for their behavior), or firm commitments to change (which they deflect by always saying, "I'll try"). The indirect nature of these social signals is what makes them so difficult to challenge, yet if they are not addressed, they function to maintain OC clients' sense of isolation by making it difficult for others to know their true beliefs.

The "don't label me" component of the enigma predicament is one reason why the use of written handouts in individual therapy is generally not recommended in work with OC clients (albeit handouts and worksheets are essential for teaching RO skills in skills training classes). After a well-intentioned therapist's attempt to speed up treatment targeting by providing a handout describing the five OC social signaling themes, one OC client asked, "Just what does this therapy pretend to be doing? I am a unique individual. This therapy doesn't allow any variations. It feels like I'm being forced into a pigeonhole."[59] From the client's point of view, it was impossible for the complexity of her inner experience to be summarized in one page. The cool thing is that the client's observation was correct, but at the same time it is unlikely that any form of written document, whether one or one thousand pages long, could adequately describe the complexity of any single human being. Despite this, our human brains are hardwired to categorize. We are highly adept at noticing and creating patterns (for example, a fluffy cloud suddenly transforms into a bunny rabbit), and this process is so automatic that most people are unaware of it when it is happening. Using one- or two-word descriptors to label complex patterns of behavior, rather than outlining every possible nuance, saves time and engenders mutual understanding when the descriptors carry shared cultural, tribal, or contextual meanings.

Interestingly, the "don't label me" component of the enigma predicament can evolve into a general avoidance of stating opinions, especially in public. As one client reported, "Whenever people ask me about my opinion, I always say, 'It depends,' and then I ask them what they think. It keeps me from ever having to take a stand and gives me time to figure out what they are up to. Once I know their perspective, I can take the heat off myself by pointing out a flaw in their perspective, without ever having to reveal what I actually believe." These disguised social signals are subtle enough to give an OC client plausible deniability or allow him to avoid direct comment from those on the receiving end.

Another manifestation of this stance appeared during the early stages of therapy with one client whenever his therapist described or reflected back what she had heard him say. The client would listen, with little expression on his face, and then he would often simply reply, "That's not my problem" and sit in silence until prompted. The therapist used the alliance rupture repair protocol to ascertain that the client's sudden silences were intended to communicate that her verbal reflections or descriptions, though broadly accurate, were not precise enough to be fully sanctioned by him. She then showed him three pebbles in a bowl and asked him how many objects he saw. The client replied that there were three objects. The therapist nodded and said, "Yes, but suppose we had a physicist in the room, and he looked at this and said there were three trillion objects, or electrons, in the bowl." She offered the client a closed-mouth smile and an eyebrow wag and then asked, "Which is the correct or more precise answer— three or three trillion?" The client, smiling sheepishly, replied, "You're trying to make a point, aren't you?" He then reluctantly admitted that, in the conditions described, there would be no correct answer. This "physicist metaphor," as it eventually came to be known, remained a playful inside joke and a reminder for the client to practice letting go of rigid insistence on precision in all circumstances. Plus, this metaphor became the impetus for major changes in how the client socially signaled disagreement; that is, he learned to do so more directly, and with humility. The following transcript provides another example of how the "don't label me" component can manifest:

Therapist: So you were feeling pretty upset, and very depressed. Do you think this could have been a time to try to use skills? (*Assesses client's engagement.*)

Client: When you're that depressed, you can't think of anything to do.

Therapist: I understand it's really hard, but my question is, do you think that it might be effective to try to use some skills? (*Holds the cue.*)

Client: What would you suggest? (*Answers question with a question.*)

Therapist: I'm not really sure (*Pauses*)…but we should definitely sort this out before we end today. (*Directly answers client's query in an open manner while maintaining the cue by not immediately providing solutions.*) My question was more about your level of commitment—whether, when you're depressed, you think it would be worthwhile to try to use skills. (*Uses "ask, don't tell" strategy; orients client to focus on the question.*)

Client: Not particularly. (*Avoids taking a stance, signaling a possible "pushback."*)

Therapist: Let's suppose you had a good friend who was depressed, just like your situation. (*Hypothesizes that client may be wanting to avoid this discussion, and decides to modify the approach by using a metaphor about a good friend.*) Would you tell her to try to do something to feel better? Or would you say, "Just be depressed—there is nothing you can do"?

Client: I haven't the faintest idea. Listen sympathetically, I suppose. *(Remains nebulous.)*

Therapist: *(Smiles)* So you actually do have a skill that you would suggest. *(Uses open curiosity, playful irreverence, and an easy manner to keep client focused on the target of assessing her commitment to use skills.)*

Client: I do? *(Implies lack of awareness.)*

Therapist: Yeah. You just said it. You said you would listen sympathetically. *(Pauses.)* So maybe if you were to use the skill of talking about problems, your depression might improve. *(Refers to client's comment in a matter-of-fact and easy manner in order determine client's level of engagement.)*

Client: Talking about problems makes matters much, much worse. *(Implies that she is not engaged in treatment.)*

Therapist: So *(Pauses slightly)*…talking about problems makes someone feel worse? *(Assesses the meaning of client's previous statement.)*

Client: For me, it does. But for others, it seems to make them feel better. At the community center, people are always talking to me about their problems.

Therapist: Do you like listening to other people?

Client: Not particularly. Eventually I decide that they're an awful bore. *(Pauses.)* For instance, there's this one person—she loves to complain, she has aches in her hands, aches in her back. *(Avoids stating a firm opinion.)*

Therapist: So you find this person annoying.

Client: No, not really. *(Maintains ambiguous stance by appearing to reverse her earlier statement.)*

Therapist: Oh, so you actually *like* talking to her.

Client: No, she is a user of people. She's like a scrawny little kitten—"poor little me." *(Avoids joining with therapist by reversing the prior implications.)*

Therapist: So you *don't* like her. Maybe we should work on skills to get her to stop talking to you! *(Uses playful irreverence; retains focus on assessing client's engagement.)*

Client: No, I'm kind of fond of her. *(Pauses.)* She's just a pitiful old thing. *(Switches her apparent perspective again.)*

Therapist: Hmmm. I am starting to notice something happening here. Have you noticed it? *(Pauses.)* I am starting to become worried that perhaps I am missing something, because it seems that every time I try to reflect back what I just heard you say, your reply seems to be the exact opposite of what I said. Can you give me a sense of what you think might be happening? *(Decides that exploration of a potential alliance rupture should take priority over discussion of any other topics.)*

In summary, the problem with the enigma predicament is that it maintains an OC client's aloofness and distance by keeping others from truly knowing the client's inner feelings, thoughts, doubts, or desires. In order to develop a close relationship with someone, it is necessary to disclose private thoughts, express vulnerable emotions, and reveal faults; indeed, genuine friendship and connectedness require vulnerable self-disclosure and being open to another person's feedback or differing opinions. Yet, despite this, a therapist is unlikely to immediately challenge or target an indirect social signal that appears to be linked to the enigma predicament, especially when first getting to know a client. As described earlier (see "Targeting In-Session Social Signaling: Basic Principles," chapter 9), an indirect social signal is targeted in session only after the maladaptive social signal has been displayed multiple times over multiple sessions. Rather than prioritizing for treatment the various emotions, moods, belief systems, or cognitive schemas associated with enigma predicament–linked responses, RO DBT targets how these internal experiences and beliefs are expressed on the outside, and the extent to which these social signals impair the client's social connectedness and interfere with his achievement of his core valued goals.

Behavioral Principles and Strategies

Behavioral principles and cognitive behavioral strategies are a core part of RO DBT. They are used both to help understand and to intervene with OC problems. Behavioral reinforcement theory is used to explain how certain maladaptive OC social signaling deficits and excesses are intermittently reinforced over time (for example, "pushback responses" function to block unwanted feedback or requests; see "'Pushback' Responses," later in this chapter). The aim in this part of the chapter is to provide a basic overview of behavioral principles and strategies, with an emphasis on those most salient in the treatment of OC problems.[60]

However, before proceeding, it may be useful to note that even though the laws of reinforcement are relatively straightforward, the technical language used to describe them is not always intuitively clear. For example, even behaviorally trained therapists often mistakenly use the term *negative reinforcement* to refer to a punisher (but negative reinforcement actually increases the probability of a response, whereas a punisher decreases it). Moreover, to make things even more confusing, professional behaviorists often use different terms to describe the same principle, or the same term to describe different principles (for example, reinforcement training is variously called *operant conditioning, behavior modification, shaping, contingency management,* and *instrumental learning*). With the aim of avoiding further confusion, the following section offers definitions of some core terminology, with clinical examples, as appropriate.

Basic Learning Principles Defined
Reinforcement

Repetitive behaviors are usually reinforced behaviors. Indeed, any behavior that occurs repeatedly does so because it functions to produce (at least occasionally) a desirable consequence (albeit the person may not be consciously aware of this). For example, compulsive fixing is reinforced when this solution works; shutting down and giving up are reinforced when someone else assumes responsibility for a problem; pretending not to hear unwanted feedback is reinforced when others stop giving it; working obsessively may be reinforced by a promotion at work.

A reinforcer is any consequential event that functions to increase the probability of an antecedent behavior occurring again in the future. Importantly, not all reinforcers are rewarding (feel good); some are relieving because they involve the removal of an aversive event (negative reinforcement). Similarly, not all factors that function to decrease a behavioral response are aversive; some are frustrating (extinction), and some are penalizing (negative punishment). Plus, what is reinforcing or punishing for one person may not be for another; for example, one person may learn to cope with unwanted feedback by pretending not to hear it, and this behavior is reinforced when others stop providing feedback, whereas for another person the same lack of feedback might function as an aversive contingency (punisher).

Reinforcement is a consequence that results, on average, in an increase in a behavior in a particular situation. Positive reinforcement increases the frequency of a behavior by providing a positive or rewarding consequence:

> **Client example:** Harsh self-criticism is positively reinforced when it elicits caregiving or soothing from others.

> **Therapy example:** After an honest and candid expression of emotion or vulnerability by an OC client, a therapist who briefly thanks the client for his candid disclosure is positively reinforcing (or attempting to reinforce) open expression of emotion.

Negative reinforcement increases the frequency of a behavior by removing or stopping an aversive stimulus:

> **Client example:** A client may learn to avoid unwanted critical feedback by pretending not to hear it (operant response), and this behavior is negatively reinforced when the other person stops providing the critical feedback (aversive stimulus).

> **Therapy example:** Since almost all OC clients strongly dislike the limelight, the removal of scrutiny or attention is a powerful (negative) reinforcer. RO DBT heat-off techniques are an example of how therapists can strategically use attention to shape adaptive behavior (see "Heat-Off Strategies," chapter 6).

Punishment

Punishment is a consequence that results, on average, in a decrease in a behavior in a particular situation. Positive punishment decreases the frequency of a behavior by providing an aversive consequence:

Client example: A client uses a hostile or blank stare ("the look") to purposefully punish feedback or criticism she does not want to hear.

Therapy example: Since OC clients dislike the limelight, therapists can strategically use heat-on techniques as an aversive contingency (see "Heat-On Strategies," chapter 6). Most often this involves some form of directed attention by the therapist, whereby the client momentarily feels scrutinized (for example, direct eye contact, repeating a request, or therapeutic teasing).

Negative punishment decreases the frequency of a behavior by removing or stopping a positive stimulus. It is penalizing because it removes a rewarding event:

Client example: A client withdraws warmth from his voice tone when someone is late for an appointment.

Therapy example: An inpatient unit removes a client's telephone privileges after a client misuses them.

Extinction

Extinction reduces the likelihood of a behavior because reinforcement is no longer provided in a particular situation. Extinction principles are used frequently in RO DBT, most often to decrease indirect social signaling and disguised demands:

Client example: A client who never acknowledges smiles from others will likely extinguish smiling behavior in other people, especially people the client encounters on a regular basis.

Therapy example: A therapist is placing a "pushback" or "don't hurt me" response on an extinction schedule when he ignores it and carries on with his agenda as if nothing has happened (see "'Pushback' Responses" and "'Don't Hurt Me' Responses," later in this chapter).

Extinction Burst

An extinction burst is a temporary increase in the frequency and intensity of a behavior when reinforcement is initially withdrawn. For most OC clients, an extinction burst involves gradual increase in the intensity of an indirect social signal or disguised demand. An extinction burst is like a social signaling temper tantrum—and the most effective way to respond to a temper tantrum is to ignore it:

Client example: A client's averted gaze (the initial indirect social signal) suddenly transforms into the client's lowered head, her slumped shoulders, and her hands covering her face, almost immediately after her therapist fails to respond to the averted gaze in the way the client desires (see "'Don't Hurt Me' Responses," later in this chapter). In this case, the extinction burst is the sudden increase in the intensity of the client's nonverbal signaling.

Therapy example: The therapist ignores the client's extinction burst until the client displays a more adaptive social signal by directly revealing what she wants or needs.

It is important to note, however, that if an extinction burst continues, and the client does not offer a more direct expression of her needs, wants, or desires, the therapist should shift to the alliance rupture repair protocol and enquire openly about what is happening. The good news is that both approaches—either continuing to ignore the extinction burst or inquiring into what is happening—will decrease the frequency of indirect social signals and disguised demands.

Shaping

Shaping is the process of reinforcing successive approximations toward a desired behavior:

Client example: Early family and environmental experiences that overvalued an appearance of control may have repeatedly reinforced the client in masking his inner feelings and constraining his expressions of emotion, to such an extent that his unexpressiveness became a source of admiration: "You appear so calm in a crisis. That is really amazing!" Unfortunately for the client, however, always being calm, nonreactive, and unexpressive is not particularly beneficial when it comes to establishing and maintaining intimate bonds.

Therapy example: A therapist who wants to encourage an overly shy OC client to give his opinions may initially reinforce anything the client expresses that even slightly resembles him giving an opinion and may then gradually shape more effective opinion-giving behavior.

Natural vs. Arbitrary Reinforcement

Natural reinforcement is innately connected to a desired behavioral response, whereas arbitrary reinforcement is not something that occurs naturally in the client's normal living environment:

Client example: A client who buys a gift for every new person she meets, or who brings cake to every meeting she attends, is using arbitrary reinforcement.

Therapy example: A therapist who says "Thank you" every time his OC client candidly reveals her inner feelings is overusing this reinforcement strategy, and it can quickly begin to feel arbitrary and contrived to the client. Instead, the therapist should prioritize using nonverbal social safety signals, such as openhanded gestures, a musical tone of voice, or eyebrow wags, since they are naturally reinforcing for most people, regardless of cultural background or learning history.

Fixed (Steady) vs. Intermittent (Variable) Reinforcement

Fixed or constant reinforcement is needed during the early phases of learning. However, once the new behavior has been acquired, a variable or intermittent schedule of reinforcement is more likely to maintain it. For example, slot machines in Las Vegas intermittently reinforce a player's continued insertion of coins by only occasionally and unexpectedly delivering the reinforcer (loud bells and whistles accompanied by the clanging of coins hitting a metal basket). Intermittently reinforced behavior is the most difficult to extinguish or change (which is why gambling is so addictive).

Parsing Behavior from Social Signaling

What is a behavior? From a radical behaviorist point of view, a behavior is anything a person does, publicly or privately, including thinking, feeling, and acting; that is, B (behavior) = R (response). Similarly, RO DBT does *not* consider private behaviors, such as thinking, sensations, urges, or emotions, to be qualitatively different from overt behaviors, since private and public responses are subject to the same behavioral principles. Yet RO DBT differs from other treatments, including so-called third wave behavioral treatments (Hayes, 2004), in its emphasis on social signaling, both as the primary mechanism of change and as the primary problem targeted for change. Why the emphasis on social signaling? The quick answer is that social signals represent a unique class of overt behaviors that powerfully impact social connectedness. Social signaling deficits are posited as the core source of OC loneliness, isolation, and emotional distress.

So what is a social signal? RO DBT defines a social signal as any behavior a person performs in the presence of another person, whether intentionally or not (for example, sometimes a yawn is just a yawn) and whether consciously or not (for example, an involuntary sigh). Actions, gestures, or expressions delivered without an audience (that is, in private) are simply overt behaviors, not social signals. Even when rehearsing in front of a mirror what you might say to your boss, you are not socially signaling; you are simply preparing your lines before you go onstage. Thus a social signal (SS) = a public R (response).

According to RO DBT, human social signaling behavior evolved not just to communicate intentions but also to facilitate the formation of strong social bonds among unrelated individuals. This facilitative advantage resulted in unprecedented collaboration among unrelated individuals—a unique human feature that to this day is unparalleled in the animal world. We are constantly socially signaling when around others (for example, via microexpressions and body movements), even when we are deliberately trying not to (for example, silence can be just as powerful as nonstop talking). As a consequence, most RO DBT behavioral interventions focus on reducing factors that interfere with social connectedness, and all of the skills in RO DBT are designed to address core OC social signaling deficits in one way or another.

Thus the key to effective treatment targeting when treating problems of overcontrol is not to focus solely on inner experience (such as dysregulated emotion, maladaptive cognition, lack of metacognitive awareness, or past traumatic memories) as the source of OC suffering. Instead, RO DBT targets indirect, masked, and constrained social signaling as the primary source of OC clients' emotional loneliness, isolation, and misery. Indirect social signals interfere with social connectedness because they make it harder to know the sender's true intentions (for example, a furrowed brow can reflect intense interest or disagreement). Plus, although words can help, words alone are not enough when it comes to forming intimate bonds. It's not what is said, it's *how* it is said (for example, a person can say the words "I love you" in a manner that leaves the recipient thinking otherwise). People trust what they observe. Therefore, targeting social signaling problems in OC clients, rather than inner experience, has the additional advantage of being undeniable because a social signal, by definition, is a publicly observable behavior, making it harder to ignore its consequences or pretend that all is well.

Essentially, when social signaling is targeted, the OC client loses his shield of plausible deniability. Even when a social signal (such as a yawn) occurs unintentionally or without conscious awareness, it should be examined as a potential target if it functions to damage or potentially damage relationships. For example, an OC client might have a habit of furrowing his brow and frowning whenever he is concentrating or listening intently; unfortunately for the client, however, most people interpret frowns and furrowed brows as signs of disapproval or dislike, and frowning often triggers reciprocal frowning in recipients as well as reduced desire for affiliation. The main point to remember is that self-reported intentions or conscious awareness of a social signal are not necessary for effective targeting; instead, the maladaptive nature of a social signal is defined by the extent to which it interferes with social connectedness and interpersonal relationships (see "Targeting In-Session Social Signaling: Basic Principles," chapter 9).

In addition, social signaling behaviors may appear on the surface to be the same or similar, but in reality they may be functionally quite different. For example, ignoring one's own needs in order to care for another might function to maintain a relationship for one person, to elicit nurturance for another, to reduce aversive emotions for a third, and to self-punish for a fourth. Thus, similar to third wave behavioral treatments, RO DBT considers psychological acts to be best understood contextually and functionally (Hayes, Follette, & Follette, 1995).

Finally, social signaling targets can be broadly classified according to whether the social signal in question is occurring too frequently (and is therefore excessive), not frequently enough (and therefore represents a deficit), or at the wrong time or place (and is therefore an outcome of faulty stimulus control; see table 10.1). Distinguishing among these three characteristics of a problematic social signal helps therapists identify what should be reinforced (or not) and determine the contingency-management principles that are most likely to be effective.

Table 10.1. Defining Social Signaling Problems Behaviorally

Problem	Description	Example
Social signaling excess	Behavior is unwanted	Walking away
Social signaling deficit	Behavior is desired but missing	Not engaging in vulnerable self-disclosure
Faulty stimulus control	Behavior occurs in wrong situation or fails to occur in right situation	Displaying a flat, nonexpressive face regardless of the situation

Discriminating Between Operant and Respondent Behaviors

An important task for therapists working with OC clients is to determine whether the maladaptive behavior is respondent or operant, since doing so helps guide the interventions to be used:

- Is the maladaptive behavior *respondent?* That is, is it controlled by a stimulus that precedes the behavior? For example, the flat, numbed, blank facial expression commonly observed among anorexic individuals often reflects a respondent reaction to prolonged starvation. Extreme undernourishment can trigger evolutionarily prepared shutdown responses designed to conserve energy and maximize survival (see chapter 2). The respondent behavior, in this case, is the numbed and flattened facial affect. It is maladaptive because a flattened affect stemming from PNS-DVC activation makes it biologically more difficult to signal genuine prosocial and friendly intentions (even when one is desperate to do so), and as a consequence it negatively impacts social connectedness. Respondent behaviors can be unconditioned (automatic) or conditioned (learned). For example, an unexpected loud sound elicits an unconditioned startle response in most humans, and the "deer in the headlights" response (see chapter 6) is an example of an unconditioned anxiety response triggered by prolonged eye contact from the therapist. By contrast, a (classically) conditioned response occurs whenever a previously neutral stimulus (such as being asked for an opinion) becomes paired with an uncon-ditioned response (extreme fear because the client's mother locked her in a closet whenever she dared to disagree). In general, respondent behaviors are not easily controlled (for example, it is hard to inhibit blushing once the process of blushing has already started). The good news is that new responses can be learned (see "Using Behavioral Exposure to Enhance Social Connectedness," later in this chapter).

- Is the maladaptive behavior *operant*? That is, is it controlled by contingencies of a reinforcing or punishing stimulus that follows the behavior? For example, pouting, a maladaptive social signal, is reinforced whenever the recipient soothes the pouter.

- Is the behavior the product of a *combination* of operant and respondent con-ditioning? For example, sometimes a yawn is just a yawn (respondent behav-ior triggered by tiredness), whereas at other times a yawn is more than a yawn (an operant response that is negatively reinforced when it functions to help the client avoid an unwanted topic).

Treatment Not Working? Think Behaviorally!

Maladaptive OC behavior persists because it gets reinforced. Yet the very same reinforcement principles that reinforce maladaptive OC behavior can equally influ-ence therapists to deliver less than effective therapy. Thus, when a therapist finds herself struggling with understanding a client, knowing what to target, or feeling demoralized about the case, she should include in her evaluation a functional analysis of her own behavior (ideally, by watching a videorecording of a session, with a supervi-sor or in a consultation team). For instance, an OC client may initially respond to a challenging question from the therapist by pouting or looking away. If the therapist then stops asking the challenging question, the pouting behavior is more likely to occur again in the future whenever the client feels challenged, since it has been rein-forced by the therapist's removal of an aversive contingency (that is, the challenging question; see "Reinforcement," earlier in this chapter). In this situation, the client is using an aversive contingency (pouting) to punish the therapist for asking a challeng-ing question, and the therapist has inadvertently reinforced pouting (via negative rein-forcement) by removing the aversive stimulus (the challenging question) and changing the topic. If this dynamic is repeated without intervention from the therapist, the most likely outcome will be an increase in the frequency and intensity of the client's pouting behavior, increased meekness on the part of the therapist, and poor treatment out-comes. The way forward is for the therapist to learn how to recognize when an indirect social signal is maladaptive and not reinforce it—in this case, by placing pouting on an extinction schedule (see "'Don't Hurt Me' Responses," later in this chapter).

RO DBT also uses reinforcement principles to shape adaptive responses (such as vulnerable self-disclosure and candid expression of emotion) that are linked to establishing and maintaining close social bonds. Unfortunately, however, the subtle nature of most OC behavioral responses can make it difficult for therapists (or others) to identify what to reinforce. Plus, high self-control is often equated with approach coping. Traditionally, avoidance coping has been associated with poor mental health outcomes and harmful activities, whereas approach coping is usually assumed to be the healthiest and most beneficial way to reduce stress. However, OC clients compulsively and excessively use approach coping, even when doing so may cause harm. For example, they are unlikely to put off an important task simply because it elicits discomfort but are more likely to work obsessively in order to complete the task, regardless of other life circumstances. Maladaptive approach coping can be both positively reinforced (for example, by a sense of pride in achievement) and negatively reinforced (for example, by reductions in arousal secondary to planning ahead), whereas maladaptive avoidance coping is primarily maintained via negative reinforcement (for example, by reductions in aversive arousal secondary to avoiding a feared stimulus; see "Reinforcement," earlier in this chapter). Thus one important distinction between RO DBT and other behavioral treatments is that approach coping is not always considered advantageous, particularly in treating problems of overcontrol.

It is also important to recognize that punishment and aversive contingencies (for example, "If you don't give me what I want, I will take you to court and sue you") are less effective than positive reinforcers (such as expressing appreciation and promising to return a favor). Punishment (or the threat of punishment) is also less likely to result in long-term changes: when the cat's away, the mice will play (that is, when the punisher is not around, old behavior reemerges). Although punishment or threats of punishment can force compliance, among humans punishment often results in resentment, grudges, desires for revenge, and/or passive-aggressive behavior directed at the punisher. The price for punishing behavior in long-term close relationships is rarely worth it. Thus, since the overarching goal in the treatment of OC is to help the client rejoin the tribe, aversive contingencies are applied judiciously in therapy and are usually mild (see "Teasing, Nondominance, and Playful Irreverence" and "Heat-On Strategies," chapter 6).

Using Behavioral Exposure to Enhance Social Connectedness

Almost ubiquitously, OC clients report social situations as mentally exhausting—and the very situations they find fatiguing, others are likely to find rewarding or reinvigorating. Thus, for OC clients, the types of stimuli they are most likely to fear are social in nature, particularly social events requiring spontaneity, joining with others, or sharing inner experiences.

For example, an OC client may have been punished for stating opinions that were not approved by his parents; now, as an adult, he experiences automatic anxiety whenever he is asked for his opinion. Nevertheless, there is little or no threat of harm to him for stating his opinion as an adult. In fact, avoidance of giving his opinion as an adult negatively reinforces his fear of stating an opinion by reducing his anxiety about it. Exposure works by repeatedly presenting the cue (such as stating an opinion, an adaptive social signal) while blocking the automatic escape response. In the absence of a harmful consequence, the link between opinion giving and anxiety is weakened.

Traditionally, behavioral exposure principles and exposure therapy have involved an individual's repeated exposure to fear-provoking stimuli in the absence of repeated aversive outcomes, However, research has shown that repeated nonreinforced exposure to conditioned stimuli (CS) does not weaken the initial association formed by the pairing of the unconditioned stimulus (US) and the CS. Instead, exposure masks the CS-US relationship, and extinction training involves the learning of new CS associations (Robbins, 1990). In this framework, behavioral exposure entails the active learning of alternative responses to stimuli that elicit unwanted internal experiences (for example, relative safety in the presence of conditioned fear cues). Thus what is behavioral exposure? It is *not* simply shaving away a learned fear association—it is new learning. With exposure, cues take on new meanings.

Brief Exposures to Tribe Enhance Reward Learning

In skills training classes, RO DBT uniquely uses exposure principles rather than habituation in order to attach experiences of consummatory reward linked to tribal participation with previously feared social cues (see the "participate without planning" practices in the skills training manual). It is the extreme brevity of the exposure to the feared social stimuli (only thirty to sixty seconds) that may be most important for the new reward learning to occur, since the brevity and the unexpected nature of the exposure make it less likely for self-consciousness to arise and more likely for natural feelings of pleasure to arise secondary to a shared tribal experience. Frequent and unpredictable "participate without planning" practices create a store of positive memories associated with joining in with others. With repeated practice, these associations begin to generalize to social situations outside the classroom. Attendance at social events is no longer motivated solely by obligation. Instead, often for the first time in their lives, clients begin to experience anticipatory reward or pleasure, as opposed to their normal dread, prior to social interactions.

Using Informal Exposure to Habituate to Feared Stimuli

In general, RO DBT exposure interventions can be differentiated from other approaches by their brevity and by their less structured or informal nature (some formal exposure sessions last from fifty to ninety minutes; see Foa & Kozak, 1986). Indeed, OC clients are posited to more likely experience long exposures (greater than five to ten minutes) or intense exposures (flooding) as overwhelming; as a consequence, such exposures can trigger a shutdown response (see the material on the "deer in the headlights" response, chapter 6). Ideally, when using informal exposure, the therapist should orient the client to the rationale and strategies used in informal exposure before applying them (albeit, as described earlier, "participate without planning" practices never include an orientation period). The client is then oriented to the specific steps involved and to how they are likely to manifest in session. The therapist and the client collaboratively agree on the cues that are most likely to elicit the feared response. For instance, a client who was fearful of personal self-disclosure agreed that at least three times during each session she would share something personal that she might normally withhold from other people. In planning informal exposure practices, whether they are to be carried out in session or in vivo (that is, in the client's social environment), it is important to structure the exposure so that old learning is not reinforced. Therefore, practices need to be carefully graduated, with an exposure hierarchy moving from least to most extreme. Table 10.2 provides a summary of the steps for informal exposure in RO DBT.

Table 10.2. RO DBT Informal Behavioral Exposure Protocol Targeting Maladaptive Social Signals

Step	Action(s)
1	The therapist is alert for subtle changes in social signaling that are discrepant, odd, or off-putting in the given context (for example, the client suddenly goes quiet and exhibits a flat face after being complimented).
2	The therapist directly asks about the client's change in social signaling, but only after it has occurred multiple times, and over multiple sessions. This step usually includes an assessment of the extent to which the client is aware of the repetitive nature of the social signaling behavior and can identify what may have triggered the change. The therapist says, for example, "I noticed just now that you seem to have gone a bit more quiet, and now you're looking down. Do you have a sense about what may have happened to trigger your less expressive face?" The therapist, with eyebrows raised, follows this question with a warm, closed-mouth smile.
3	The therapist asks the client to label the emotion associated with the maladaptive social signal and assesses the client's willingness to experience the emotion without engaging in the maladaptive social signal (that is, response prevention).*
4	The therapist and the client collaboratively identify the stimulus (such as a compliment) that triggered the maladaptive social signal.
5	The therapist briefly orients the client to the principles of behavioral exposure and obtains the client's commitment to practice using these principles in session as the first step.

6	The therapist provides the emotional cue or trigger. For example, the therapist compliments the client and then encourages the client to practice going opposite to her automatic social signaling urges and/or delivering the context-appropriate prosocial signal, such as smiling and saying "thank you" rather than frowning, looking down, and saying nothing in response to the compliment.
7	The therapist repeats the cue multiple times during the session, ideally using the same or nearly the same facial expression and voice tone each time: "Well done. Let's try it again. Remember to go opposite to your automatic social signaling urges, such as exhibiting a flat face and avoiding eye contact, by doing the opposite, such as using a closed-mouth smile and engaging in direct eye contact. Instead of resisting or avoiding any internal emotions or sensations, allow them, without seeing them as good or bad—they just are."
8	The therapist avoids prematurely removing the cue and instead provides it repeatedly, multiple times and across multiple sessions, allowing the client sufficient time to practice her newfound social signaling skills until the client is able to engage in the appropriate response most often associated with the cue (for example, saying "thank you," making direct eye contact, and using a warm, closed-mouth smile and an eyebrow wag in response to a compliment).
9	The therapist reinforces the client's participation and encourages her to practice the same skills whenever she encounters the eliciting stimulus (such as a compliment) during the coming week. The therapist explains that behavioral exposure requires multiple experiences with the eliciting stimulus. The therapist also obtains the client's commitment to continue this type of work in future sessions.

* For skills linked to identifying emotions, see "Four Steps to Emotion-Labeling Bliss!" in the skills training manual, chapter 5, lesson 6.

Although careful orientation to exposure principles is often ideal, sometimes spontaneous or less planned exposure can be at least equally effective, depending on the nature of the problem. For example, one OC client strongly believed that any form of self-soothing was both selfish and decadent. For her, wanting two scoops of ice cream rather than one, sleeping until lunchtime, and reading for pleasure were unnecessary indulgences that, if allowed, could only lead to an increasingly immoral and unproductive existence. Though her frugality and strong work ethic were admirable, she herself recognized that her insistence on frugality and prudence, combined with her fear of being perceived as decadent, was exhausting and oftentimes prevented her from joining in fun activities (such as partying or celebrating with others). For her, even hearing the word "decadence" was sufficient to trigger automatic disgust and revulsion. With this as a backdrop, her therapist suggested that informal exposure could be used to help her learn the art of enjoying life and celebrating with her tribe. For example, during a session, her therapist might suddenly and without warning ask his client to repeat, loudly and proudly, the word "decadence" at random times, with her back straight and her head held high and, ideally, with a smile. The therapist also obtained agreement from the client that he would unexpectedly say the word "decadence" or other similarly feared words ("indulgence," "pleasure," "fun," "lazy") in session, to further augment informal exposure practices. For example, during the middle of a chain analysis on redoing others' work, the therapist might suddenly and loudly say "decadence" three times in a row, then briefly check in with the client regarding her experience of hearing the word, while reminding her of their goal of increasing her pleasure in life, and then quickly return to the chain analysis. For another OC client, who feared blushing, an RO DBT therapist used a similar strategy by exposing the client to words and phrases such as "embarrassment," "humiliation," "red face," and "flushing," a strategy that culminated in multiple practices over multiple individual sessions, with the therapist unexpectedly asking the client to stand up, whereupon both of them together would raise their hands toward the ceiling and proudly exclaim, in a loud voice, "Public humiliation, I love you! Public humiliation, I love you! Public humiliation, I love you! Public humiliation, I love you!" This sequence was then repeated multiple times over multiple sessions; the key to success was repetition and the short duration of each exposure (each mini-exposure lasted thirty to sixty seconds at most). These brief exposures would most often end with mutual spontaneous giggling and laughing, and later the client identified this work as a seminal step in becoming freer to participate more fully in interactions with others. In both of the examples just discussed, the therapists were careful to raise their eyebrows and smile during the exposure practices, to signal affection and playfulness to their clients. Thus, in contrast to therapists using most other exposure techniques, RO DBT therapists are likely to combine brief exposure to nondangerous stimuli with prosocial nonverbal signals (smiling and eyebrow wags) in order to viscerally signal that self-discovery and trying out new things call for celebration, not seriousness, and that having fun is okay. Clients' informal exposure to the value of disinhibition represents one of the core reasons why it is important for therapists to practice RO skills themselves.

In the following transcript, the therapist first orients the client to the idea of using informal exposure and then uses informal exposure techniques to help the client learn to be more receptive to praise and compliments:

Therapist: So I just want us to notice that whenever I compliment you, it seems that you are likely to change the topic or somehow avoid the experience. Any praise on my part seems to invalidate how you see yourself, as if you're not worthy—as if you're a piece of crap. Yet at the same time *(Pauses)*…I somehow feel like it's not right for me *not* to express a genuine positive feeling I might have toward you, especially since you've let it slip that you actually don't want to feel like a piece of crap for the rest of your life. *(Ties praise to problematic beliefs that the client has regarding himself.)*

Client: Well, I've been trying to absorb this. But it takes a conscious effort for me to absorb the praise. Last night I was thinking about some of the positive things you've said. The relationship…the idea of you caring…it takes a conscious effort for me to absorb that. It doesn't come natural.

But, to some extent, I'm doing it…to some extent. I think, you know, the trouble—I guess I don't believe it, because I don't believe it about myself. I just figure "This guy doesn't know anything. He doesn't know what he's talking about." *(Free self-disclosure indicates client's engagement in therapy.)*

Therapist: I see your point. It's like a dance that you do with me and with other people. What I'm trying to get you to understand is that the dance you've learned is exhausting, and it's keeping you stuck. I know this is hard, but we need to practice some different steps and go opposite to proving to others and yourself that you're a piece of crap. That's the old dance that keeps you from ever getting close to others. You reject other people before they can reject you, to the tune of "See, I'm Right—No One Likes Me." *(Pauses.)* There is a way out of this, though. *(Pauses.)* Would you be interested in knowing about this? *(Highlights problem of avoidance, using a metaphor; asks for commitment to try something different.)*

Client: Yeah. I guess it is about time.

Therapist: Okay, good. So the question is, what is the way out of this self-made trap? First it will involve a lot of practice on your part that will probably be hard. *(Pauses slightly.)* Plus, it will involve learning to accept kindness and positive feelings from others, and going opposite to your natural tendency to avoid hearing nice things about yourself, while letting go of that inner voice that is always self-critical. It will mean learning the steps of a new dance. *(Takes a long pause.)* The actual name for this approach is "behavioral exposure." It's a well-tested way to lay down new learning about old fears. *(Smiles.)* Actually, my grandmother used the same principle whenever she told me to get back on my horse after a fall and ride again. Does this seem to make sense? *(Uses a metaphor to introduce the idea that client's behavior is a learned habit; introduces principles of change associated with exposure; checks in with client to determine client's response to this approach.)*

Client: Yeah, sure. Exactly.

Therapist: So, assuming you are agreeable, we'll experiment together, and I'll be mindful that any praise or compliment on my part may be experienced as painful for you, but I will not stop providing praise unless we both decide that something needs to change. That is, we will be practicing getting back on the horse, with the idea that horseback riding is something you can do, and that it's important for you to have a decent life. Do you think you would be willing to try this out? *(Summarizes contingencies associated with praise, and dialectically suggests that client needs to be aware of the pain that praise can elicit; says that in order for behavioral exposure to work, it is important not to remove the cue; asks for commitment.)*

Using Informal Exposure to Grieve

Successful grieving requires the brain to learn that what was before is no longer. Grief work means feeling the loss and then letting it go (practicing regulation). Over time, the brain adjusts to the changing circumstance; that is, we give up searching for the lost object and begin to build a new life (see the skills training manual, chapter 5, lesson 29).

OC Behavioral Chain and Solution Analyses: Broad Principles

Conducting an effective behavioral chain analysis means being a good detective. Good detectives are curious—they want to see for themselves the scene of the crime, they want to know every possible detail leading up to the crime, and they also want to know what the consequences were after the crime was committed. As a result, more often than not they are able to solve the crime. The same goes for a behavioral chain analysis, though I feel compelled to say that OC social signaling deficits are not a crime (they most often reflect social skills deficits). The detective metaphor can be useful when orienting clients to chain analysis: "Let's be detectives together!" For one thing, good detectives are open-minded, yet when they first enter a crime scene they are likely not to talk to anyone until after they have examined the scene on their own (this helps them avoid having their perceptions biased by the opinions of others who arrived before them). Similarly, the best chain analyses are those that are done with open curiosity; thus, before you even begin a chain analysis, check in with yourself and ask the following questions:

- Do I have any energy about my client, or about the chain analysis I am about to conduct?

- Do I have a pet theory about my client?

- To what extent is this influencing my behavior at this moment?

- How open am I to radically considering an alternative perspective?

- Is there something here for me to learn?

A brief check-in like this (it only takes a couple of seconds) should give you a sense of whether you might be bringing into your chain analysis (and into the session) a bias or personal edge that might interfere with the ideal stance of open curiosity (later on, you can share any bias you discover with your RO consultation team or use it as part of a personal self-enquiry practice).

> The best chain analyses are those that are done with open curiosity.

A chain analysis can be conducted around any behavior of interest that a therapist or a client wants to understand better, whereas a solution analysis is used to identify alternative behaviors or skills that might prevent similar social signaling problems in the future. Occasionally a chain analysis can be conducted in order to understand the chain of events leading to a failure to complete a homework assignment or practice a new skill that was assigned as homework. However, the vast majority of chain analyses should be focused on social signaling targets that are being monitored via a diary card; in RO DBT, chain analyses are rarely used as an aversive contingency to motivate an OC client to try harder or be more serious. (Recall that OC clients are already too serious, and so there is no reason to encourage more seriousness, with the sole exception of life-threatening behavior). Instead, the aim of chain analyses when working with OC clients is to help them learn how to be their own detectives in order to discover a life worth sharing.

There is no need for a long-drawn-out chain analysis. In fact, when working with OC clients, short chains are often the best (recall that OC clients dislike the limelight). In RO DBT, then, chain and solution analyses should be relatively short (ideally, around twenty minutes, although an effective chain and solution analysis can be completed in seven to twelve minutes) and should be conducted in a manner that encourages self-enquiry rather than more self-control. A short chain analysis also leaves time for other agenda items, such as didactic teaching and informal behavioral exposure. I have found that most therapists, with practice, can learn the skill of conducting short chain and solution analyses. The key is not to get distracted by the other potentially relevant targets that frequently emerge, and instead to take note of them for later discussion. My general rule of thumb (there's that rule thingy again) is to find two to four new solutions per chain.

Appendix 6 uses a clinical example to illustrate how to set the stage for a chain analysis. Appendix 7 uses a clinical example to illustrate the protocol for conducting a chain analysis and a subsequent solution analysis.

Conducting a Chain Analysis, Step-by-Step

An RO DBT chain analysis is made up of six basic steps. Strive to complete each step in the order in which they are presented in the following sections.

Step 1. Clearly Describe the Problem

Start with a clear description of the social signaling problem behavior (that is, the context), and, if possible, ask the client to demonstrate, in session, what the social signaling behavior looked like. The description should include the context, the frequency, the intensity, and the duration of the problem behavior.

Step 2: Determine the Contributing Factors

Identify the distal contributing factors (also known as *vulnerability factors*) that may have made it more likely for the client to engage in the problem behavior on a particular day (for example, exhaustion stemming from compulsive cleaning or working).

Step 3. Determine the Prompting Event and Its Relevance

Identify the event that may have prompted or cued the problem behavior, and confirm that this event is indeed relevant. The idea is to discover what occurred to trigger the chain reaction leading to the problem behavior (that is, the event without which the social signaling problem probably would not have occurred).

Step 4. Get a Detailed Description of Events

Obtain a detailed description of the chain of events that led up to the problem behavior, with each link in the chain consisting of an emotion, an action, a thought, or a sensation. It is important to note that actions should be described to clients as social signals, unless an action (overt behavior) has occurred in isolation (for additional clarity, see "It Takes Two to Tango: Social Signaling Defined," chapter 9).

A useful aide-mémoire is the acronym EATS, where each letter stands for a different behavior or function (E = emotions, A = actions, T = thoughts, S = sensations). By the way, EATS functions as a therapeutic tease when working with OC anorexic clients. It can be changed, of course, if the client reports disliking it, to FAT (F = feelings, A = actions, T = thoughts). Anyway, where was I? [Editor's note: Off the deep end, or so it seems to us.] [Author's reply: Right. Okay, then…coming up for air…]

After obtaining the prompting event, ask the client, "What happened next? What next?" And, again, "What next?" This process continues until all the links connect to the problem behavior. Record all the links in the chain of events, moment by moment, no matter how minuscule, and be careful not to clump differing functions together (for example, by making the mistake of combining thoughts and emotions into one link). It can sometimes be useful to write a chain out on a whiteboard, in order to facilitate a sense of mutual problem solving, with an overall idea of being very specific; the process is similar to writing a movie script. For each link in the chain, ask whether there is a smaller link, and whether the link makes sense in the overall story. Each link should logically follow the one before. For example, if a client indicates that immediately after thinking *He's selfish and lazy* (thought link) she experienced sadness (emotion link), encourage her to explore with you how this might have occurred, since most of the time judgmental thoughts about other people are associated with emotions other than sadness. This line of questioning can help you and your client see that the client actually experienced anger first (emotion link), and that the sadness she initially reported had come after a sensation of exhaustion (sensation link), which was then followed by the thought *I'm never going to get any help, because I don't know how to ask for it* (thought link), which in turn led to the client's slumped shoulders, downcast eyes, and frown (social signaling link). The point is this: the chain should make sense; each link should be logical or understandable and connected to both the preceding link and the link that follows. Interestingly, most often it is areas of discrepancy (when something doesn't seem to fit; think of a jigsaw puzzle) that, pursued rather than ignored, result in the most important learning.

When Suddenly "Everything's Fine" on a Diary Card

Diary cards, as we've seen, are used in RO DBT to monitor social signaling targets and progress over time. Therefore, when you don't seem to have any targets—that is, when a client appears not to have recorded any maladaptive social signaling behaviors on the diary card over the previous week—you should take that as a social signal in itself. The question to ask yourself is *What is my client trying to tell me?* That said, it may just be that the client had a fantastic week, but if the same pattern is repeated the following week, then you should begin to look for evidence of an alliance rupture and also start looking for some new social signaling targets—pronto!

The major point is this: if you find yourself repeatedly struggling to identify a social signaling target in order to conduct a chain analysis, then assume first and foremost that your treatment targeting has been ineffective or not relevant to the core social signaling deficits that are keeping your client out of the tribe, and then out yourself to your client. That is, practice radical openness and willingness to question yourself by pointing out to the client that it is your job to find relevant targets, even though this work is, ideally, collaborative. When outing yourself about this, it is important to actively block any attempts on the client's part to soothe you, make excuses, or change the topic. Simply raise your hand, palm forward, and say, "Stop. This is not your job. It's mine. But I appreciate your willingness to help." (Finish with a warm closed-mouth smile.) Interestingly, the more a client tries to pull you off the topic, the more likely it is that the client may have something to hide.

Regardless, it is important to keep an open mind because the more willing you are to genuinely signal readiness to take responsibility for your own actions—without falling apart, or signaling that you are blaming the client (in this case, for possibly not being effective in locating a social signaling target)—the more able you are to send a powerful message of caring and equality while simultaneously modeling core RO skills. This RO stance does not imply that you have done something wrong, but simply that you practice what you preach; that is, you are not going to ask your client to do anything that you would not be willing to do yourself.

After having signaled (hopefully) genuine willingness on your part to engage in self-examination, you can (*should*, ideally) flip immediately to the opposite dialectic (playful irreverence). Thus, instead of refusing offers of help, directly ask for help by saying, "But you know what? Now that I think about it, I could really use your help." Finish with a warm closed-mouth smile and a slight wink. The smile, combined with the quick wink, is a therapeutic tease. It signals to the client that you are not upset about not being perfect at locating relevant social signaling targets (an important message for hyperperfectionist OC clients) and simultaneously implies (via the smile and the wink) that you suspect there might be more going on behind the scenes than your client has been willing to reveal, but you are not going to rub the client's nose in it and instead will wait for the client to take the first step toward you.

Either way, the entire process provides an opportunity for both you and the client to practice radical openness. What's important is to recognize that when you use a dialectical stance in this manner, you signal trust, respect, and kindness to your client by giving the client the benefit of the doubt. If this polarity could speak, it would be saying, "I trust you to do the right thing. I believe in your competence, and I have faith in your ability to follow through with prior commitments." And yet the dialectical stance itself, as a whole, retains a dash of healthy skepticism or teasing. I sometimes refer to this strategy as "therapeutic induction of guilt" because, either way, it functions to help the client. For example, if the client is being candid and forthcoming, then the client will find the stance of trust validating, and this will likely reinforce further honest self-disclosure. If, by contrast, the client is purposefully concealing or pretending, then the client is likely to find your blind faith somewhat disconcerting because it will seem undeserved (the client will start to feel guilty), and it will be more difficult for the client to fall back into old habits of blaming others or fatalistic thinking. In general, you should remain in a stance of unqualified trust until the following conditions are present:

- You have concrete evidence suggesting that your trust is unwarranted, at which point you reveal what you know to the client and encourage the client's candid disclosure.

- The client outs himself and is more candid. In this case, immediately reinforce the client's candor by saying, "Wow. Thanks for telling me." Offer a warm closed-mouth smile and say, "You know, I sort of had an idea that something like that might have been going on, but I wasn't sure, so I just figured that I would wait to see if you might tell me. How does it feel now that I've said that?"

- The client appears to be less engaged, or blames you, after you've made a kindhearted attempt to take responsibility for the lack of a relevant target. This suggests the possible existence of an alliance rupture and triggers an alliance rupture repair.

Step 5. Describe the Consequences

Describe the consequences that immediately followed the problem behavior, with particular emphasis on any reinforcing or punishing consequences as well as on reactions from others in the social environment. For example, one client reported that he experienced a sense of pride after redoing a coworker's spreadsheet (notice that pride reinforces future redoing behavior), yet immediately afterward he experienced exhaustion and resentment, linked to the thought *Why do I always have to be the one to make it right?* In this case, the client also noticed that the coworker had left work uncharacteristically early. The therapist helped the client use self-enquiry to examine the possibility that his coworker's response (leaving work early) might have represented a potentially negative social consequence linked to the client's compulsive urges to redo other people's work. Be alert for ways to influence reinforcing or punishing consequences in order to help change the problem behavior (see Farmer & Chapman, 2016, for a review of principles of contingency management). Most important, work to help your OC clients recognize the impact their behavior has on the social environment, and explore whether their behavior and its impact fit with their valued goals.

Step 6. Conduct a Solution Analysis

Look at each link in the chain after you write it down. Solution analyses are either conducted after a chain analysis or woven in during a chain analysis, emphasizing skills that, had they been used, would likely have prevented the problem behavior. Each potential solution or alternative behavior should be linked to a specific maladaptive link that led to the problem behavior. For example, you might ask, "Is there something else you might have said to yourself or something else you might have done that might have been more effective? What skill might you have used at this link if you desired to change this behavior?" It can sometimes be helpful to imagine yourself in a predicament or situation similar to the client's and ask yourself, *What would I have done if I were in this client's shoes?* This can facilitate creative and practical problem solving. You should gain the client's commitment to use identified solutions, and you should troubleshoot factors that might make it difficult for the client to engage in those solutions. Preferably, clients should keep a written copy of solutions nearby at all times. Copies of chain and solution analyses are given to clients to keep as reminders. Clients are encouraged to develop the skill of doing their own chain analyses, without the aid of a therapist. Whenever possible, look for opportunities for clients to practice new skills in session (via role playing); the idea in treating OC clients is not to talk about what to do but to practice doing. Finally, do not overwhelm clients with too many solutions; the emphasis should be on quality, not quantity (in general, only two to four new solutions per chain analysis are recommended). As an individual therapist, your role is that of an informal skills trainer, meaning that you should not wait for a skill to be taught in skills training class before recommending its use; instead, during individual therapy sessions, teach informally whichever new skill may be needed.

Targeting Maladaptive Social Signals: The Big Picture

It is imperative for therapists to keep in mind that the primary reason for conducting a chain analysis is not simply to gain insight but to generate alternative ways of coping and social signaling in order to help the emotionally lonely and isolated OC client get back to the tribe. Similarly, when it comes to generating alternative ways of coping and social signaling, the emphasis is on generating solutions that help the client reestablish social connectedness with others, not necessarily on changing how the client feels inside (albeit this might be a consequence of improved social signaling).

Yet the sheer number of possible social signaling alternatives available to a therapist is staggering. For example, it is estimated that modern humans can make over ten thousand different facial expressions, and when these are combined with the enormous number of body postures, movements, and gestures at our disposal for expressing ourselves, the number of possible solutions becomes exponential. (As a reminder, see appendix 5 for a clinical example of just how much nonverbal social signaling takes place within milliseconds during interpersonal interactions.)

Innate Biological Social Signals vs. Culturally Bound Social Signals

Fortunately, therapists do not have to be cognizant of each and every possible social signaling combination in order to be effective. A few basic principles can be used to guide solution analyses and can perhaps be distilled down to one overarching recommendation: *social signaling solutions should prioritize social signals that are universally perceived by all humans as prosocial*—that is, innate biological social signals.

But how can a therapist be certain that a social signaling recommendation is truly universal? After all, there are enormous numbers of gestures, and they vary by culture and region. For example, the circle sign formed with the thumb and the forefinger of one hand means "okay" to an American, but the same sign, unless accompanied by a smile, means "zero" or "worthless" to an Italian, and it may mean "money" in the Japanese culture (Morris, 2002). Cultural influences on emotional expression are often discussed in terms of what are called *display rules* (Ekman, 1972; Friesen, 1972), defined as values and attitudes pertaining to the appropriateness of emotional expression that are passed down from generation to generation. For example, in nonstressful situations, both Japanese and American research participants exhibited the same facial expressions when viewing emotional films (Ekman, 1972); however, this changed when the same films were viewed a second time in the presence of a higher-status individual, with the Japanese participants tending to cover up or mask their expressions of disgust by smiling, and with the American participants tending to display the same emotions, albeit in a somewhat more downregulated form than had been the case earlier. Thus, when it comes to how certain emotions are expressed, cultural experience matters. Although people in all cultures downregulate certain emotions (such as disgust) when around high-status individuals, the means by which this downregulation is achieved appear to vary by culture. Interestingly, differences in cultural expressivity appear to be most influenced by two dimensions: the extent to which the culture or society values individualism over collectivism, and the extent to which the culture or society values hierarchy, status, and power differences among its individual members (see Matsumoto, 1991). Thus Americans tend to be highly individualistic but somewhat less concerned than people from Mexico or the Philippines about hierarchy, status, and power (Hofstede, 1983).

The good news is that, although it's important for therapists to be sensitive to cultural differences in expression, and to take such differences into account when devising social signaling strategies, RO DBT therapists are not the final arbiters or decision makers when it comes to what is to be done about deficits in social signaling. The client always has the final say (though this does not mean that the client is not sometimes teased, cajoled, or debated by the therapist). Fundamentally, RO DBT therapists consider it arrogant to tell others how to live (the only exception to this has to do with life-threatening behavior). Rather than telling their clients what is wrong with them, RO DBT therapists encourage their clients to discover for themselves what ails them and then to learn to value the rewards that can occur via the practice of self-enquiry. That said, an RO DBT therapist is far from a pushover; sometimes the most caring act someone can perform for another person is to tell a painful truth in order to help the person achieve a valued goal, and to tell this hard truth in a manner that acknowledges the truth teller's potential for fallibility. Thus it is up to the client, not the therapist, to determine (most often via practices involving self-enquiry) whether a particular behavior represents a violation of a culturally specific social norm or convention. (See "The Need for More Insight," chapter 9, for examples of self-enquiry questions that a client can be encouraged to ask after reporting social signaling behavior that the therapist considers maladaptive.)

> Rather than telling their clients what is wrong with them, RO DBT therapists encourage their clients to discover for themselves what ails them and then to learn to value the rewards that can occur via the practice of self-enquiry.

Despite the influence of culture and learning, there is also an enormous amount of research supporting the universality of those nonverbal social signals that emotion theorists and evolutionary paleoanthropologists posit as having been essential to the survival of our species and to individual well-being. For example, regardless of culture, we raise our arms high with our palms facing outward when we celebrate success, almost as if we were embracing the world; as we saw in chapter 6, congenitally blind athletes, whether they win or lose a competition, display the same facial expressions and gestures as winning and losing athletes who are not blind (Matsumoto & Willingham, 2009). The many universal or cross-cultural facial expressions, voice tones, and body movements that have been proposed and researched include smiling, frowning, laughing, staring, glaring, shrugging, pouting, wincing, blushing, bowing, gazing, winking, nodding, beckoning, and waving. Research suggests that innate emotional expressions can be classified into three broad functional domains—those related to status, to survival, and to intimacy—each one identifiable by a primary channel of expression specific to that domain (App, McIntosh, Reed, & Hertenstein, 2011). For example, emotions related to social status (embarrassment, humiliation, shame, pride) are expressed through the body, emotions related to survival (anger, disgust, fear, enjoyment or happiness, sadness) are expressed through the face, and emotions related to intimacy (love, sympathy) are expressed through touch.[61] However, in the long run, what matters most, in my opinion, is not so much what one feels inside but whether there is anyone in your life who actually gives a damn about how you feel—the extent to which you feel part of a tribe. Which brings us full circle: to get into a tribe (that is, to form a close social bond) and stay in it, you must be able to signal to your fellow tribe member(s) that you, too, give a damn about someone other than yourself. Reciprocity matters greatly when it comes to caring relationships.

It is the universality of emotional expression that binds us together as a species. Revealing intentions and emotions to other members of our species was essential to creating the types of strong social bonds that are the cornerstone of human tribes. Thus, regardless of our cultural background, social status, personal beliefs, or skin color, when the going gets tough, what matters most is the extent to which we feel part of a tribe or connected with another. Everything else simply falls away; just ask people closely involved in the 9/11 crisis in New York City about the extent to which they were worried about whether the people they were helping were homeless or millionaires, religious or atheists, black or white. Altruistic acts are culturally nonspecific and most powerful when performed without forethought. Indeed, it is our fundamental tribal nature that makes us suddenly blind to individual differences when we lend a hand to a stranger or make self-sacrifices for someone we may hardly know, without ever expecting the favor to be returned. From my perspective, the ability to experience others as the same as ourselves is one of the core evolutionary survival advantages of our species and the source of a great deal of pleasure. Essentially, from an RO DBT perspective, when it comes right down to it, we are all the same, no matter what our individual or cultural differences may be; we are better together, and each one of us inwardly knows this, regardless of how much we may have been hurt or may have attempted to persuade ourselves otherwise. This is why we fear social exclusion, care so much about what others think about us, are upset when others disapprove of our behavior (despite often trying hard to pretend otherwise), love to gossip, and feel self-righteous about punishing those who have harmed or deceived other tribal members for personal gain. We all desire to be loved and respected; we all want to be treated fairly, believe in equity, and desire to be perceived by others as impartial—and, as a species, we uniquely believe in fairness (Shaw & Olson, 2012).

For example, unlike most species, humans do not automatically side with their allies or kin (DeScioli & Kurzban, 2009).

Plus, research shows that we can viscerally tell whether we like or trust others, based on their social signaling. We trust what we see, not what is said. For example, appearing too controlled, too self-possessed, or too accepting can send the wrong message in circumstances that call for open and uninhibited expression of emotion (for example, discovering that your friend has just been diagnosed with cancer, dancing at a party, asking someone to marry you, praising a child for a job well done, going out for a beer with coworkers, or arguing with your spouse). A calm exterior can be (and often is) misread by others as expressing arrogance, indifference, manipulativeness, or dislike. Research shows that we like people who freely express their emotions, even when those emotions are negative, more than we like people who habitually suppress their emotions. Thus the key to effective solution analyses when working with OC clients is to continually ask yourself, in session, *How might my client's social signaling impact his social connectedness?*

Fortunately, even if the answer to this question is that the impact of the client's social signaling is not very positive, the good news is that, with a little training and practice, it is relatively easy to change social signaling habits. There are three basic principles that can be used to guide both a solution analysis and the alternative social signals that are proposed as solutions to the client's social signaling deficits:

1. They should be relevant to the client's social signaling deficits.

2. They should be linked to the client's valued goals.

3. They should be unambiguous (that is, the solution analysis itself should be clear, and the alternative social signals that are proposed as solutions should be unlikely to be misinterpreted by recipients).

Social signaling solutions should also be collaboratively obtained, individualized, and, whenever possible, practiced in session (the latter possibility will be specific to the client's circumstances).

One rather useful way to enhance the specificity and creativity of social signaling solutions (that is, to think outside the box) is to get into the habit of imagining yourself in the exact same situation (social context) being described by your client during the behavioral chain analysis and then silently ask yourself, *If I were in this exact same situation, how would I behave? What would I do differently from my client in order to achieve the valued goals expressed by my client?* This does not mean that you should then try to get the client to become your Mini-Me (that is, to start acting or behaving like you, even though that might be fun). Nevertheless, assuming that you have been successful (to some extent, at least) in obtaining and maintaining close and intimate ties with others in your own life, placing yourself in your client's shoes and asking silently, *What would I do if I were in this situation?* can lead to some surprisingly novel solutions. Ideally, when you are deriving solutions in this manner, you should model or demonstrate what the alternative social signal might look or sound like, via role playing, rather than talking about it or attempting to describe it.

The following transcript shows how these principles can be put into practice. The client has sought treatment for her chronic depression. She and her therapist are in the seventeenth session and have already experienced several alliance ruptures and repairs, a fact that suggests a decent therapeutic alliance. The therapist has completed the chain analysis of a maladaptive social signal labeled "walking away," and so he already knows when, where, and how this social signal has occurred, and he also knows the contributing factors, thoughts, emotions, and actions leading up to it, as well as the consequences that occurred afterward. The transcript begins in the middle of the solution analysis. In this scenario, the RO DBT therapist recognizes that if he were in the same situation the client has described—that is, receiving unwanted feedback—he would not walk away without saying a word; instead, in addition to using core RO skills designed to enhance openness to critical feedback, he would try to find a way to slow down the pace of the interaction in order to give himself and the other person time to consider how best to proceed (the therapist creatively labels this social signaling intervention a "stalling tactic"):

Therapist: (Expresses open curiosity) So, Anna, when you think about openness, what's the signal? What's the message you want to get across to her at this time? You're just about to go into a big meeting with your colleague, one that will have important outcomes for your company, and you need to be on the same team with her. (Summarizes the circumstances.) Despite your disagreement with some of what she has just said, how do you want both of you to walk into this meeting?

Client: In a relaxed, calm, professional manner.

Therapist: Yeah, like a team. Teammates. (Smiles warmly.)

(Client nods.)

Therapist: And so, to get that across to her, you're going to have to signal…what? I mean, she's just told you that she doesn't believe you know the budgets when it comes to the project, and one of our solutions we just came up with is for you to use the Big Three + 1 next time that happens, so that you are signaling to her that you are open and listening to her feedback. But how can we go even further—to get a slam dunk, so to speak? Do you have a sense? (Expresses open curiosity; offers a warm closed-mouth smile.)

Client: Something that I could say to her? (Client is engaged.)

Therapist: Yeah. (Uses easy manner.) I mean, when you think about one of our other solutions—using Flexible Mind ADOPTS—like we said earlier, at some point you are going to want to find some time to answer those twelve questions…

(Client nods.)

Therapist: ...to know whether to accept or decline the feedback. But in the heat of the moment...(*Pauses slightly; looks toward client.*)

Client: I won't have time at all.

Therapist: Yeah. So what I'm thinking—and tell me if this resonates with you—is to kind of slow things down a bit. To do a stalling tactic of some sort that signals to her that you are open-minded to her comments, but that also gives you the time you need to consider how you might want to respond, rather than just walking out of the room and leaving her, perhaps, with an impression that you would prefer not to have occur. So when I say that to you, what comes to mind? How does that fit for you? (*Checks in before moving on.*)

Client: Yes. I can really see, from our company's point of view—the company Claire and I work for—how it would be much better if we go into the meeting...like you say, as a team. And in terms of my future potential in the company, it's really important for me to get along with Claire. Although she's young, she's a rising star, so it's really important to get along with her. She's going to be picking the next team, and I want to make sure she wants me on the team. (*Client is engaged, earnest.*)

Therapist: Yeah. (*Pauses very slightly; uses an easy manner.*) So the other thing about openness is that it's not just about signaling it nonverbally. It's also important that we combine our nonverbals with what we say with our words. We could practice right now. Tell me if this fits. What if you said something like "You know, Claire, I can really hear what you're saying." (*Pauses.*) You might even add that you can see some truth in what she said. (*Pauses.*) That is, of course, if you *do* see some truth. (*Pauses slightly.*) Do you think there might have been some truth in the feedback she gave you? (*Before proceeding, therapist checks in with client about whether there might have been some truth in the feedback she received from her colleague, to help ensure client's engagement and avoid assumptions; offers warm closed-mouth smile, eyebrow wag.*)

Client: Yeah...with hindsight. She does know the budgets better than me on this project. I really haven't been involved so much with this project, so there is some truth in what she was saying. (*Client is engaged, earnest.*)

Therapist: Yeah...at the very least, you could say to someone in a situation like this something like "You know, Claire, I can see that you have a point. I'll tell you what—would it be okay with you if we talked about this some more a bit later? Because I really would like to go into this meeting together as a united front—as a team." And then you could check in with her to make sure she was in agreement, by saying something like "Would that work for you?" Or something along those lines. (*Offers warm closed-mouth smile.*) How do you think that might work? (*Continues closed-mouth smile; leans back in chair, eyebrows raised.*)

Client: *(Writes down in her self-enquiry journal the statement therapist has just made)* Yeah, I think that might work. *(Client is engaged, earnest.)*

Therapist: Okay—great. Why don't we practice it right now? *(Expresses open curiosity.)*

Client: Okay, so…you want me to practice it now? *(Client is engaged, earnest.)*

Therapist: Yeah. *(Uses easy manner.)* As best you can. *(Offers warm closed-mouth smile.)*

Client: Okay. *(Looks down at her notes, leans forward, begins role playing.)* So, Claire, I can hear what you're saying, and I think what's important is that we go into this meeting as a team. So, um, I can see that you have a point here, and what I would like to do is just hold it for the moment, and then maybe we can talk about it after the meeting. *(Client is engaged, earnest; her voice is serious and slightly monotonic; client leans forward, makes direct eye contact.)*

Therapist: Great. *(Offers warm closed-mouth smile.)* Try it one more time…only this time, lean back in your chair a bit. *(Reinforces client by saying "great" with a warm closed-mouth smile, then simply asks her to practice again, this time with a change of posture.)*

Client: *(Leans back in chair, face relaxed)* Okay, I can really hear what you are saying now, and I think what's important is that we go into this meeting as a team, and then what I would like to do is talk about it after the meeting, if it's okay with you. *(Client is engaged; her voice is softer, and her affirmative head nods increase.)*

Therapist: That's great. I think that's really excellent. *(Offers warm closed-mouth smile to reinforce client's progress.)* For me, just your leaning back somehow changed your voice tone. It made me feel like you weren't criticizing me, or something like that. *(Offers warm closed-mouth smile; leans back in chair with slight shoulder shrug and openhanded gestures.)*

Client: *(Nods)* It felt like it took the edge off my voice a bit. *(Client is engaged.)*

Therapist: Yeah, it really seemed to do just that. Well done! *(Offers warm closed-mouth smile.)* So we've come up with three things today that you can do to be more open to feedback instead of just walking away. Two of them are things you can do in the heat of the moment—the Big Three + 1 and the stalling tactic we just talked about. What's nice about the stalling tactic is that it kind of slows things down a bit, without your losing your chance to disagree later if you decide the feedback doesn't make sense, like after doing the twelve questions from Flexible Mind ADOPTS. Plus, when the relationship is an important one, like with Claire, it says to the other person, "I can see merit in your feedback, but if it's okay with you, I'd like to think about what you just said before I respond." At the very least, it signals to the other person that you are taking their comments seriously. *(Offers warm closed-mouth smile; uses easy manner.)*

(Client nods.)

Therapist: So why don't you write down "stalling tactic" in your journal, as a reminder. And the third solution was to remember to start your day with an LKM practice, to get you in your safety zone. How does all of that sound to you? *(Offers warm closed-mouth smile; checks in with client.)*

The interaction shown in the preceding clinical example took less than ten minutes. The social signaling solutions were demonstrated in session, via mini–role playing, with no attempt to find the perfect example. Finally, the therapist summarized the three solutions he had come up with, checked in to confirm the client's engagement, and—rather than dwelling on other possible solutions or attempting to further refine the three solutions he had identified—took the heat off the client (after confirming her engagement) by turning to another topic (recall that OC clients dislike the limelight, and heat-off strategies can be used to reinforce new adaptive behaviors). In addition, as seen in the clinical example, solutions often involve helping a client remember to practice one of the RO skills taught in the skills training class—in this instance the Big Three + 1 (skills training manual, chapter 5, lesson 3), Flexible Mind ADOPTS (skills training manual, chapter 5, lesson 22), and loving kindness meditation, or LKM (skills training manual, chapter 5, lesson 4). Thus individual therapists, not just RO skills trainers, must become highly familiar with all the RO skills and personally practice them if they are going to effectively recommend them to their OC clients. (Imagine going to a scuba diving instructor who has never been in the water.) It is also important to place yourself in the shoes of your client and imagine yourself trying to practice the social signaling solution you are recommending. This can help prevent you from sending clients out to practice a new skill that would never work in the client's actual context. For example, you would not recommend that a client practice the Awareness Continuum (skills training manual, chapter 5, lesson 12) when she is in conflict with her boss. At first blush, it sounds like great RO DBT, but when you take a moment to actually think about what it would look like in real life, it quickly loses its benefits. Imagine your client saying to her boss, "I am aware of a feeling of anger" or "I am aware of a sensation of heat in my chest." It is most likely to quickly end with your client telling her boss something like "I am aware of imagining you think I'm crazy" (since her boss has neither any idea of what the Awareness Continuum is nor the time and desire to find out).

Note also that the therapist, after asking the client to practice once again what she might say to her colleague, did not go overboard with his praise, although his manner signaled warmhearted appreciation. This type of restraint should not be considered a rule in work with OC clients, but in general they dislike the limelight, and so praise delivered too dramatically can often be read as phony and manipulative, or as just a technique. That said, sometimes change—especially when it goes several steps beyond what might have been expected from a client, or when the client initiates it—really does deserve a big celebration (as mentioned earlier, reciprocity matters). Plus, when the therapist asked the client to practice again, he signaled that he considered her already capable of taking feedback, and he knew that any adverse response on the client's part would be an additional opportunity for growth, perhaps for both of them, through an alliance rupture repair.

Effective social signaling solutions (such as the stalling tactic suggested in the clinical example) are not always in this book. Therefore, therapists are encouraged to use their own social signaling experience as a guide to developing solutions that work for their clients in specific circumstances.

Finally, practicing radical openness, self-enquiry, and outing oneself function as social safety signals; they enhance relationships because they model humility and willingness to learn from what the world has to offer. Indeed, openness and cooperative intentions are evaluated through actions—facial affect, voice tone, rate of speech, eye contact, body posture, and gestures—not through words. When we feel attached to others, we feel part of a tribe; we feel safe; our social safety system is activated. Our body is relaxed, and our breathing and heart rate are slower. We feel calm yet playful. We are less self-conscious, and we desire to socialize. We can effortlessly make eye contact and flexibly communicate, using our facial muscles. We have a musical tone of voice. We enjoy touching and being touched. We are open, receptive, curious, and empathic toward the feelings of others. However, as noted multiple times throughout this book, OC biotemperamental biases (for high threat sensitivity and low reward sensitivity) make it more likely for an OC client to feel anxious and depressed than safe and secure. Thus therapists should also encourage strategies that function as protective, or that can reduce emotional vulnerability, and when clients struggle practicing social signaling skills, therapists should encourage self-enquiry before moving to problem solving, by asking, "What is it that you might be trying to signal to me, or yourself, by behaving this way? Is it possible that you want to tell me something? What is it that you might need to learn?"

For a summary of important points covered up to this point in the chapter, along with some additional suggestions, see "RO DBT Solutions: Focus on Changing Indirect Social Signals."

In summary, indirect social signaling and indirect speech are powerful—they allow a person to influence others or make requests of others and yet deny doing so. A recipient positively inclined to a request can simply agree to it, whereas an antagonistic recipient is unable to argue against it (Lee & Pinker, 2010). Unfortunately, indirect speech often leads to misunderstanding and distrust because it is hard to know the true meaning or intentions of the sender. Yet being discreet, indirect, or economical with the truth is not always maladaptive; for example, tactfully turning a person's attention to a blunder or error he has made, without rubbing his nose in it or publicly making a big deal of it, can serve as an act of kindness. Indeed, the core concept known as *smuggling* in RO DBT is essentially a form of indirect communication. Plus, sometimes we don't say what mean, out of politeness, yet when we're among friends or family, our body gestures and facial expressions are more expansive, and our language is less formal and more colorful because we are less worried about impression management. Thus we therapists should be delighted (rather than appalled) when our OC clients use colorful language, tease us, crack jokes, give us a hard time, or openly disagree without preamble, because their lack of self-consciousness might mean that they consider us friends or members of their tribe (a great compliment, in my eyes). It also suggests the possibility of the existence of a strong therapeutic alliance, and permission from the therapist for candid disclosure (essential in close social bonds) and for playful teasing (a common way that friends give each other feedback). RO DBT incorporates these theoretical observations into treatment interventions in several ways:

- By teaching clients how to be context-appropriate in expressing emotions and in using nonverbal social signaling strategies that have been shown to enhance social connectedness

- By targeting overcontrolled biotemperamental deficits and excesses via skills designed to activate areas of the brain associated with the social safety system, and encouraging clients to use these skills prior to engaging in social interactions (enabling overcontrolled clients to naturally relax facial muscles and nonverbally signal friendliness, thus facilitating reciprocal cooperative responses from others and fluid social interactions)

- By teaching therapists how to take advantage of mirror neurons and proprioceptive feedback in order to elicit activation of the social safety system in their overcontrolled clients through deliberate employment of gestures, postures, and facial expressions that communicate relaxation, friendliness, and nondominance (this strategy underlies the emphasis in RO DBT on therapists' practicing and modeling self-enquiry and radical openness skills themselves)

Yet perhaps the most important questions to keep in mind when collaboratively working with OC clients on alternative ways of social signaling are the ones that clients should ask themselves:

- What would I like to communicate to this other person?

- How do I want to be perceived by this person?

- Does my social signaling accomplish this?

- To what extent does my social signaling reflect my valued goals?

The last question is important because a person might desire to bend the truth for personal gain, and yet doing so would go against a valued goal for honesty and integrity. It is important to demonstrate and practice a new social signaling solution in session (via mini–role playing), not just talk about it. Therapists should avoid assuming they know what a client means when the client speaks in vague terms or uses indirect language. Rather than ignoring this lack of clarity, therapists should reveal

RO DBT Solutions: Focus on Changing Indirect Social Signals

- Encourage clients to get in the habit of using social signals (for example, eyebrow wags and closed-mouth smiles) that are universally prosocial.

- Help clients determine what they want to express, and link it to a valued goal. Make sure a solution is practical by imagining yourself using it in similar circumstances. Don't give clients solutions you would never use yourself. Ask yourself, *How would I signal my intentions or valued goals if I were in the same situation?* But remember that how you signal may not always be effective or right for your client.

- Show, don't tell. Demonstrate and practice new social signaling solutions in session (for example, how to lean back in a chair, affirmative head nods, shoulder shrug combined with openhanded gestures to signal nondominance and openness).

- Remind clients to activate the social safety system prior to social interactions.

- Encourage clients to match the social signaling of those with whom they are interacting, to enhance social connectedness. The exception is when the other person has a flat face; in this situation, encourage clients to go opposite by using big gestures, eyebrow wags, and closed-mouth smiles.

- Make sure that social signaling recommendations are unambiguous.

- Encourage and reinforce candid self-disclosure and uninhibited expression of emotion in a manner that takes into account the needs of others. Be aware of the contexts clients are in.

- Remind clients that being open to another person's point of view socially connects, without the need to say a word.

- Write solutions down, to help clients remember to use them.

- Conduct frequent check-ins to assess engagement.

- Encourage self-enquiry when clients appear uncertain. Don't try to convince them.

- Less is more. Don't overwhelm clients with too many solutions in one session. Build slowly over time, with three to four new solutions, at the most, per chain analysis.

- Teach specific RO skills that are relevant to clients' social signaling problems. Don't depend on RO skills classes to cover relevant skills that your clients need now.

their failure to understand (that is, out themselves) and ask (not tell) the client to practice being more direct. Finally, everything gets easier when both the therapist and the client know the RO skills inside and out (this is most important for therapists, so they can model RO skills and serve as guides for their clients). Therapists should also be highly familiar with the material covered in chapter 6 of this book and, ideally, should be practicing self-enquiry on a regular basis.

Indirect Social Signals and Disguised Demands

- "I do what I do because that's the way I am." (Hidden message: "Don't expect me to change.")

- "I am not like other people." (Hidden message: "I am better than other people.")

- "No, really. It's okay. I'm fine with the decision. Let's do it your way." (Hidden message: "I disagree totally and will make you pay.")

Most OC clients signal indirectly. They tend to mask, hide, or deamplify their inner feelings, making it harder for others to know their true intentions. For example, when an OC client says "maybe," he may mean "no," or when he says "hmmm," he may really mean "I don't agree." The problem for the therapist (and others) is that OC social signaling has plausible deniability ("No, I'm fine—I just don't feel like talking" or "No, I'm not angry—I'm just thinking"), which makes direct confrontation of potentially maladaptive behavior more difficult. Hidden intentions and disguised demands negatively impact relationships. For example, OC clients are experts at unobtrusively avoiding unwanted feedback in two apparently dissimilar ways; a "pushback" response looks very different from a "don't hurt me" response, yet both function to block unwanted critical feedback. What is most important from an RO DBT perspective is how these behaviors impact the social environment: they are posited to be problematic primarily because they represent social signaling deficits. Both responses function primarily to prevent or stop painful feedback, to allow OC clients to avoid engaging in a behavior, or to help OC clients achieve a desired goal.

"Pushback" Responses

A "pushback" response usually involves two components:

1. "I'm not telling you what to do…"

2. "…but you'd better do what I want." (Essentially, the message here is "If you were wise, you would immediately stop challenging me, asking me questions, or giving me feedback, because I will make your life miserable if you don't comply with my wishes, and I'll do it in a way that no one will ever be able to prove.")

"Pushback" responses are signaled nonverbally as well as verbally, as in the following examples:

- Flat and stony facial expressions

- The silent treatment

- Scowling

- Hostile stares

- Walking away

- Contemptuous expressions

- Eye rolls

- Disgust reactions

- Cold, sharp, sarcastic, patronizing, and monotonic voice tones

- Callous smiles

- Burglar smiles

- Dismissive gestures

- Sneering, snickering, mockery, scornful giggling, and disdainful laughter

"Pushback" responses trigger the recipient's threat system and defensive arousal (the recipient is likely to want to flee or fight—to run away or punch the sender).[62] The "I'm not telling you what to do…" component usually allows the sender to avoid taking responsibility for trying to control the other person or the situation. As one client put it during a chain analysis of a tension-filled social interaction, "I was perfectly fine doing it the way they wanted, as long as they did it the proper way, so any tension that arose was their responsibility." Although the statement is technically agreeable, it places blame on others for the conflict because it implies that they did not abide by the rules that the client had decided beforehand were required for genuine agreement.

This apparently cooperative behavior can sometimes be embedded in statements implying that the other person is free to choose. One OC client, after being queried about an interaction that appeared to have triggered anger or frustration, adamantly insisted, "I was not angry." Her therapist gently asked for clarification, whereupon the client stated, "I told you—I don't *do* anger! And if you ask me one more time about this, I am going to get up and walk right out of this room!" The words "if you ask me one more time" offered the illusion of choice to the therapist: if the therapist chose to keep asking, then the client could blame him when she walked out of the session; alternatively, the therapist could choose to stop asking, and the client would thereby avoid discussion of an unwanted topic. In this scenario, it was difficult for the therapist not to reinforce the client's behavior, to some extent, since the client was in the early stages of therapy. Nonreinforcement would have required the therapist not to remove the cue, by not changing the topic and by continuing, at least to some degree, to discuss what was happening in the moment. Instead, the therapist realized that the client's behavioral response suggested the likelihood of an alliance rupture. Therefore, the therapist dropped his agenda and focused instead on understanding the apparent rupture in the therapeutic relationship, thus modeling radical openness and using the misunderstanding as an opportunity to practice interpersonal skills with the client. Interestingly, repairing the alliance rupture required further discussion of anger, including understanding what anger meant to the client. The therapist discovered that the client believed anger meant losing control and fits of rage. Since the client rarely lost control or exhibited intense rage in public, admitting to anger would have seemed inaccurate to her. By using the RO DBT alliance rupture repair protocol, the therapist was able to learn more about the client's worldview while simultaneously avoiding removing the cue (the discussion about anger) and blocking automatic abandonment of a relationship as the solution to a misunderstanding. This became an important turning point for the client, who was able to use self-enquiry to examine her adamant rejection of anger, whereupon she started to notice low-level anger and hostility (including resentment and desires for revenge) that in the past she had denied experiencing or avoided labeling, but that were negatively impacting her relationships. The ability to acknowledge her previously hidden anger and its impact on others (family members) proved to be a pivotal point of growth for her.

Another type of "pushback" behavior, which on the surface may appear to be non-avoidant, involves declarations of responsibility or dutifulness. One client reported, "Rather than dismiss criticism, I do exactly the opposite. I take it *all* on myself. It's my entire fault. I embrace *all* the criticism." The therapist encouraged the client to reevaluate her public declarations of responsibility by suggesting, "Although it can feel safer for all of us to criticize ourselves rather than have someone else do it, our intentions may not always be so noble. Do you think it might ever be possible for someone to assume all the responsibility for something in order to achieve something else?" This line of questioning became an important step for the client toward a better understanding of the possible functions served by her previously unquestioned behavioral responses.

Apparently nonavoidant "pushbacks" can be manifested in many other ways, too, such as in a quick retort or comeback, a personal attack, a defensive rebuttal, a refusal to comply, or an act of putting the other person on the spot. These "pushbacks" can be difficult to identify because they often appear to be signaling willingness to participate or engage with what is happening. For example, when a therapist asks a client to show her what it looks like when he feels sad, the client's immediate response may be "Why do you want me to do that?" Answering a question with a question is a common OC "pushback" behavior. On the surface, it appears engaged and nonavoidant, yet in reality it functions to turn the tables by putting the other person on the defensive (since the other person must now justify the question) or by diverting the discussion from an unwanted topic. When this type of response has been observed on multiple occasions, the therapist should start to highlight the behavior when it occurs and should also encourage the client to do the same and then use self-enquiry to determine whether this way of behaving has brought him closer to or taken him farther away from his valued goals (for example, to form more intimate relationships).

Another client appeared to engage in a "pushback" after his therapist asked about his feelings in the moment. He said, "This sounds more about you than it does about me." In response, the therapist modeled radical openness by nondefensively addressing his comment, without removing the cue (that is, without allowing herself to get distracted from the importance of knowing about how the client was feeling):

Therapist: Hmmm. I can see that you might think this. Let me think about what you said…(*pauses*) I don't know, but somehow it seems important that I ask you about your experience, especially after giving you what I am now aware of imagining was experienced as critical feedback. To *not* ask—to me, at least—would be uncaring. What is it that I am doing that leads you to believe that my asking about your feelings is more about me than about you?

Because the therapist did not apologize, change the topic, or defend herself, this approach avoided reinforcing the potentially maladaptive behavior (the "pushback"). Instead, the therapist signaled genuine caring and used "ask, don't tell" strategies to encourage the client to reveal his inner experience. This approach also allowed the therapist to take the client's observation seriously while also encouraging the client to more directly reveal what he meant (that is, go opposite to masking his inner feelings). This interaction was an important part of helping the client learn how to openly express difficult emotions and how to block his automatic tendencies to blame others for his emotional reactions.

"Pushbacks" can also be communicated solely via relatively subtle nonverbal channels (a scowl, an unexpected awkward silence during a conversation, a rolling of the eyes, frowning, or a disinterested expression), or they can be more obvious (a controlled temper tantrum, hitting a desk with a fist). One client described her mother this way:

> When she was in one of her moods, everyone in the family knew it, but you weren't allowed to comment about it. She didn't yell. She just would have this look about her that would send people scurrying. If you were wise, you knew to be quiet, do whatever you were supposed to do, and avoid crossing her at all costs until the mood passed, which might not happen for days.

Another client described a work colleague:

> I used to respect this guy at work for his tough, no-nonsense approach. I now see he was more overcontrolled than I am! For example, I've noticed that whenever he walks into a room, people freeze—they stop talking and joking, or they change the topic. It's almost like they're waiting to see what mood he's in, or maybe they're waiting for him to leave, because as soon as he does, they all seem to relax—and he's not even their boss! This really makes me wonder whether I sometimes have the same effect on people.

These two examples illustrate how "pushbacks" can powerfully influence other people, including therapists. Despite appearing innocuous, cordial, restrained, or proper on the surface, the implied threats woven into many "pushbacks" send a strong message to the social environment ("Don't mess with me"). Moreover, direct attempts to confront "pushbacks" can be easily rebuffed because the behavior has plausible deniability: "What—me, angry? No. I was simply expressing my opinion." Thus many OC clients who habitually engage in "pushback" behavior may have little experience with direct challenges to such behavior.

The therapist must remember that "pushbacks" are most often overlearned responses, frequently delivered without malicious intent and often with little conscious awareness. They are part of a set of behaviors that functions to help the client avoid unwanted feedback or suggestions for change, and the "pushbacks" have been intermittently reinforced. As such, a "pushback" has become a dominant automatic response to stress. Remembering this can help the therapist retain a compassionate stance when "pushbacks" occur. That said, the therapist needs to be alert to his own inner emotional experience when working with "pushback" responses, to ensure that he is not inadvertently reinforcing them. For example, most people are acutely aware when a person is behaving in a hostile manner, even when the hostility is delivered with a smile. Covert expressions of hostility tend to elicit similar feelings in recipients (people dislike being coerced or aggressed upon). Thus the therapist can use his internal experience as a guide to uncovering a hostile "pushback." However, the therapist should not assume that his emotional response necessarily signals a problem with the client; instead, these moments signal opportunities for growth—sometimes for both the therapist and the client—that, when explored collaboratively, help the OC client experience belonging to the tribe rather than being an outsider.

The following example illustrates how a therapist might challenge "pushback" behavior:

Therapist: I noticed that you changed the topic. We were discussing whether it might be possible that you actually experience anger sometimes but have learned to avoid labeling it as an emotion. What are you feeling right now? (*Maintains the cue—in this case, the discussion about anger.*)

Client: Nothing.

Therapist: Any sensation in your body?

Client: No. I don't see how this is relevant. I told you that I rarely experience anger.

Therapist: What are you feeling right now?

Client: (*Looks away*) Nothing…uncomfortable. Why does this matter? (*Signals "pushback."*)

Therapist: I don't know. (*Pauses.*) I'm aware of thinking that maybe your avoidance of this topic suggests that there is actually something important for us to understand. Just how adamant are you not to discuss this? (*Ignores "pushback" and directly assesses behavior.*)

Client:	(Looks down; pauses) I don't know.
Therapist:	Hmmm. (Uses soft voice.) Perhaps you feel emotions more often than you care to admit. (Pauses.) What do you think? (Ignores nondescriptive behavior; encourages honest expression of emotions and thoughts.)
Client:	It could be. I do not like emotions—never have. I've worked to avoid ever feeling them. (Reengages; exhibits adaptive behavior.)
Therapist:	Thanks for letting me know about this. I think talking about your avoidance might be important. (Reinforces adaptive behavior and honest expression of emotions and thoughts.)

As mentioned earlier, a "pushback" can be difficult to address because it may imply that the problem is not about the "pushback's" sender but rather about its recipient. Accusations of blame (direct or implied) and expressions of hostility trigger defensive arousal and often defensive actions in other people. Therapists are not immune to these normal responses. In addition, "pushbacks" can elicit apologetic or capitulating behavior from others, and analogous acquiescent responses by therapists can reinforce "pushbacks." And yet the aversive emotions triggered in session by "pushbacks" can be confusing, particularly if the therapist believes that she should rarely experience strong emotion during sessions with clients, or that she should always behave in a caring manner when working with clients. The therapist can become demoralized or angry when her attempts to explicitly target these often subtle and deniable behaviors, or to join with a client by revealing her own vulnerable emotions, are repeatedly rebuffed, dismissed, or considered manipulative. As a result, the therapist may completely avoid targeting possible "pushback" behavior. At the same time, premature confrontation of a "pushback" can reinforce the behavior, since the ensuing discussion of the "pushback" behavior directs attention away from the very topic that the client wanted to avoid in the first place (that is, it removes the cue). Consultation teams should be alert to these factors and help therapists find a middle ground.

The overall goal when working with "pushbacks" is for the client himself to identify them as problem behaviors. The therapist should look for opportunities to reinforce direct and open expression of emotions or opinions while ignoring or compassionately confronting indirect or disingenuous expressions that may be maladaptive. Prior to obtaining commitment, "pushback" responses are usually best managed by placing them on an extinction schedule that ignores indirect expressions of needs and desires and responds only to direct expressions of the same. The therapist behaves as if the "pushback" is not present, with the result that the client is required to make his wishes known explicitly if he is going to have a chance of obtaining what he may want. Thus the therapist, ideally, continues to behave in a positive, prosocial manner that signals affection and appreciation for the client's perspective. This approach is useful because it requires the OC client to be more direct if he is going to get the therapist to take him seriously, and it simultaneously provides opportunities for the client to practice candid self-disclosure (that is, to engage in adaptive behavior that can be reinforced). Once commitment has been obtained, "pushbacks" can be monitored on diary cards and incorporated into chain analyses. Learning to let go of "pushback" behavior, and instead to directly express desires, often becomes the cornerstone of successful treatment for many OC clients.

"Don't Hurt Me" Responses

"Don't hurt me" responses are operant behaviors that function to block unwanted feedback or requests to join in with a community activity. They are typically expressed nonverbally, via behaviors (lowering the head, covering the face with the hands or hiding the face from view, slackening and shrinking the posture, lowering the eyelids, casting the eyes downward, avoiding eye contact, and slumping the shoulders) that, collectively, are associated with self-conscious emotions. The underlying message of a "don't hurt me" response is as follows:

> You don't understand me, and your expectations are hurting me, since normal expectations for behavior do not or should not apply to me because of my special status or talents, my exceptional pain and suffering, my traumatic history, the extreme efforts I have made to contribute to society, my hard work, or my self-sacrifices for the benefit of others. As such, it is unfair of you to fail to recognize my special status and expect me to participate, contribute, or behave responsibly, as other members of my community are expected to behave. Consequently, if you were a caring person, you would stop pressuring me to change, behave appropriately, and conform to norms.

In other words, "Stop expecting me to complete my homework, stop asking questions I don't like, and stop expecting me to participate in skills class." The final hidden or indirect message in a "don't hurt me" response is "And if you don't stop, I will fall apart, and it will be your fault."

A "don't hurt me" response can be hard to identify, for one or more of the following reasons:

- Although it is an operant behavior, it may be subtly disguised to look like a respondent reaction to physical or emotional pain, as when a client cries out after twisting her ankle or expresses sadness or grief after the loss of a friend.

- It may take the form of an unwarranted expression of self-consciousness or shame, as when a client lowers his head or averts his gaze after an appropriate self-disclosure in class.

- It may occur habitually, without the client's conscious awareness.

It is possible, however, to distinguish a "don't hurt me" response from a respondent reaction:

- A "don't hurt me" response has a long duration and may last for an entire skills training class or family meeting, whereas a respondent reaction (such as the pain of a stubbed toe) fades quickly and independently of others' behavior once the eliciting stimulus is removed.

- The intensity of a "don't hurt me" response increases if a desired response (such as soothing, withdrawal of a question, a change of topic, or an apology) is not forthcoming, whereas a respondent reaction matches the intensity of the eliciting stimulus.

Another way to understand the maladaptive nature of "don't hurt me" responses is to examine the behavior from the perspective of the tribe, family, or community group, since the "don't hurt me" response always occurs within a social context (although its cousin, self-pity, often occurs alone and frequently precedes "don't hurt me" social signaling). What can often be missed by the recipients of a "don't hurt me" response is that the sender has almost always willingly chosen to be part of the community, group, or tribe in which this behavior is exhibited (that is, the sender has not been forced to participate), and yet the sender expects special treatment. Usually an OC client's "don't hurt me" responses have been intermittently reinforced by family members and others in the community (including therapists and treatment programs), most often through well-intentioned attempts to avoid upsetting the client by soothing her, taking care of her, or helping her avoid apparently distressing topics—in other words, walking on eggshells around the client. And yet "don't hurt me" responses can engender social ostracism of the client when they are long standing, pervasive, or nonresponsive to attempts by others to offer assistance. Similar to pouting, "don't hurt me" responses are maladaptive because they function to signal disagreement and nonengagement indirectly. As a consequence, over the long term, they negatively impact the client's sense of self and interfere with her ability to form close social bonds.

The difficulty for the therapist is in knowing whether to reinforce (soothe) or not to reinforce (ignore) a "don't hurt me" response (see Farmer & Chapman, 2016). This can be tricky because OC clients need to learn how to express and signal vulnerable emotional reactions (such as sadness following the death of a parent) to others in a genuine manner, and yet "don't hurt me" responses are social signals that mimic expressions of vulnerability in order to influence the social environment. Thus "don't hurt me" responses masquerade as justified or warranted reactions to distress, yet in reality they function to help the client avoid or prevent feedback or requests for change.

In the following clinical example, during a session targeting a client's rigid belief that he can tell what others are thinking from their reactions to him, the therapist has been using logic and "ask, don't tell" strategies to lead the client toward the reluctant admission that his belief is unlikely to be literally true. Now, at a critical point in this discussion, the client has suddenly reported, with his head down and a sad expression, "No one has touched me for twenty years." This utterance might be interpreted differently in a different context, but in this case the therapist hypothesizes that it represents a possible "don't hurt me" response and is intended to change the topic. Consequently, the therapist notes the new information and proceeds as follows:

Therapist: Wow, John. (*Pauses.*) That sounds like something we will need to talk about. However, before we go there…(*Pauses; leans back in chair; breaks eye contact; slows pace.*) I have a question for you. (*Pauses; offers a half smile and an eyebrow wag; looks at client.*) Did you notice that you just changed the topic?

Using "ask, don't tell" strategies, the therapist was able to help the client recognize and reveal that he had purposefully changed the topic in order to avoid further discussion of the possibility that his previously held conviction might be a fallacy. Using this as a template, the therapist and the client were able to notice not only how he used similar avoidance tactics in other situations but also the impact this might have been having on social relations, which became a major point of growth for the client.

Another example of a "don't hurt me" response can be seen in the following transcript from the eleventh session with a forty-five-year-old OC client who has long-standing chronic depression, lives alone, and, although on disability, manages her instrumental needs (such as shopping and traveling to medical appointments) without assistance. The "don't hurt me" response occurs during a chain analysis of the client's noncompletion of a homework assignment (to visit her brother, who lives in the same town):

Client: I figured out the bus route I would need to use online, but I couldn't go, because I didn't have anyone to go with me.

Therapist: (*Leans back in chair*) Hmmm. Is there a law in your brother's neighborhood requiring people to travel with an escort? (*Offers an eyebrow wag and a half smile; uses irreverence to challenge maladaptive behavior.*)

Client: (*Pauses; looks down; lowers voice volume*) No, but I just can't do things like that.

Therapist: (*Hypothesizes that client's statement is a possible "don't hurt me" response*): So why do you think I asked the question about a law in your brother's neighborhood? (*Offers an eyebrow wag with slight smile; ignores the "don't hurt me" response by behaving matter-of-factly, bringing client back to the original question, and not removing the cue.*)

Client: I don't know. (*Looks down; slumps shoulders; frowns.*) I just can't do this. I'm just so tired…and I have a headache, too. (*Changes the topic.*)

Therapist: Gosh, Sarah, this could be really important. Whatever is happening right now, in how you are talking about this with me, could be a key factor in your depression. What do you think is happening right now? (*Highlights the importance of the in-session behavior; uses "ask, don't tell" strategy to encourage self-enquiry.*)

Client: I don't know. (*Glances briefly at therapist.*)

Therapist:	*(Retains the cue; leans back)* Well, let's think about it. If there is no neighborhood law requiring escorts, and if we also know that you travel alone by bus twice a week to come here for therapy, then what does that tell us?
Client:	That I'm avoidant? *(Makes eye contact with therapist.)*
Therapist:	Or maybe you don't really like your brother. *(Smiles gently.)*
	(Client appears to be reengaging.)
Therapist:	*(Pauses slightly)* Either way, we know it's not a capability deficit. You can ride buses without escorts. But there is something else I have noticed that seems to occur whenever we encounter a difficulty—usually, from what I can tell, when new behaviors are required. It involves both what you say with your words, and what you do with your body. Do you have any idea what I am talking about? *(Uses "ask, don't tell" strategy.)*
Client:	Hmmm…that I don't look at you? *(Looks at therapist.)*
Therapist:	Yeah, that's part of it. You were doing it just a minute ago… Something happens, and then it seems that you shift into a slumped position, with your head down. And, like you said, you don't look at me, and you start using words like "I can't" or "It's not possible." I think it's great that you have noticed this, too. What do you think you are trying to communicate when you do this?

The therapist used this interaction to introduce the concept of "don't hurt me" responses and to gain the client's commitment to monitor them on the diary card, with the initial goal of discovering the frequency of the behavior and whether it was linked to other targets. The therapist smuggled the idea that the "don't hurt me" response might be keeping the client stuck in her chronic depression because it signaled to the social environment that she was fragile and incompetent. Plus, when others took her off the hook by lowering their expectations or stopping important feedback, they inadvertently reinforced future "don't hurt me" responses. The client agreed to allow the therapist to highlight possible in-session "don't hurt me" behaviors and to use them as moments for the client to practice taking responsibility for her emotional reactions instead of expecting others or the environment to change or take care of them. It was also agreed that the client would begin practicing going opposite to her nonverbal "don't hurt me" behaviors by lifting her head up instead of lowering it, putting her shoulders back rather than slumping, and speaking with a normal voice tone and volume instead of whispering.

Similar to how "pushback" responses are treated, the goal of treating "don't hurt me" responses is to reinforce direct communication of emotions and thoughts and not reinforce indirect or passive expressions of emotion or thoughts (that is, the therapist does not remove the cue, blocks soothing, and ignores the behavior). Sometimes it can be helpful for the therapist, using a matter-of-fact tone, to ask a nonresponsive client (one who is avoiding eye contact, has slumped shoulders, and is whispering) to put her shoulders back and, while making eye contact with the therapist, repeat what she has just said, without whispering. This encourages the client to socially signal competence while also providing her an opportunity to practice direct expression of her thoughts and emotions. If a "don't hurt me" response intensifies (that is, if the client puts her head down lower) or continues unabated, then the therapist, with an open mind, should directly ask the client about the function of the behavior:

Therapist: I don't know about you, but I've been noticing that something has changed or shifted in how you are responding to our discussion. *(Leans back; offers an eyebrow wag and a half smile.)* Have you noticed anything different?

If the behavior is respondent, then the client will most likely answer the query nondefensively, freely continue discussing her experiences, and actively engage the therapist in a manner that does not change the topic. If the behavior is operant, then the client will typically freeze, change the topic, exaggerate the "don't hurt me" response, or engage in "pushback" behavior (for example, by implying that the therapist's question is inappropriate). In the following clinical example, the client has been repeatedly shifting in her chair, looking away, and attempting to change the topic, and the therapist is seeking to determine whether the client's behavior is operant or respondent:

Therapist: *(Notices change in client's behavior)* Hmmm…I am aware of imagining right now that you don't want to talk about this anymore. How do you want me to behave? *(Directly asks about the function of this change in client's behavior.)*

Client: I want you to be nice to me.

Therapist: *(Notices possible "don't hurt me" response; uses an easy manner)* Really? *(Pauses.)* Just be nice? *(Pauses.)* I don't know…somehow it seems like something else. *(Does not remove the cue.)*

Client: Like what?

Therapist: Like maybe you don't want me to give you any feedback. Do you think this might be partly true? *(Confronts possibility that client's behavior is operant.)*

Client: *(Pauses; looks down)* Yeah…maybe so. *(Exhibits adaptive behavior.)*

Therapist: *(Uses quiet, gentle voice tone)* Yeah…that's honest. *(Pauses.)* Thanks. And, by the way, it's also effective behavior.

(Client looks up.)

Therapist: What I mean is that acknowledging to me and to yourself that you were avoiding the previous topic actually took some courage. Somehow, this type of expression is what I think we need to work to have happen more often. *(Pauses.)* What do you think? *(Reinforces adaptive behavior.)*

In summary, therapists must become adept at noticing subtle signals of nonengagement or avoidance. "Pushback" and "don't hurt me" responses function to block unwanted feedback or requests to join the community, or they may indirectly signal nonengagement. A "pushback" response usually functions to elicit acquiescence, avoidance, or submission from others, whereas a "don't hurt me" response functions to elicit soothing, caregiving, or nurturance. Both of these OC operant behaviors are usually experienced as aversive by others in the social environment and often result in recipients' feeling confused or unsure about their own perceptions or motives. Therapists can use their personal emotional reactions to help differentiate between "pushback" and "don't hurt me" responses. A sudden desire to warmly validate, sympathize, or soothe a client may suggest the presence of a "don't hurt me" response, whereas a sudden desire to back off, apologize, or justify one's actions is more likely to reflect the presence of a "pushback" response.

The overarching goal when working with these maladaptive OC behavioral patterns is to not reinforce indirect or passive expressions of needs or desires and to reinforce open, honest, direct expressions instead. When these maladaptive patterns occur, the initial response by the therapist should be to place the behavior on an extinction schedule by continuing the discussion as if the social signal had not been observed (that is, continue to cheerfully discuss the topic at hand). If the client more directly reveals his intentions or inner experience, the therapist should reinforce the disclosure (for example, by thanking the client for candidly revealing his inner experience). However, if the behavior continues unabated or increases in intensity, without the client's more direct expression of his needs, wants, or desires, then the therapist should use the alliance rupture repair protocol and ask with an open mind about what is happening. This helps the client take responsibility for his emotional reactions and personal preferences rather than automatically denying them or blaming them on factors outside his control—and, ideally, it leads to new self-discoveries.

Review: Intervening with "Pushback" and "Don't Hurt Me" Responses

How should you intervene with "pushback" and "don't hurt me" responses?

1. Place the behavior on an extinction schedule by ignoring it. Act as if it never happened, and carry on in a nonchalant manner with the agenda for the therapy session.

    - There is an exception to the approach of simply ignoring the behavior. If the client is displaying a *prolonged* "don't hurt me" response— for example, if he is bowing his head, covering his face, averting his eyes, and exhibiting postural shrinkage—then ask him, in a matter-of-fact way, to sit up straight and look at you. Remember, the person who is socially signaling in this way has almost always chosen to be included in the community, group, or tribe; no one is forcing him to participate, and yet he still expects special treatment.

2. If the behavior continues, and if the client doesn't express his needs, wants, or desires more directly, then shift to the alliance rupture repair protocol. With an open mind, ask the client about what is happening.

Now You Know…

▸ In RO DBT, dialectical thinking allows for the simultaneous presence of two seemingly opposite points of view and can be very helpful with OC clients, who often tend toward rigid, absolutist thinking.

▸ In work with OC clients, there are two key dialectical polarities regarding the stance of the RO DBT therapist: nonmoving centeredness versus acquiescent letting go, and playful irreverence versus compassionate gravity.

▸ Among other dialectical dilemmas, many OC clients have fallen into some form of the enigma predicament, which has to do with their general belief that they and their problems are so special and so complex that no one else can ever hope to understand them, a conviction that functions to discourage expectations for them to change their maladaptive behavior.

▸ When it comes to emotional health, RO DBT takes a collectivist, interpersonal approach, focusing on clients' social signaling as a way to reduce factors that interfere with their social connectedness and to build explicit skills designed to enhance their social connectedness.

▸ RO DBT uses chain analysis and solution analysis to target clients' maladaptive social signaling.

▸ In targeting OC clients' maladaptive social signaling, RO DBT therapists are careful to distinguish between clients' respondent behavior and such operant behavior as "pushback" and "don't hurt me" responses, which function to help clients avoid taking responsibility for changing their maladaptive social signaling and thus improving their social connectedness.

CHAPTER 11

Final Remarks, Practical Questions, and Treatment Adherence

The primary aims of this final chapter are to answer a few commonly asked questions, interject a final tease or two, provide a self-assessment adherence checklist for clinicians, and end with a few concluding remarks.

Some Commonly Asked Questions

How Do I Know I Am Doing Adherent RO DBT?

This question pertains primarily to issues of treatment adherence and fidelity. There are several things that can help with this. For one, supervision by a certified RO DBT clinical supervisor—that is, having an RO DBT expert rate one of your sessions to adherence—is probably the best way. Therapists can also use the RO DBT adherence self-assessment checklist in appendix 8. The checklist is designed to be used flexibly, depending on setting, and can be rated either by the therapist or an independent rater. Ideally, the ratings reflect the entire session, with a higher number of checkmarks in relevant sections suggesting higher treatment adherence.[63]

Adherence ratings are also always improved when therapists stick to the manual. Broadly speaking, adherent RO DBT therapy is identifiable by its emphasis on social signaling targets and solutions and a therapeutic stance that is collaborative, humble, kind, playful, structured, and challenging. My experience over the years has revealed that the first big hurdle most therapists need to get over when first learning RO DBT is learning to see the client from a social signaling perspective and to let go of other models that prioritize other targets or mechanisms of change (for example, internal experience, emotion dysregulation, maladaptive schemas). Other common misunderstandings or errors that are seen when therapists are first learning the treatment are to assume that "flexible" means "unstructured"; to mistake "easy manner" to mean "always smiling and being nice"; taking too long reviewing a diary card; and not conducting a chain analysis. RO DBT is both highly structured and highly flexible, and it is highly relationship-focused. Finally, RO DBT can be distilled down to four core components (Wow, did I just say that?):

1. Ensuring the client stays alive, thus necessitating the monitoring of life-threatening behavior

2. Identifying and repairing alliance ruptures

3. Targeting social signaling deficits

4. Practicing radical openness skills (clients as well as therapists)

How Do I Know I Have a Strong Working Alliance with My OC Client?

Recall that because OC clients are overly cautious and hypervigilant for threat, they tend to be slow to warm up and trust other people (including therapists). Thus, in contrast to most other therapies, RO DBT is more conservative about how long it takes to establish a strong working alliance (that is, it tends to take about fourteen weeks before a working alliance is considered to be possibly present). Three factors can be used as part of a self-assessment regarding a strong working alliance:

1. There have been multiple alliance ruptures *and repairs.*

2. The client's social signaling is reciprocal (when the therapist laughs, the client laughs, and vice versa) and less formal or polite (the client's body language is more laid back and his use of language is less formal).

3. The client directly challenges or disagrees with the therapist with an open mind and without abandoning the relationship.

Thus therapists should be delighted (rather than concerned) when an OC client uses colorful language, teases them, cracks a joke, or openly disagrees, because the client is sending a powerful social signal suggesting that she trusts you and considers you part of her tribe. Yet perhaps the most powerful means of making genuine contact with an OC client is to practice what you preach. That is, practicing radical openness naturally brings humility into our lives, and your OC clients are likely not to be the only ones who benefit.

> Perhaps the most powerful means of making genuine contact with an OC client is to practice what you preach.

Do I Really Have to Practice Radical Openness? I Mean, Really?

Of course you don't. I mean, it's your life, right? It would be arrogant of me to tell you that you absolutely have to practice radical openness or develop a personal self-enquiry practice in order to effectively model the core principles of RO DBT. But do it anyway—again, your clients will not be the only ones who benefit.[64]

How Do I Know the Right Questions to Ask When Practicing Self-Enquiry?

Self-enquiry means finding a good *question*, one that brings you closer to your edge (your personal unknown), not a good answer. Similarly, the self-enquiry facilitator practices letting go of needing to find the right question, as that implies that there *is* one and also assumes that the therapist is somehow responsible for fixing the issue (because the therapist must find the right question). Thus there are no right questions to ask, other than some of the classics—for example, "What is it that you might need to learn from this situation?" or "What have you done to contribute to this event?" or "Are you at your edge, or have you regulated?" Finally, notice and block the anti-self-enquiry behaviors listed here:

- Soothing: "Don't worry—everything will work out."

- Validating: "I would have found that hard, too."

- Regulating: "I think we should both take a deep breath."

- Assessing: "Do you know where you learned this?"

- Reassuring: "Remember, you are a really caring person."

- Problem solving: "You need to confront this person about…"

- Encouraging acceptance: "You need to accept that you cannot fix this problem."

- Cheerleading: "You can do this!"

Final Remarks

Our species has not only survived—we have thrived. But how did we do it? Our physical frailty is proof that our survival depended on something more than individual strength, speed, or toughness. We survived because we developed capacities to form long-term social bonds with unrelated others, work together in tribes, and share valuable resources. But perhaps what makes us uniquely human is not just safety in numbers but instead our willingness to make self-sacrifices to benefit another or contribute to our tribe. RO DBT contends that human emotional expressions evolved not just to communicate intentions but to facilitate the formation of strong social bonds and altruistic behaviors among unrelated individuals. Our facilitative advantage required our species to develop complex social signaling capabilities that allowed for a quick and safe means to evaluate and resolve conflict and that resulted in unprecedented collaboration among unrelated individuals, a unique human feature that to this day is unparalleled in the animal world.

Indeed, we are a hypercooperative species, more so than any other animal species. We engage in highly complex and coordinated group activities with others who are not kin and comply without resistance to requests from complete strangers. Research shows that most humans, rather than falling apart or running amuck when disaster strikes, are calm, orderly, and work together to help others. During times of extreme crisis, we forget about our individual differences, backgrounds, and beliefs and unite for a common cause (ask people closely involved in the 9/11 crisis in New York City the extent to which they were worried about whether the people they were helping were homeless or millionaires, religious or atheists, black or white). According to RO DBT, our mirror neuron system and capacities for micromimicry of facial affect both make it possible for us to literally experience the pains and joys of nearby others and make empathy and altruism a reality. This helps explain why we are willing to risk our lives to save a stranger from drowning, or to die fighting for our nation.

RO DBT differs from most other treatments by positing that individual well-being is inseparable from the feelings and responses of the larger group or community. Thus, when it comes to long-term mental health and well-being, what a person feels or thinks inside or privately is considered less important in RO DBT, whereas what matters most is how a person communicates or social signals inner or private experience to other members of the tribe and the impact that social signaling has on social connectedness. Feeling happy is great, but when you are lonely it's hard to feel happy, no matter how much you might try to accept, reappraise, or change your circumstances, keep busy, exercise, practice yoga, or distract yourself. In the long run, we are tribal beings, and we yearn to share our lives with other members of our species. Essentially, when we feel part of a tribe, we naturally feel safe and worry less.

Finally, although our evolutionary heritage may compel us to instinctively care for our children or members of our family, this is not what makes us different from other animal species. From my perspective, our humanity is not about our superior intellectual capacities or opposable thumbs. What makes us unique is our capacity to love someone different from ourselves. Indeed, our capacity to form long-lasting bonds and friendships with genetically unrelated individuals is posited to have been a key part of the evolutionary success of our species. Yet our capacity for love is not an instinct (reflex); it doesn't just happen or suddenly appear on our eighteenth birthday. It is a predisposition, not a given. It is something that must be both earned and learned and then chosen again and again over the course of our lives. It can grow or wither, depending on what we decide and what we do, and there is no easy way out. That said, it is a joy to engage, if one enters the room with humility.

To close…perhaps Kowock of Tribe Roc may have put it best when he explained to his tribal chief how they could join forces with Tribe Clog to defeat a pride of ferocious, voracious lions:

> We must signal vulnerability. We must wash our faces clean of war paint and freely expose our bellies. We must not hide behind our shields but instead walk freely toward Tribe Clog with an open heart and a willingness to reveal our fears and joys. Only then will Tribe Clog know that we are their brothers, and only then can we band together with them and defeat the lions.

In my opinion, the risk is worth it.

Assessing Styles of Coping: Word-Pair Checklist

Instructions: Read the pair of words or phrases in each row under columns A and B. For each row, place a checkmark in the box next to the word or phrase that is more descriptive of you. Check only one box for each of the paired words or phrases (that is, use only one checkmark per row). If you are not sure which of the two choices better describes you, imagine what your friends or family members might say about you. To get your score, add up the number of checkmarks in each column. The column with more checkmarks represents your *overall* personality style, with a higher score for column A indicating a tendency to be more undercontrolled, and a higher score for column B indicating a tendency to be more overcontrolled, but a high score for either column does not necessarily indicate *maladaptive* undercontrolled or overcontrolled coping.

A	B
◻ impulsive	◻ deliberate
◻ impractical	◻ practical
◻ naive	◻ worldly
◻ vulnerable	◻ aloof
◻ risky	◻ prudent
◻ talkative	◻ quiet
◻ disobedient	◻ dutiful
◻ fanciful	◻ realistic
◻ fickle	◻ constant
◻ act without thinking	◻ think before acting
◻ animated	◻ restrained
◻ changeable mood	◻ stable mood
◻ haphazard	◻ orderly
◻ wasteful	◻ frugal
◻ affable	◻ reserved
◻ impressionable	◻ not easily impressed
◻ erratic	◻ predictable
◻ complaining	◻ uncomplaining
◻ reactive	◻ unreactive
◻ careless	◻ fastidious
◻ playful	◻ earnest
◻ intoxicated	◻ clearheaded
◻ self-indulgent	◻ self-controlled
◻ laid back	◻ hardworking

A	B
☐ unconventional	☐ conventional
☐ dramatic	☐ modest
☐ brash	☐ unobtrusive
☐ obvious	☐ discreet
☐ vacillating	☐ determined
☐ unrealistic	☐ sensible
☐ gullible	☐ shrewd
☐ unpredictable	☐ dependable
☐ dependent	☐ independent
☐ improper	☐ proper
☐ chaotic	☐ organized
☐ susceptible	☐ impervious
☐ unstable	☐ steadfast
☐ volatile	☐ undemonstrative
☐ excitable	☐ stoical
☐ lax	☐ precise
☐ unsystematic	☐ structured
☐ thoughtless	☐ thoughtful
☐ inattentive	☐ attentive
☐ short-lived	☐ enduring
☐ perky	☐ despondent
☐ passionate	☐ indifferent
☐ immediate gratification	☐ delay gratification

The Clinician-Rated OC Trait Rating Scale

Form 3.1. Descriptions of Traits for Assessors/Clinicians

Instructions: Read the following descriptions of traits, and then rate each trait on the 1–7 scale in form 3.2. A score of 6 or 7 denotes "caseness" (that is, the individual closely matches the predicted OC trait pattern). When totaling scores, make sure you reverse scores for *Openness to experience, Affiliation needs,* and *Trait positive emotionality* (see ** next to item); a score of 40 or higher suggests OC "caseness."

**Openness to experience: Refers to the degree to which a person is receptive and open to new ideas and change, novel situations, or unexpected information, including the degree to which a person is willing to listen to critical feedback before making a judgment and is willing to admit when he or she is wrong.
**Affiliation needs: Refers to the degree to which a person values giving or receiving warmth and affection and enjoys intimate and close social bonds with others.
Trait negative emotionality: Refers to the degree to which a person is vigilant and cautious in life, concerned about making mistakes, and focused on what went wrong rather than what went right; also refers to the degree to which a person experiences anxiety, worries, or is overly concerned about the future.
**Trait positive emotionality: Refers to the degree to which a person feels excited, enthusiastic, energized, or passionate about what is happening in the current moment.
Inhibited emotional expressivity: Refers to the degree to which a person attempts to control, inhibit, restrain, or suppress how he or she expresses inner feelings or emotions; individuals scoring high on this trait tend to be understated in how they express emotions and/or may report that they rarely experience emotions.
Moral certitude: Refers to compulsive desires to plan for the future, extreme dutifulness, hypermorality, and hyperperfectionism; individuals scoring high on this domain set high standards and lack the flexibility to loosen these standards when appropriate.
Compulsive striving: Motivated to act according to what may happen and/or in order to achieve a long-term goal rather than according to how they are feeling in the moment; they delay immediate gratification or pleasure in order to achieve long-term goals and may persist in stressful activities in order to achieve a desired goal, despite feedback that persistence may be harmful to them; compulsive immediate fixing occurs, whereby any problem is treated as urgent, and this behavior leads to immediate yet ill-timed and detrimental results.
High detail-focused processing: Refers to superior detail-focused as opposed to global processing, insistence on sameness, hypervigilance for small discrepancies, and preference for symmetry over asymmetry; an OC client high on this trait might tend to notice grammatical mistakes that others miss, or to quickly detect a missing data point in a complex chart.

Note: Clinicians are encouraged to use individual trait ratings to guide treatment planning (for example, high scores on *Inhibited emotional expressivity* highlight the importance of targeting this feature in treatment).

Form 3.2. Clinician-Rated OC Trait Rating Scale

OC Trait	Low						High
**Openness to experience	1	2	3	4	5	6	7
**Affiliation needs	1	2	3	4	5	6	7
Trait negative emotionality	1	2	3	4	5	6	7
**Trait positive emotionality	1	2	3	4	5	6	7
Inhibited emotional expressivity	1	2	3	4	5	6	7
Moral certitude	1	2	3	4	5	6	7
Compulsive striving	1	2	3	4	5	6	7
High detail-focused processing	1	2	3	4	5	6	7

Note: When totaling scores, it is important to reverse scores for *Openness to experience, Affiliation needs,* and *Trait positive emotionality* (see ** next to item).

The Overcontrolled Global Prototype Rating Scale

Form 3.3. The Overcontrolled Global Prototype Rating Scale

Instructions: This postinterview prototype rating scale assesses four core OC deficits (each category of deficit has two subheadings):

1. Receptivity and openness

2. Flexible responding

3. Emotional expression and awareness

4. Social connectedness and intimacy

After completing a clinical interview, the interviewer should read the description under each of the eight subheadings and then, rather than counting individual symptoms, should rate the extent to which the client matches the description as a whole, using the following 0–4 scale:

0 = little or no match (description does not apply)

1 = some match (some features apply)

2 = moderate match (has significant features)

3 = good match (has the majority of features)

4 = very good match (exemplifies features)

Ratings should be done after the client has left the interview room. Add up the eight subheading scores, and then use the scale at the end of form 3.3 to determine the extent to which the client represents the OC prototype.

Notes

1. Average time to complete all ratings is approximately five minutes.

2. OC subtypes are rated only if the client has scored 17 or higher on the global rating scale.

3. The summary scoring sheet provided at the end of form 3.4 can be incorporated into the client's medical record.

1. Deficits in Receptivity and Openness

a. Is hypervigilant for stimuli perceived to be threatening, critical, discrepant, disorganized, or lacking in symmetry

1. Is more alert to the potential for harm than to the potential for reward when entering new or unfamiliar situations; is less likely to find uncertainty or ambiguity enjoyable, stimulating, or potentially profitable. For example, will avoid taking unplanned risks (that is, risks for which he has not had time to prepare) and/or dislikes scrutiny and the limelight (because it might invite criticism), despite desiring appreciation or recognition for achievements.

2. Tends to avoid new, uncertain, or novel situations for which he has not been able to prepare, especially if he can avoid them without calling attention to himself. Tends to prefer situations where rules or prescribed roles are preordained (for example, he will prefer a business meeting to a picnic). Will tend to chastise himself whenever he perceives himself as making a mistake, not living up to his values, or not behaving properly.

Prototype Rating for This OC Feature

Place a checkmark in the relevant box, and record the total score in the box below.

- ☐ Little or no match (description does not apply) score = **0**
- ☐ Some match (some features apply) score = **1**
- ☐ Moderate match (has significant features) score = **2**
- ☐ Good match (has the majority of features) score = **3**
- ☐ Very good match (exemplifies features) score = **4**

Score for this feature = ☐

---

b. Tends to discount critical feedback or new information

1. When confronted with feedback with which he disagrees, will tend to automatically refute it (albeit often this is done silently), minimize it, or avoid it and/or pretend to agree with it as a means of preventing further criticism. For example, may respond to feedback by ruminating about a rebuttal, searching for disconfirming evidence, shutting down, refusing to listen, counterattacking, changing the topic, and/or behaving as if bored.

2. May secretly harbor resentment and/or plans for revenge if challenged, questioned, or frustrated or may feel thwarted, overwhelmed, or hopeless about achieving a desired goal.

3. To avoid critical feedback, may be reluctant to reveal true beliefs or feelings.

4. May reject a differing opinion on the basis of minor inaccuracies or "inappropriate" word usage (or other perceived inconsistencies) rather than on the basis of logic or reason.

5. May automatically go on the offensive or the defensive when feeling criticized (for example, by answering a question with a question, by counterattacking, by behaving as if he has not heard the feedback, by denial, or by providing a vague answer).

6. May attempt to beat an imagined critic to the punch by criticizing or minimizing his own accomplishments first.

Prototype Rating for This OC Feature

Place a checkmark in the relevant box, and record the total score in the box below.

☐ Little or no match (description does not apply) score = **0**

☐ Some match (some features apply) score = **1**

☐ Moderate match (has significant features) score = **2**

☐ Good match (has the majority of features) score = **3**

☐ Very good match (exemplifies features) score = **4**

Score for this feature = ☐

---

2. Deficits in Flexible Responding

a. Has compulsive needs for structure and order

1. Is hyperperfectionistic (for example, sets high standards for himself and others).

2. Is compulsively rule-governed and tends to hold strong convictions and/or have high moral certitude (for example, believes that there is a right way and a wrong way to behave, or believes that there is only one correct answer). May feel compelled to follow rules of etiquette even when the rules do not make sense in a given situation. Tends to prefer highly structured or rule-governed games (such as chess).

3. May compulsively hoard information or, oftentimes, relatively meaningless objects "just in case" they may be needed in the future.

4. Likely to attribute his actions to rules, not to his current mood or anticipated rewards. For example, when asked why he went to a party, will tend to answer, "Because I thought it was the right thing to do."

5. Compelled to "fix" a problem (even a minor one) immediately rather than giving himself time to think about it or obtaining a much-needed rest before beginning work.

Prototype Rating for This OC Feature

Place a checkmark in the relevant box, and record the total score in the box below.

☐ Little or no match (description does not apply) score = **0**

☐ Some match (some features apply) score = **1**

☐ Moderate match (has significant features) score = **2**

☐ Good match (has the majority of features) score = **3**

☐ Very good match (exemplifies features) score = **4**

Score for this feature = ☐

---

b. Engages in compulsive planning and/or rehearsal

1. Works beyond what is needed in order to avoid being seen as incompetent (for example, overrehearses a speech).

2. Has difficulty altering a planned course of action or revising a prior solution after circumstances have changed, or after feedback that the prior way of doing things will not be useful in the current context.

3. May engage in apparently high-risk sports or other activities (such as scuba diving, skydiving, or stock trading), but the risk taking is always carefully planned or premeditated (that is, the activity is not performed on a whim).

4. Exhibits compulsive persistence (for example, continues to engage in a difficult task in order to achieve a long-term goal, even if persistence may prove damaging). Will persist in an activity (working, running, striving) despite feedback that doing so could result in harm to himself or others (such as physical injury or a damaged relationship). May find it difficult to rest (by taking a nap, for example) or ask for help when it is obvious that persisting in his current course will not prove beneficial.

Prototype Rating for This OC Feature

Place a checkmark in the relevant box, and record the total score in the box below.

☐ Little or no match (description does not apply) score = **0**

☐ Some match (some features apply) score = **1**

☐ Moderate match (has significant features) score = **2**

☐ Good match (has the majority of features) score = **3**

☐ Very good match (exemplifies features) score = **4**

Score for this feature = ☐

3. Deficits in Emotional Expression and Awareness

a. Has diminished emotional experience and awareness

1. Has low awareness of emotions and bodily sensations (for example, may report difficulty labeling and distinguishing between emotions and bodily

sensations). When depressed or anxious, may report feeling tired or fatigued rather than using emotion words to describe mood. May adamantly insist that he does not experience certain emotions (such as anger). May feel numb or empty when experiencing intense emotions (especially anger). When asked about feelings, tends to report thoughts rather than using emotion words. May use idiosyncratic and/or peculiar language when describing emotions (for example, "I feel like plastic").

2. Tends to be stoic and uncomplaining and to minimize or discount emotional experience (such as anger, pain, or excitement), both publicly and privately (even with family members, for example). Reports mood states as stable and static, with little variability or contrast in intensity. May hold idiosyncratic beliefs about certain emotions (for example, may report never experiencing anger because to him anger means being out of control and having fits of rage, or because he may believe that showing fear or feeling sad is a sign of weakness or cowardice). Tends to underreport emotions. For example, may habitually say "I'm fine" when queried about how he feels, regardless of current mood state (even when highly distressed, for example). Exhibits high distress tolerance; is able to tolerate pain or discomfort without complaint for long periods and may ignore injuries or medical problems. When angry, becomes quieter (rather than louder), as in the silent treatment; may pout when angry but deny doing so when queried. When an outburst of anger occurs, it tends to occur in private (for example, only in the presence of immediate family members or a therapist), not in public places (such as at a train station or in the street). May communicate a stance that devalues the importance of emotions (for example, may change the topic when emotions are discussed, or may quickly attempt to "fix" the emotional distress exhibited by another person by giving that person advice).

Prototype Rating for This OC Feature

Place a checkmark in the relevant box, and record the total score in the box below.

- ☐ Little or no match (description does not apply) score = **0**
- ☐ Some match (some features apply) score = **1**
- ☐ Moderate match (has significant features) score = **2**
- ☐ Good match (has the majority of features) score = **3**
- ☐ Very good match (exemplifies features) score = **4**

Score for this feature = ☐

b. Masks inner feelings (via facial expressions, gestures, and actions)

1. Strives to keep up appearances and be seen as in control.

2. Exhibits facial expressions or body posture that may not match inner experience, or that may be incongruent (for example, may smile when afraid or angry, may cry when angry, may sit upright in a rigid position with tightly clasped hands while smiling).

3. May exhibit little variability in the expression or intensity of positive or negative emotional experiences. May tend to inhibit the expression of both negative and positive emotions. May rarely show extreme excitement or demonstrate joy.

4. Rarely describes himself as excitable or enthusiastic; tends to be serious, and rarely engages in spontaneous laughter or giggling, although may rehearse jokes and may be able to entertain or make others laugh. May pride himself on being witty.

5. Exhibits expressions that tend to be flat, impassive, or restrained (for example, may exhibit a flat face when angry or amused) and that tend to be disingenuous and/or incongruent with inner experience (for example, may smile when distressed or show an expression of concern when angry).

6. Is rarely demonstrative in gestures, facial expressions, or actions (for example, is less likely to make large or big gestures and less likely to use hand or arm gestures while talking).

7. May consider masking of emotions to be a sign of maturity.

Prototype Rating for This OC Feature

Place a checkmark in the relevant box, and record the total score in the box below.

☐ Little or no match (description does not apply) score = **0**

☐ Some match (some features apply) score = **1**

☐ Moderate match (has significant features) score = **2**

☐ Good match (has the majority of features) score = **3**

☐ Very good match (exemplifies features) score = **4**

Score for this feature = ☐

---

4. Deficits in Social Connectedness and Intimacy
a. Has an aloof/distant interpersonal style of relating

1. In general, is cautious, restrained, and reserved during interactions.

2. Is conflict-avoidant; may abandon a relationship rather than deal with conflict.

3. In general, finds social interactions fatiguing, mentally exhausting, or unrewarding.

4. Attends social activities out of a sense of duty or obligation, not because of genuine desire to participate (anticipatory reward).

5. Dislikes non-goal-focused social interactions that involve joining with others or sharing inner experiences, that lack prescribed roles, and/or that involve free-flowing conversation (such as picnics, parties, group celebrations, and team-building activities).

6. Is slow to warm up to another person and less likely to reveal his opinions until he gets to know the person better. May be proud that he is not easily impressed, or that it takes a long time to get to know him. Tends not to talk about himself (for example, rarely brags overtly about himself or spontaneously describes an adventure in detail and is less likely to reveal doubts or past failures). Is low in vulnerable self-disclosure (for example, tends only rarely to reveal socially unacceptable beliefs or emotions, or may tend to ask others questions rather than reveal personal information).

7. Will generally behave prosocially, but without revealing much personal information. For example, tends to be polite and cordial during most interactions, especially during greetings or when ending a conversation (will shake hands, smile, nod, and ask appropriate questions). May spend a great deal of time rehearsing the "appropriate" response and/or carefully planning what he might say or how he might behave prior to a social engagement, and his interactions can appear stilted, awkward, or insincere when the prepared script doesn't fit the situation. May appear to be actively engaged in a conversation without revealing personal information. When asked personal questions, may give long-winded answers that are intellectual or vague, may change the topic, or may turn the question back on the questioner (for example, may quickly answer and then ask the other person the same question). More likely to discuss nonsocial topics (such as politics, the weather, and the news) or provide opinions about nonemotional topics (for example, the taste of a meal). After a prolonged social interaction, may yearn for sensory deprivation (for example, reduces external stimuli by closing all window shades, putting in earplugs, advising family members to leave him alone, taking a headache remedy, and retiring to bed).

Prototype Rating for This OC Feature

Place a checkmark in the relevant box, and record the total score in the box below.

☐ Little or no match (description does not apply) score = **0**

☐ Some match (some features apply) score = **1**

☐ Moderate match (has significant features) score = **2**

☐ Good match (has the majority of features) score = **3**

☐ Very good match (exemplifies features) score = **4**

Score for this feature = ☐

b. Highly values achievement, performance, and competence (or at least the appearance of competence)

1. In relationships, what takes precedence for him is avoiding feelings of vulnerability, humiliation, or embarrassment (for example, may be willing to damage a relationship in order to avoid being discovered as incorrect, incompetent, or vulnerable).

2. Makes frequent social comparisons and relies on downward social comparisons to boost self-esteem.

3. May hold on to grudges or past hurts, and may experience periods of high envy and/or bitterness.

4. May secretly harbor ill will toward rivals or those he perceives as having an unfair advantage over him.

5. May view himself as a social misfit, an outsider, and a loner, or as different or awkward.

6. May develop a cynical view of relationships and come to believe that love and genuine caring are either false or impossible.

7. May feel unappreciated or unrecognized for his talents, hard work, or self-sacrifices, and these feelings can lead to resentment and bitterness and may have a negative impact on his relationships. May desire recognition for his efforts but seldom directly request it.

8. Has low skills in empathy and validation. May struggle to understand the importance of understanding another person's perspective. May actively make self-sacrifices to help others but does so from a sense of duty or obligation rather than from strong feelings of warmth, sympathy, or compassion. May believe that only outstanding performance is worthy of validation or appreciation. Even when he achieves outstanding performance, may allow himself little time to rest or bask in glory. May be more likely to say no to new ideas or suggestions. May find it difficult to compliment, praise, or help others (or be praised or helped by others). May find it difficult to admit when he has made a mistake. May apologize only rarely for wrongdoing, or may apologize excessively in order to avoid social disapproval. May frequently provide unsolicited advice to others.

Prototype Rating for This OC Feature

Place a checkmark in the relevant box, and record the total score in the box below.

- ☐ Little or no match (description does not apply) score = **0**
- ☐ Some match (some features apply) score = **1**
- ☐ Moderate match (has significant features) score = **2**
- ☐ Good match (has the majority of features) score = **3**
- ☐ Very good match (exemplifies features) score = **4**

Score for this feature = ☐

Notes

_____

_____

_____

_____

_____

Add up the scores from each of the eight subfeatures, and then use this scale to determine the degree to which the individual meets the criteria for OC.

OC Clinical Rating Scale total score = ☐

0–7 = unlikely to be OC

8–16 = low to moderate OC features

17–24 = good match for OC

25–32 = exemplifies OC

Form 3.4. Overcontrolled Subtype Rating Scale

Instructions: Complete the two items in form 3.4 *only if the client has scored 17 or higher* on the Overcontrolled Global Prototype Rating Scale (form 3.3). These two items should *not* be completed if the client is not overcontrolled.

Overly Disagreeable Subtype

1. Motivated to be perceived as competent but not compliant.

2. Less concerned about social approval, politeness, or social correctness. Willing to appear unfriendly, bad-tempered, or disagreeable in order to achieve an objective, even if it harms interpersonal relations.

3. Tends to appear businesslike or serious in public. May display flattened or inhibited emotional expression during social interactions.

4. Behavior usually driven by a sense of duty, obligation, or ambition. For example, may display friendly, polite, or affable expressions because these are customary or expected according to rules of etiquette (at a wedding, for example, or when greeting a friend or acquaintance or purchasing something from a salesclerk), or may do so in order to achieve a personal goal (for example, during a business meeting), not simply because of feeling particularly warmhearted or kindly toward someone.

5. When an important personal goal or rule is thwarted or violated, may quickly lose prosocial persona and behave in an indifferent, cold, detached, or critical manner.

6. May consider himself strong-willed, and may value his ability to resist social pressure or to remain unaffected by interpersonal issues or conflict.

7. May genuinely struggle with communicating positive emotions and/or with feeling easy or laid back while interacting with others. May find it difficult to communicate desires for affiliation or express vulnerable emotions to others. May resist or avoid a public display of affection, even when the situation clearly calls for it.

8. May find it difficult to apologize, praise, or offer help to others (or may find it difficult to believe that apologies from others are genuine, and may have difficulty accepting help or praise from others).

9. May be described by others as aloof or arrogant. Tends to value competence over relationships. May believe genuine love or intimacy is false or a waste of time.

Prototype Rating for This OC Feature

Place a checkmark in the relevant box, and record the total score in the box below.

- ☐ Little or no match (description does not apply) score = **0**
- ☐ Some match (some features apply) score = **1**
- ☐ Moderate match (has significant features) score = **2**
- ☐ Good match (has the majority of features) score = **3**
- ☐ Very good match (exemplifies features) score = **4**

Score for this feature = ☐

Overly Agreeable Subtype

1. Motivated to be seen as competent and socially acceptable.

2. Tends to be preoccupied with monitoring himself internally for signs of anxiety, and with monitoring others for signs of disapproval.

3. Likely to display disingenuous or incongruent expressions in order to avoid social disapproval (for example, may smile when distressed, laugh while not finding something amusing, or express concern and caring while not feeling concern or caring). May believe that removing his mask of acceptability would lead to extreme social rejection.

4. May adopt a style of behaving that avoids personal self-disclosure but appears intimacy-enhancing. For example, may be highly adept at steering a conversation away from himself by asking apparently compassionate questions about the other person's life. May also feign interest (for example, by pretending to take notes during a conversation), express artificial concern (via polite expressions of sympathy), and exhibit false humility (for example, by criticizing himself before others can).

5. May quickly express agreement or concede defeat despite inwardly disagreeing, or may flatter or praise a rival to conceal envy

6. May feel resentful when his overly solicitous, socially considerate manner is not recognized, appreciated, or reciprocated, but will work hard to conceal any hostile feelings.

7. May work hard to convince his therapist that he is okay or "normal."

8. May obsessively rehearse how he will behave or what he might say prior to a social event. Avoids situations requiring spontaneous behavior. Desires recognition but not the limelight.

9. May report feeling exhausted after a social event because it is draining to keep up his façade of social acceptability for long periods of time. His need for rest after social interactions may be so intense that it leads to abnormal periods of social isolation (for example, he may turn off all the lights and go to bed in the middle of the afternoon or may have no contact with others for several days) and even to states of shutdown or collapse (for example, he may take frequent sick leave).

Prototype Rating for This OC Feature

Place a checkmark in the relevant box, and record the total score in the box below.

☐ Little or no match (description does not apply) score = **0**

☐ Some match (some features apply) score = **1**

☐ Moderate match (has significant features) score = **2**

☐ Good match (has the majority of features) score = **3**

☐ Very good match (exemplifies features) score = **4**

Score for this feature = ☐

OC Prototype Rating Scale: Summary Score Sheet

		Little or no match (description does not apply)	Some match (some features apply)	Moderate match (has significant features)	Good match (has the majority of features)	Very good match (exemplifies features)
1. Deficits in receptivity and openness	Hypervigilant for stimuli perceived to be threatening, critical, discrepant, disorganized, or lacking in symmetry	0	1	2	3	4
	Tends to discount critical feedback or new information	0	1	2	3	4
2. Deficits in inflexible responding	Has compulsive needs for structure and order	0	1	2	3	4
	Engages in compulsive planning and/or rehearsal	0	1	2	3	4
3. Deficits in emotional expression and awareness	Has diminished emotional experience and awareness	0	1	2	3	4
	Masks inner feelings (via facial expressions, gestures, and actions)	0	1	2	3	4
4. Deficits in social connectedness and intimacy	Has an aloof/distant interpersonal style of relating	0	1	2	3	4
	Highly values achievement, performance, and competence (or at least the appearance of competence)	0	1	2	3	4
	Add up scores for each feature 0–7 = unlikely to be OC 8–16 = low to moderate OC features 17–24 = good match for OC 25–32 = exemplifies OC					

Rate the level of OC subtype (only if score on form 3.3 was 17 or higher)

Overly disagreeable subtype		0	1	2	3	4
Overly agreeable subtype		0	1	2	3	4

RO DBT Semistructured Suicidality Interview

A script for introducing a discussion of life-threatening behavior with an OC client is outlined in chapter 5, in the section titled "Assessing OC Life-Threatening Behaviors." The following questions, derived from clinical experience, are recommended as a guide for conducting the discussion. The therapist should expect to ask more questions and spend more time on this topic as warranted by the degree and severity of self-harm and suicidal problems that have been or are present in the client's life.

Questions preceded by an asterisk (*) are indicators of high risk and should always be asked.		
1. Have you had thoughts that life is not worth living? *If the client says yes, ask:* What have you thought about? When was the last time you thought this way? *Notes*	YES	NO
2. Do you sometimes wish you were dead or think that people or the world would be better off if you were not around? *If the client says yes, ask:* When was the last time you thought this way? *Notes*	YES	NO

3. Have you ever wanted to harm or kill yourself in order to punish others (for example, thinking *They'll be sorry when I'm gone* or *This will teach them*)? *If the client says yes, ask:* Whom do you wish to punish? When was the last time you thought this way? *Notes*	YES	NO
*4. Have you ever come up with a specific plan to kill or harm yourself? *If the client says yes, ask:* What was your plan? Have you ever told anyone about this? *Notes*	YES	NO
*5. Have you ever deliberately hurt yourself without meaning to kill yourself (for example, have you cut yourself, burned yourself, punched yourself, put your hand through windows, punched walls, banged your head)? *If the client says yes, ask:* How often do you deliberately self-harm? When was your most recent self-harm event? What did you do? Where did you do it? Were other people in the immediate area (for example, in the same house), or were you alone? If others were nearby, who were they? Did you hope you might be discovered? What happened afterward? Did you require medical treatment? *Notes*	YES	NO
*6. Have you ever intentionally tried to kill yourself? *If the client says yes, ask:* When was your most recent attempt? What did you do? What happened afterward? Did you require medical treatment? Had you planned it in advance? Did anyone know about your plans? How many times in the past have you attempted suicide? *Notes*	YES	NO

*7. Do you have urges, thoughts, or plans to kill or harm yourself in the near future? *If the client says yes, the therapist should identify the events that have triggered the client's response and then work collaboratively with the client to reduce high-risk factors before ending the session. Plus, ideally, the therapist should obtain a commitment from the client that he or she is willing to work on eliminating self-harm or suicidal behaviors during the course of treatment.* *Notes*	YES	NO
*8. Would you be willing to commit to me to not self-harm or attempt to kill yourself between now and our next session? *If the client says no, see "The RO DBT Crisis-Management Protocol," in chapter 5 of this book.* *Notes*	YES	NO
The following questions should be asked only if a client has endorsed suicide and self-harm as a problem.		
9. When you self-harm, do you plan it ahead of time (for example, by scheduling when and where you will self-harm and ensuring that the means are available)? *If the client says yes, ask: How long do you plan beforehand?* *Notes*	YES	NO
10. How many people know about your self-harm or suicidal behavior? *If at least one person, ask: Who are they? What have you told them? How have they reacted?* *Notes*	(Write number)	NOBODY
11. Have you been psychiatrically hospitalized following a self-harm or suicide attempt in the past? *If the client says yes, ask: Did you want to be hospitalized? How long did you stay in the hospital? How many times have you been hospitalized?* *Notes*	YES	NO

12. Why do you think you want to harm or kill yourself?		
If the client is unsure, use the following questions as prompts.		
a. Have you often self-harmed because you were angry with yourself?	YES	NO
b. Do you self-harm to change an emotion—for example, to deal with feelings of unbearable misery and despair?	YES	NO
c. Do you self-harm in order to punish yourself?	YES	NO
d. Have you ever self-harmed or attempted suicide to prove a point, make someone feel sorry, as payback, or to teach someone a lesson?	YES	NO
e. Other reasons?		
Notes		
f. If there is more than one reason, which one do you think describes your motivations the best?	YES	NO
Notes		

Targeting Indirect Social Signals: In-Session Protocol

1. Highlight potential maladaptive social signaling behavior in session, but only after it has occurred multiple times and over multiple sessions.

Therapist: You just yawned…did you notice that?

Therapist performs eyebrow wag, signals an easy manner.

Client: Yeah. I'm just tired.

Client shrugs shoulders slightly, uses flat tone of voice.

The client's nonverbal behavior may signal Fatalistic Mind thinking (see the skills training manual, chapter 5, lesson 11) or a low-level "don't hurt me" response (see the material on "don't hurt me" responses, chapter 10).

2. Assess the extent to which the client is aware of the repetitive nature of the social signaling behavior.

Therapist: Oh, okay…you're just tired. But have you ever noticed that you seem to get tired at certain time points but not others in the same session? For example, whenever we talk about diary cards? Like now, for instance? You seem to yawn more. Have you ever noticed that?

Therapist offers warm closed-mouth smile, signals an easy manner, displays open curiosity.

Client: Not really…but now that you mention it…

Volume of client's voice drops slightly; client offers slightly inhibited smile, averts gaze.

The client is sending a complex social signal that may indicate her mixed emotions and/or her attempt to deamplify her emotions or conceal her true intentions. For example, the client may be experiencing embarrassment, a prosocial self-conscious emotion (as evidenced by her inhibited smile and averted gaze), low-level shame (as evidenced by her lowered voice volume and averted gaze, but not her inhibited smile), or secret pride, a nonengagement signal of dominance (as evidenced by her inhibited smile, also known as a *burglar smile*).

3. Reconfirm the client's commitment to targeting social signaling.

Therapist: Sure, that makes sense…but what's cool is that your willingness to think about it suggests to me that you remain committed to targeting social signaling as a core part of our work together, based on the idea that how we behave around others really impacts our relationships. Is that something you remain committed to working on?

Therapist offers warm closed-mouth smile, signals an easy manner.

The therapist's use of the word "cool" is intentional, simultaneously signaling friendship (friends use less formal language during interactions) and that it's okay for the client not to have noticed yawning.

Client: Yeah, sure…I think social signaling is important.

Client maintains eye contact, nods affirmatively.

The client is engaged.

4. Ask the client directly about the social signal, without assuming that you already know the answer.

Therapist: Great. So what do you think you might be trying to tell me when you yawn like that? What's the social signal?

Therapist offers warm closed-mouth smile, performs eyebrow wag, displays open curiosity.

Client: Nothing, really…I'm just tired.

Client uses mildly exasperated tone of voice, shrugs shoulders minutely, emits low-intensity sigh.

The client, despite having just admitted to yawning as a possible social signal, has now reverted to her original position (she is "just tired"). Her exasperated tone of voice, combined with her low-level appeasement signal (a minute shoulder shrug), suggests possible nonengagement and/or the presence of a low-level "don't hurt me" response (see the material on "don't hurt me" responses, chapter 10).

Therapist: Oh, okay…you're tired. Are you tired right now?

> *Therapist offers warm closed-mouth smile, raises eyebrows, uses playful and curious tone of voice, makes direct eye contact.*

The therapist recognizes the client's sudden reversal, but instead of challenging her, he gives her the benefit of the doubt while also showing disbelief by engaging in a low-intensity therapeutic tease and using playful irreverence.

Client: Umm…yeah, a little bit.

> *Client slightly shrugs shoulders, shuffles feet, briefly breaks eye contact.*

The client may be experiencing warranted (justified) low-level guilt or shame because she is not being fully truthful about her current state of tiredness.

5. Stay focused on the social signaling target; avoid getting distracted by other potential targets.

Therapist: Yeah, okay, you're just tired…but have you ever noticed that you seem to get tired at certain time points but not others in the same session? For example, whenever we talk about diary cards—like now, for instance— you seem to yawn more. Have you ever noticed that?

> *Therapist offers warm closed-mouth smile, displays open curiosity.*

The therapist ignores the client's possible deception and models kindness first and foremost, keeping the focus on the social signaling target (yawning). The only exceptions to keeping the focus on the social signaling target are the presence of imminent life-threatening behavior and a possible alliance rupture.

Client: I think it's just one of the problems of depression—you just feel tired.

> *Client uses gloomy tone of voice, slightly slumps shoulders, turns gaze slightly downward.*

The client's tone of voice, downward gaze, and slumped shoulders are highly suggestive of a "don't hurt me" response (see the material on "don't hurt me" responses, chapter 10). The client also does not actually answer the therapist's question.

6. Demonstrate the potentially maladaptive social signal to the client.

Therapist: Yeah, okay. Well, let's think about it differently. Let's see if this might help… Tell me about your weekend—I think you mentioned that you spent some time with your husband—and I will use your story to demonstrate something about what we have just been discussing. But make sure you keep your eyes on me while you're talking.

> *Therapist intermittently offers warm closed-mouth smile; uses open, curious, matter-of-fact tone of voice.*

The therapist places the potential "don't hurt me" response on an extinction schedule by behaving as if all is well, via his lighthearted request for the client to talk about her weekend, which also keeps the focus on the social signaling target of yawning (see the material on "don't hurt me" responses, chapter 10). The therapist does not explain in advance what is going to happen (see the material on the RO mindfulness practice of "participate without planning" in the skills training manual, chapter 5, lesson 12).

Client: Okay. So this weekend was our once-a-month big shopping day, and Ben always comes with me...

Client sighs briefly, uses monotonic voice.

The client's willingness to comply with the therapist's request to speak about her weekend suggests engagement. Her sigh occurs at the very beginning of her verbal statement, most likely signaling her resigned engagement (that is, her acceptance that her earlier attempts to avoid discussing the social signaling target are not going to work) and thus indicating therapeutic progress.

Therapist begins to yawn visibly.

Client pauses and stares briefly upon noticing therapist's yawn.

Client: ...and so when we got in the car, and the rain was absolutely pouring down—it was really wet...

Therapist yawns again.

The therapist purposefully exaggerates his yawn to ensure the client notices it.

Client stops talking.

Client: Hmmm...I think I can see what you might be getting at.

7.   Assess the client's response to the social signaling demonstration.

Therapist: So what did you think when I started yawning like that while you were telling me about your weekend? I mean, I guess that first off I should ask if you even noticed that I was yawning.

Therapist offers warm closed-mouth smile and broader smile, giggles slightly, displays open curiosity.

Client joins therapist in giggling, slightly covers mouth.

The client's behavior suggests slight embarrassment, acknowledgment of yawning as a potential problem, and engagement.

Client: I did!

Client makes direct eye contact, uses animated tone of voice, performs eyebrow wag.

The client is engaged.

Therapist: Yeah…so how did it impact you?

> *Therapist offers warm closed-mouth smile, performs eyebrow wag, uses warm tone of voice, slowly nods in affirmation, slightly slows pace of speech, slightly lowers voice volume.*

The therapist, by slowing his pace (rate) of speech, slightly lowering the volume of his voice, and combining these prosocial signals with others (a warm closed-mouth smile, an eyebrow wag, and affirmative head nodding), signals noncritical appreciation and warmth. The therapeutic use of slower speech and lower voice volume mimics the way we speak in our most intimate moments to those we love and functions as a powerful social safety signal and positive reinforcer that can be delivered in seconds (see the material on compassionate gravity, chapter 10).

Client: It made me feel uncomfortable. I thought I was boring you.

> *Client maintains solid eye contact; her voice tone is animated.*

The client is engaged.

8. Reinforce the client's engagement.

Therapist: Yeah. That kind of makes sense, doesn't it?

> *Therapist performs eyebrow wag, smiles playfully.*

> *Client nods.*

Therapist: And yet it can be both disconcerting and amazing that something so seemingly trivial as a yawn can pack within it such a capacity to influence a social interaction, oftentimes in ways that may never have been intended.

> *Therapist nods in affirmation.*

The therapist, recalling that OC clients dislike the limelight, is taking the heat off the client—but without removing the target—by broadening the topic to include people in general rather than just the client, thus further reinforcing the client's engagement.

> *Client nods.*

Client: Yeah. Actions speak louder than words.

> *Client chuckles, makes direct eye contact, uses animated tone of voice, performs eyebrow wag.*

The client is engaged.

9. Remind the client of the definition of a social signal, and then return to the social signaling target.

Therapist: That's for sure!

Therapist chuckles with client, displays playful curiosity, signals an informal and easy manner, offers warm playful smile combined with slight wink.

Therapist: Remember, as we have discussed before, any action that can be observed by another person—say, yawning or burping—

Therapist feigns a burp.

Therapist: Oops! Pardon me. As I was saying, any action that can be observed by someone else, or our tone of voice, as well as the words we speak, can serve as a social signal, whether it was intended or not. So sometimes a yawn is just a yawn, but then again sometimes a yawn is more than a yawn.

Therapist smiles and winks.

The therapist's playfulness (for example, the feigned burp) is essential in order to signal to the hyper-threat-sensitive, overly serious OC client that she is not assumed to be doing something wrong (that is, it is up to the client to decide whether the way in which she socially signals reflects her core valued goals, and it is the therapist's job to facilitate this decision). The therapist's silliness, smiling, and winking send a powerful message of friendship and equality that mirrors the type of easygoing teasing and lighthearted joking often seen among close friends as well as in healthy families and tribes.

Therapist: The question we want to figure out is whether you ever yawn with the intention of sending a message other than that you're just tired. What comes to mind when you hear me say that?

Client: Hmmm… Yeah, I'm just thinking that my daughter often says that you can always tell when Mom doesn't like what you're doing, because she starts to get tired, and my husband is always asking if I'm bored with him. I don't like admitting it, but I think it's possible that I'm yawning when they say those things. I just never made the connection before.

Client uses earnest tone of voice, slightly bows head, slightly shrugs shoulders, offers barely discernible smile, touches face quickly and nervously.

The client is engaged. With her statements of open enquiry and her nonverbal signaling of what is most likely low-level embarrassment, the client signals openness to considering that her yawning may be a maladaptive social signal.

10. Link the social signaling target to the client's valued goals.

Therapist: Those are great observations. I am guessing that behaving in a bored or disinterested way with your daughter and your husband is not necessarily a core value of yours—

Therapist signals an easy manner, offers warm closed-mouth smile, performs eyebrow wag, uses warm tone of voice and slightly slower pace of speech, displays open curiosity.

The therapist is purposefully choosing not to highlight the client's display of embarrassment because this could imply that the client is doing something wrong by revealing her vulnerability. Focusing on the client's embarrassment would also pull the discussion away from its primary purpose (that is, identifying a new social signaling target).

Client nods.

Therapist: —and perhaps not even something you want to signal to other people as well.

Client: No, it's not what I want to do, and I think it gets me into trouble. I think I might even yawn during business meetings.

Client uses earnest tone of voice, bows head, and shrugs shoulders when making comment about business meetings; combines these nonverbal behaviors with slight smile and eye gaze directed toward therapist.

The client is signaling engagement and prosocial embarrassment. Although displays of embarrassment most often involve gaze aversion, the client maintains eye contact, possibly because she is trying to gauge the therapist's response to her self-disclosure.

11. Agree to monitor the social signal on the client's diary card.

Therapist: Yeah… It's great that you are noticing these things—and I think it's fantastic that you were able to share them with me…because it's how I get to know you better, and also maybe how you get to know yourself better. But, as we both have previously agreed, you can be pretty tough on yourself, and we also know that when you find a problem, *watch out*, because you're going to try to fix it right away. But we also have both agreed that sometimes your problem-solving spirit can get you into trouble, and that it's exhausting to try and fix everything—

Therapist pauses, smacks hand on forehead.

Therapist: Wow! And here we are, talking about you being exhausted!

Therapist smiles warmly, winks slightly, slows pace.

Therapist: So if it's okay with you, what I would like to do is slow things down just a bit and not immediately assume that yawning is necessarily a problem, without getting some more data to prove our case. How does that sound when I say that to you?

Therapist signals an easy manner, displays open curiosity, slightly bows head, slightly shrugs shoulders, makes openhanded gesture, offers warm closed-mouth smile, raises eyebrows, makes direct eye contact.

The therapist is signaling nondominant cooperative friendliness in order to encourage the client's candid disclosure by combining appeasement signals (a slightly bowed head, a shoulder shrug, openhanded gestures) with cooperative-friendly signals (a warm closed-mouth smile, raised eyebrows, direct eye contact). The therapist checks in with the client to confirm her engagement before proceeding.

Client: Yeah, I agree… I think sometimes I rush in too fast to fix something that I find out later never needed fixing.

Client uses thoughtful, earnest tone of voice.

The client is engaged.

Therapist: Okay, cool. So here's my thought. Why don't we begin by simply monitoring yawning for a week or so, without trying to change it. That way, we can find out just how often it is happening, and whether there are particular times or topics where you find yourself yawning more, or whether it only happens with certain people, like your husband and your daughter—or, say, someone at work. I mean, it's not as if you are yawning all the time—like right now, for instance, you're not yawning. How does that sound to you when I say that?

Therapist signals an easy manner, displays open curiosity.

The therapist checks in with the client to confirm her engagement before proceeding.

Client nods.

Client: So that means I should put it on my diary card, and I'll just note how frequently I yawn and when it happens. Should I just count the number of yawns?

Client uses animated tone of voice, displays open curiosity.

The client is engaged and is already working on how to operationalize the therapist's suggestion to monitor her yawning behavior.

12. Agree on how the new social signaling target will be monitored.

Therapist: Yeah, you could do a frequency count—how many yawns per day—and then, in that little box on your diary card labeled "Notes/comments/chain analysis," you might make a note of whether you were with someone or alone when you yawned, and if you were with someone, who it was, and what the topic was.

Therapist offers warm closed-mouth smile, wider smiles, and compassionate expressions of concern (see the material on expressions of concern, chapter 6).

13. Identify one or two non–social signaling behaviors (involving emotions, thoughts, medication use, or restricted eating, for example) that might be related to the social signaling target.

Therapist: Plus, it would be cool to see if any of the non–social signaling targets we have already been monitoring, like resentment or thoughts about not being appreciated, are linked to yawning. Finally, I also think it would be useful to add a new non–social signaling target when it comes to yawning, and—tell me if you disagree—I think we should also start recording each day, using our 0 to 5 scale, how rested you felt when you woke up in the morning. It might be cool to see how your degree of tiredness comes into the picture, considering that was one of your original hypotheses for what might be triggering the yawns.

14. Remind the client that the goal of radical openness is to practice being open, more flexible, and socially connected, not to practice being perfect.

Therapist: Finally, what's important is that you not try to do this perfectly. Our aim is to see if we can understand this social signal better, not be perfect at it. If we are doing a good job with this, then it should be sort of fun to see what we discover.

15. Remind the client to alert you if she finds herself struggling with completion of the diary card, no matter what the reason.

Therapist: And to help with this, just as we're trying to do with other targets we are monitoring, if you start to find yourself not wanting to monitor yawning or anything related to it, don't keep it a secret!

Therapist smiles.

Therapist: Let me know, and we will sort it out together because, remember, as we have talked about before, when you don't complete diary cards, or partially complete them, or pretend to complete them, you are not only making it harder for us to get you out of the hole you sometimes describe yourself as being in, you're also sending me a big social signal!

Therapist smiles widely.

The therapist is signaling both the seriousness of the client completing the diary card and the importance of the client letting the therapist know if she struggles with completing the diary card. The therapist is attempting to convey these points in a manner that communicates his kindhearted appreciation as well as his genuine willingness to consider other options.

Therapist: Fortunately for you and for me, at least so far this has not happened. But you never know what might happen, and I for one would like to know. How does that sound to you?

Client confirms agreement.

Therapist: Okay. Before we change topics, let's make sure we have the new targets recorded on your card.

Client nods agreement.

Setting the Stage for Effective RO DBT Chain Analysis: In-Session Protocol

Use the diary card to identify the social signaling target that will become the focus of the session's behavioral chain analysis.

Therapist: Okay, I can see here on your diary card that it seems like Sunday may have been your worst day. It appears that you walked away, and also on Sunday you reported smiling while angry and refusing help—though smiling while angry also occurred on Monday. Plus, on Sunday you reported experiencing both high Fatalistic Mind signaling and thinking and high Fixed Mind signaling and thinking on the same day. I also see that you had high shame, self-critical thoughts, and high urges for revenge that day. You've done a great job of filling this out. There are several places we could go today, but Sunday really stands out. I know we had a special homework assignment last week that involved asking a particular person out on a date, using your Match + 1 skills.

Therapist displays open curiosity, uses a matter-of-fact voice tone, scans client's diary card.

The therapist is looking for the previous week's most seriously problematic day that was linked to a social signaling target (in this case, the target is the behavior labeled "walking away"). Therapists should avoid spending too much time reviewing the diary card; ideally, the review of the diary card should take approximately six or seven minutes (see "Individual Therapy Structure and Agenda," chapter 4). Diary cards provide a quick overview of the client's preceding week. The aim is to identify the problematic behavior that will become the focus of the session's chain analysis. Most often this problematic behavior should be one of the social signaling deficits (that is, the "biggest," or most conspicuous, maladaptive social signal of the week). The only exception is that imminent life-threatening behavior takes precedence. (For an explanation of Match + 1 skills, see the material on Flexible Mind ALLOWs in the skills training manual, chapter 5, lesson 21.)

Therapist: So…I'm curious. Was Sunday also the day you chose to ask Mary out on a date?

Therapist offers a warm closed-mouth smile.

The therapist is checking out her personal hypothesis by asking the client whether the social signaling target labeled "walking away" was linked to the homework assignment of asking someone out on a date.

Client: Yeah, it was. Um…I just felt so completely miserable after asking her. It just obviously was never going to work out. I don't know…I just got to this place where I just started thinking *Why bother?* So I just walked out.

Client maintains eye contact.

The client is engaged, although it is not exactly clear what happened.

Link target to valued goals (determine the most impactful social signaling problem when there is more than one on the same day).

Therapist: Yeah…Okay. Well, that makes sense and seems important, especially considering your goals to establish a long-term romantic relationship with someone. Plus, we decided together last session that Mary might be someone you would really like to get to know better—at the very least as a friend. So something must have happened for you to walk away from all that, and I am aware of imagining that is not what you wanted to socially signal.

Therapist signals an easy manner and continues to display open curiosity.

Instead of asking for clarification of the client's preceding statement, the therapist remains focused on the immediate goal of identifying a social signaling target for chain analysis and then setting the agenda for the remainder of the session. A common mistake during agenda setting is to ask for more information than is really needed; this can make review of the diary card take much longer than intended and can eat into valuable session time. When there is more than one maladaptive social signal recorded on the client's diary card for a single day—a very common occurrence—the therapist should pick the one that probably caused (or could have caused) the most damage to the client's relationship(s).

> *Client nods.*

Therapist: Plus, we always want to work on the biggest social signal. So of the three social signaling problems that occurred on Sunday—smiling while angry, refusing help, and walking away—which one do you think was the most powerful social signal that made it more likely, not less likely, for you to continue to feel alone and isolated from others?

Client: Walking away. The refusing help happened afterward, and so did the smiling when angry. But if I hadn't screwed up and walked away, probably none of the other issues would have happened, at least on that day… She probably won't speak to me again.

> *Client's voice tone is gloomy; client's eyes are slightly averted.*

The client remains engaged but may also be signaling Fatalistic Mind thinking or a low-level "don't hurt me" response.

Avoid getting distracted by other potential targets, storytelling, or premature problem solving—save it for the chain analysis.

Therapist: So it sounds like walking away would be the best target for us to take a more in-depth look at, after we finish setting the rest of the agenda. How does that sound to you?

> *Therapist signals an easy manner.*

The therapist avoids the temptation to problem solve or explore the issue further and instead confirms the client's agreement to target "walking away" as the social signaling problem that will be targeted via chain analysis. The therapist also checks in with the client to confirm the client's agreement before moving on.

Client: Yeah, that sounds good.

> *Client has a matter-of-fact voice tone, makes direct eye contact.*

The client is engaged.

The therapist and client ultimately complete setting the agenda, and the therapist briefly checks in with the client about RO skills training classes before conducting the actual chain analysis (see appendix 7, "Using RO DBT Chain and Solution Analysis: Principles and In-Session Protocol").

Using RO DBT Chain and Solution Analysis: Principles and In-Session Protocol

Determine the context in which the problematic social signal occurred (the *who, what, when, where,* and *intensity* of the signal).

Therapist: Okay, so…well done. It sounds like we are now ready to begin our chain analysis. Let's see if you and I can figure this out together. So, first off, where were you and what time of day was it on Sunday when you walked away from Mary?

Therapist offers a warm closed-mouth smile, displays open curiosity.

The therapist reinforces the client's engagement, then focuses on identifying the contextual features surrounding the maladaptive social signal. In this case, some of the contextual information has already been obtained (that is, Mary was the recipient of the client's maladaptive social signal).

Client: It was around nine in the morning. As you know, my bird-watching club always has a little gathering over coffee for the guides, where we plan who will go with which group and the routes that will be taken. Mary was there, just like always, along with the typical collection of volunteer nature guides—probably twenty of them altogether.

Client's voice tone is earnest.

The client is engaged and staying on topic.

Identify the contributing factors (also called vulnerability factors).

Therapist: What about contributing factors? Was there anything going on just prior to the prompting event, or the day before, that may have made it more likely for you to walk away? For example, had you eaten that day? How was your sleep? Any interpersonal conflict the day before, or just prior to the event?

Therapist signals an easy manner, uses matter-of-fact voice tone, displays open curiosity, performs eyebrow wag.

The therapist's questions are aimed at establishing contributing factors that may have made it more likely for the maladaptive social signal to occur on that particular day. This should not take more than one or two minutes; it is important not to spend too much time on contributing factors. These are sometimes important areas for solution analysis, but therapists should spend the majority of their time focusing on the links in the chain that were triggered by the prompting event. In this case, the therapist and the client—now in the twenty-first session of therapy, or the late phase of treatment—have already conducted multiple chain analyses, and so there is no need for the therapist to define what she means when she talks about contributing factors or the prompting event. Therapists should look for prompting events that are temporally close—ideally, no more than thirty minutes prior to the maladaptive social signal (in reality, prompting events or triggers most often occur within seconds to a few minutes prior to the problem social signal). This helps prevent unnecessarily long chain analyses.

Client: Well, I was actually feeling pretty tired. I was…um…the night before, I had started to obsess about what might happen, so I went online and started to research tips on dating.

Client's voice tone is earnest.

The client is engaged and staying on topic.

Client: I ran across some interesting research that you would probably like.

Client offers quick, slight smile.

Client: I decided that even though we had discussed the importance of not over-planning, it would be best if I rehearsed everything. I gave myself a limit, though—only ten rehearsals.

Client smiles slightly.

Client: The problem is, this took longer than I had anticipated. So I didn't get to bed my usual time and had a pretty restless night's sleep. I suppose it's possible that I was more concerned about the homework assignment than I realized.

Therapist: Well, hmmm…at least we know you give a damn!

Therapist gives a quick wink, offers a warm closed-mouth smile, gives a low-level chuckle, displays a slight shoulder shrug.

Therapist: Recall, it wasn't so long ago that you were adamantly trying to convince me that you didn't really care much about anyone or what others thought about you.

The therapist is signaling playful irreverence. Her use of the word "damn" is intentional and signals friendship (friends use less formal language during interactions).

Therapist: At one time, you thought you might not really care about anybody—but now you are losing sleep over them! Wow.

Therapist offers a warm closed-mouth smile, performs eyebrow wag.

The therapist suggests that losing sleep over another person is proof of caring, thus providing corrective feedback without having to rub the client's nose in it. This is a therapeutic tease (see "Teasing, Nondominance, and Playful Irreverence," chapter 6). A therapeutic tease can also be used to lighten the mood (without making a big deal of it) and, ideally, to signal to a client that he has not done anything wrong. In this case, the client, even though he struggled with his homework, did practice The Match + 1 skills; he also completed his diary card and is engaged in the session. This is important when working with hyper-self-critical OC clients—actions often speak louder than words.

Therapist: What comes to mind when I say that to you?

Therapist leans back in chair, offers warm closed-mouth smile, emits slight therapeutic sigh.

By leaning back in her chair and offering a closed-mouth smile and a therapeutic sigh (see "Therapeutic Sighs," chapter 6) while checking in with the client, the therapist signals to the client that she is not "on his case" (gloating or criticizing) but is instead really interested in his experience.

Client: Yeah…I guess I'm starting to see your point—though I hate to admit it.

Client grins sheepishly, slightly shrugs shoulders, maintains eye contact; client's head is slightly bowed.

This is a complex social signal. The client is most likely signaling a blend of emotions (prosocial embarrassment, genuine pleasure, and friendly cooperation). The embarrassment is evidenced by the slight shoulder shrug, bowed head, and verbal acknowledgment of being wrong. The sheepish grin is a mixture of an inhibited smile (most often seen in displays of embarrassment) and a genuine smile of pleasure (see chapter 6). The client is acknowledging that his prior insistence on not caring about what others think may not have been fully accurate; the sheepish smile and the shoulder shrug function as a nonverbal repair (see appeasement gestures). Thus the client is engaged.

Client: I am starting to think that maybe I do care…at least more than I thought in the past.

The fact that the client has joined in with the therapist suggests that his experience of her observation is positive. If he had not lightened up, the protocol would have been for the therapist to move immediately to compassionate gravity by leaning back in her chair and, with a warm closed-mouth smile and an eyebrow wag, asking, "So why did you think I just said that?"

Therapist: Yeah, that makes sense to me—and thanks for letting me know.

            Therapist signals an easy manner, offers a warm closed-mouth smile, performs eyebrow wag.

The therapist reinforces the client's self-disclosure but purposefully chooses, in this case, not to make a big deal of it (for example, by praising it more intensely or exploring more deeply). Instead, she silently notes what the client has said and files it away to be discussed at another time (such as in a future session). This functions to keep the focus on the chain analysis, and the client may also experience it as more reinforcing (recall that OC clients dislike the limelight). It is important to note, however, that there is no right answer here.

Therapist: Plus, I am aware of imagining that walking away was not something you had planned in advance—and we know from our prior work together that, for you, walking away is something that, from what we can tell, seems to most often serve two purposes—one, to punish someone for doing something you don't like, and, two, to avoid conflict. Is that right?

            Client nods.

Identify the prompting event.

Therapist: So when you think back to Sunday, what do you think might have happened to trigger your walking away?

            Therapist displays open curiosity.

Client: Well, when I arrived, instead of being behind the sign-in desk, like she's always been in the past, I was surprised to find her sipping a cup of coffee and talking to some new guy who I heard had just moved up from Boston—a retired academic, if I recall correctly. This was not what I had planned.

            Client's voice tone is earnest, although with some sarcasm as he says "a retired academic, if I recall correctly."

The client's slightly sarcastic tone of voice suggests possible jealousy or envy. The client is engaged.

Confirm that the prompting event is relevant (that is, confirm that the maladaptive social signal essentially would not have occurred if the event had not occurred).

Therapist:	So here's my question for you. Do you think you would have still walked away if Mary had not been talking to this new guy?

Therapist uses matter-of-fact voice tone, displays open curiosity.

The therapist is using the RO DBT strategy of asking rather than telling in order to confirm that the prompting event identified by the client is relevant. The therapist ignores the potential new target possibly related to envy and bitterness. Instead, she silently notes what the client has said and files it away for later (for solution analyses, or as another possible target). This keeps the therapist and the client focused on the chain analysis.

Client:	No. When you put it that way, I'm pretty sure it wouldn't have happened.

Client's voice tone is earnest.

Identify the chain of events (actions, thoughts, feelings, sensations) leading up to the maladaptive social signal.

Therapist:	Okay, so you saw this new guy with Mary… So what happened next? What did you think, feel, or do right after seeing this?

Therapist displays open curiosity.

Client:	I remember thinking *She's not the woman I thought she was.*

Client's voice tone is earnest but gloomy.

The client is engaged, although the thought he reports is somewhat ambiguous. In general, therapists should get into the habit of asking for clarification whenever an OC client is indirect in his social signaling; for example, "When you say she's not the women you thought she was, what does that mean?" This provides an opportunity for the client to practice being direct, open, and candid when revealing his inner experience (a core part of healthy relationships) and to take responsibility for his perceptions and actions by publicly declaring them. It can also help the therapist avoid making erroneous assumptions about the client; however, further clarification at this stage is not a requirement.

In general, I use three broad principles to guide me in deciding whether or not to ask for additional clarification. First, I consider the phase of treatment—the earlier the phase, the more likely I am to ask for clarification. Second, I consider the time available for the chain analysis—the less time I have, the less likely I am to focus on internal behaviors (thoughts, emotions, and sensations) so that I have sufficient time to focus on social signaling deficits. Third, I remind myself that any link in the chain, if it's especially relevant, can always be explored again later, during the solution analysis.

Links in the chain that pertain to ambiguous thoughts often present excellent opportunities for a client to practice self-enquiry on his own rather than having the therapist do the work for him. In this case, the therapist might encourage the client to use self-enquiry to sort out what his intended meaning might be. This is especially helpful when a client reports, "I don't know" or struggles with knowing what a particular statement means for him. Self-enquiry can be assigned as homework, and the question of the statement's meaning can be revisited during the next session.

Therapist: Okay, so you thought *She's not who I thought she was.* Was there an emotion or sensation linked to this thought?

        Therapist displays open curiosity.

The therapist has moved to the next link in the chain—in this case, guessing that the client's thought was linked to some sort of emotion.

Client: I felt betrayed—and threatened by this other guy. He's one of those smooth talkers. So I guess anger, or maybe even envy or jealousy. We were just studying that in skills class.

        Client uses earnest voice tone, makes direct eye contact.

The client is engaged. Plus, his ability to come up with several emotional alternatives most likely reflects the late phase of his treatment (he has already gained a great deal of knowledge about emotions, both in individual therapy and in skills training class).

Therapist: Okay, well done. I'm not sure we need to necessarily know the exact emotion you felt. But I agree that anger, jealousy, or even envy might fit. Plus, I can see now why you recorded high urges for revenge on your diary card, plus both Fatalistic Mind thinking and Fixed Mind thinking. We can decide together later, if it seems important. Or, if you like, you might want to take a look at that worksheet we've used before—"Using Neural Substrates to Label Emotions"—as a homework assignment.

        Therapist signals an easy manner, offers a warm closed-mouth smile.

The therapist is modeling flexibility, thus taking heat off an engaged client, while remaining focused on social signaling, which is the primary focus of treatment. Therapists should get into the habit of pulling out the skills training manual and turning to worksheet 6B when a client struggles to identify an emotional link in the chain. This worksheet uses body sensations, urges, and social signals to help OC clients learn to label different emotions.

Client writes therapist's suggestions in his self-enquiry journal.

Therapist: But what I'm really curious about is how all this internal stuff started to influence your social signaling. What happened next? How did you get from this anger to actually approaching Mary to ask her out for a date?

Therapist displays open curiosity, offers a warm closed-mouth smile, performs eyebrow wag.

Client: I just thought *Well, let's just get it over with.* But I wasn't about to go up and ask her out for a date when she was talking to *that* clown. So I waited and watched, and…

Client's voice tone is earnest, but with a pronounced sarcastic edge.

The client is engaged and staying on topic, and he is answering the therapist's questions directly.

Therapist: How long did you wait?

Therapist displays open curiosity, performs eyebrow wag.

The therapist is looking for evidence of warranted (justified) jealousy. She is also choosing not to comment on the client's use of the word "clown," for several reasons. First, to highlight this word as judgmental would itself be judgmental. Second, the client may be signaling friendship by allowing himself to use more colorful language. Third, highlighting the word "clown" would move them away from the chain analysis and its focus on the behavior labeled "walking away." The therapist does note the client's use of the word "clown," as well as the fact that this is the second time in the last few minutes that he has used a sarcastic tone of voice. But even though sarcasm is a potentially important maladaptive social signal linked to the OC theme of envy and bitterness, she chooses to collect more data before discussing it with her client, and her choice keeps them focused on completing the chain analysis. Sarcasm most often is linked to envy, bitterness, disdain, and/or contempt (that is, to social status–related emotions that are themselves linked to the desire to dominate). It is a power-ful indirect social signal that can negatively impact a client's social connectedness and go against his core values for fairness or kindness. If sarcasm appears repeatedly over multiple sessions, then the therapist will move to address this indirect social signal (see appendix 5, "Targeting Indirect Social Signals: In-Session Protocol").

Client: Oh, I don't know…I suppose it wasn't that long. Someone came along in a few minutes and interrupted their conversation, and the guy just wandered off with that person. So I just marched right up to Mary—but I think by then I had forgotten everything I had planned to say.

Client uses matter-of-fact voice tone.

The client is engaged, as evidenced by his direct answer to the question. The short duration of the interaction between Mary and the other man suggests that the client's jealousy was not warranted.

Therapist: Do you remember what you were thinking about or feeling when you started to walk toward her?

Therapist displays open curiosity.

Client: I was thinking *She's cold and calculating. She just wants to hurt me.*

Client presents a flat face, uses monotonic voice tone.

Therapist: What exactly did you say to her?

Therapist displays open curiosity, offers a warm closed-mouth smile.

The therapist is focused on obtaining a detailed description of any potentially problematic behavior.

Client: I just said, "Hey, would you like to go out sometime?"

Client uses matter-of-fact voice tone, stares at therapist.

Therapist: Really...? In exactly that tone of voice?

Therapist raises eyebrows, but without an accompanying smile; her voice tone is questioning; she tilts her head slightly to one side and performs a lip curl (a quick upward movement of the upper lip on one side), which is followed almost immediately by a warm closed-mouth smile and a slight shoulder shrug.

The therapist's nonverbal behavior—a complex social signal—takes place in less than one second. It is a classic therapeutic tease, and I refer to it as the "Oh really...?" response. The lip curl is a very interesting part of this tease because it normally is associated with disgust; thus many therapists find it very difficult (at first) to use in therapy, even when they fully recognize its therapeutic value and easily deliver the "Oh really...?" signal to their friends and family members all the time. But this is an important social signal for therapists to give themselves permission to use when working with hyper-threat-sensitive OC clients. It allows a therapist to informally point out flaws, but without being too heavy-handed about it.

Client: Yeah, I figured she wouldn't want to anyway. I was like, well, you know...I don't know. I just wasn't thinking.

Client's voice tone is gloomy; client has slightly downcast eyes, slumped shoulders, slight postural shrinkage.

The client appears to be signaling low-level guilt or shame; his words don't directly imply that he believes he has done anything wrong, but his nonverbal social signaling does. Guilt stems from one's negative evaluation of oneself, which arises whenever one fails to live according to one's own values or one's idealized self, by contrast with shame, which arises in connection with real or imagined evaluations by others (see "Fun Facts: Shame Differs from Guilt" in the skills training manual, chapter 5, lesson 8). Unlike shame, however, guilt has no facial, bodily, or physiological response associated with it, and research shows that people distrust an expression of guilt (such as saying, "I'm sorry") if it is not accompanied by a bodily display prototypical of shame. In this case, the client's bodily displays—postural shrinkage, lowered gaze—are prototypical of shame, suggesting that he values the therapeutic relationship and that it is important to him to try hard to complete his homework assignments.

Therapist: So what did she say when you asked her out?

  Therapist displays open curiosity.

The therapist is staying focused on the chain analysis rather than moving to address the client's possible feelings of guilt or shame or attempting to regulate the client.

Client: She said, well, she wanted to think about it.

  Client's voice tone and facial expression are flat.

Therapist: So what did you do?

  Therapist displays open curiosity.

The therapist is focused on finding the important links in the chain—thoughts, actions, and emotions.

Client: I just said, "Okay, that figures." And then I just turned around and marched over to the coffeemaker. I didn't say anything more.

  Client's voice tone and facial expression remain flat.

Whenever possible, ask the client to demonstrate the maladaptive social signal; don't assume that you know what it looks like.

Therapist: So can you show me what it looked like when you walked away? I mean, did you storm out or sneak away? When you marched over to the coffeemaker, was it with military precision? I guess what I am asking is this—do you think it was clear to Mary that you were not happy about what was going on?

  Therapist shifts to more upbeat/musical voice tone, offers a warm closed-mouth smile and slight wink.

427

Client stands up and walks briskly across the office.

Therapist displays open curiosity, offers a warm closed-mouth smile.

This step is not always possible to perform, because sometimes it simply doesn't make sense or isn't possible to demonstrate a social signal in session. Yet it can be very important to do so; for example, a client may report having expressed rage, but when he demonstrates what he actually did, it becomes clear to the therapist that the way the client behaved would not be considered maladaptive by most people. Performing this step can prevent the therapist from inadvertently targeting adaptive behavior (recall that OC clients tend to assume any expression of emotion is maladaptive). Sometimes this step is best performed at the very start of a chain analysis (for example, when the therapist is reviewing the diary card and attempting to ascertain which social signal to target). The general rule is that if the maladaptive nature of the social signal depends on its intensity (for example, at a very low or high intensity of expression, it might be seen as adaptive), or if the therapist for any reason doubts whether it may be maladaptive, then the therapist, before beginning the chain analysis, should have the client demonstrate what he did. However, this is usually not necessary, because the maladaptive behavior is so obviously maladaptive.

> *Client smiles.*

Client: I just said, "Okay, that figures," but with a flat voice—not sure if I can get it right just now...'cause you're doing that thing again...

> *Client giggles slightly, smiles, makes direct eye contact.*

The client is engaged. The client's statement "you're doing that thing again" refers to an inside joke with the therapist (recall that this is their twenty-first session). In this case, "that thing" is therapeutic teasing. In earlier sessions, the client has reported that he finds it hard to act depressed or upset when the therapist teases him. This became an important area of discussion for the client because it helped him come to grips with the fact that most often (but not always) his hurt or sad-looking behavior is phony and is used to control people; see the material on "don't hurt me" responses, chapter 10; see also worksheet 16.A ("Flexible Mind REVEALs") in the skills training manual, chapter 5, lesson 16.

Client: I guess it sounded something like this...

> *Client deepens voice:*

Client: "Okay, that figures." I forgot to raise my eyebrows...and I'm pretty sure I wasn't smiling.

> *Client smiles sheepishly, then attempts to regain composure.*

Identify the consequences of the problematic social signal, including possible reinforcers.

Therapist:	Hmmm…so you said, "Okay, that figures" with a flat voice tone and flat face.

Client nods.

Therapist:	So what happened after you walked away?

Therapist signals an easy manner, uses serious voice tone, slows pace of speech.

The therapist has moved from playful irreverence to compassionate gravity (see "Playful Irreverence vs. Compassionate Gravity," chapter 10).

Client:	I don't know. I went over to the coffeemaker, and I just poured myself a coffee. I just stood in the corner and I started thinking *Well, everyone has hidden motives, and they are going to manipulate me if given the opportunity.* After that, I decided to get out of there. I left the room and sat outside on a bench. At the time, I felt almost righteous. But when I got home, I started thinking that I was acting like a child… I just stomped off—and then left early. I don't know…it feels like I'm doomed for failure.

Client's voice tone is earnest but gloomy; client makes direct eye contact, but his head is slightly bowed.

The client is engaged and likely feeling moderate shame, which may be partly justified.

Therapist:	So the consequences for you were that you felt terrible. And yet what happened is highly understandable—I mean, you hardly had any sleep the night before. Plus, you haven't really ever dated anyone your entire life. So it makes sense that you might have struggled a bit the first time you tried to put Match + 1 skills into action. So my self-enquiry question for you is…

Therapist offers a warm closed-mouth smile.

Therapist:	…are you using this as another opportunity to prove to yourself and maybe others that you'll never get out of this depression?

Therapist pauses; places hand up in the air, palm forward, signaling "stop."

Therapist:	But stop right there. You're not allowed to answer that question, because it is a self-enquiry question.

Therapist smiles warmly and giggles.

Client smiles.

Therapist: So one of the things we might want to think about today is, are you being too hard on yourself again?

Therapist pauses.

Client is alert.

Therapist: For example—although your behavior may have not been at its best—it's not like you went up and punched the guy she was talking to, or yelled at her. Plus, I haven't heard much yet about something very important…

Therapist pauses for effect.

Therapist: Do you know what I am thinking?

Client shakes his head no.

Therapist: Well, as far as I can tell, she actually hasn't said no to going out on a date with you. The good news is that there is a wide range of things we can do to reverse the damage—assuming there was any in the first place.

Therapist uses warm voice tone, offers a warm closed-mouth smile and slow affirmative head nod, slightly slows pace of speech, and lowers voice volume.

The therapist's slowed pace (rate) of speech, combined with a slight lowering of her voice volume, signals noncritical appreciation and warmth when used along with other prosocial signals, such as a warm smile, an eyebrow wag, or affirmative head nodding. The therapist also encourages self-enquiry, but in a playful manner, thus moving between compassionate gravity and playful irreverence.

Client: Yeah…I guess. We don't really know.

Client shrugs.

Therapist: Has anything else happened since? For example, have you tried to contact Mary and repair any damage done?

Therapist displays open curiosity.

The therapist is starting to move toward solution analysis (see chapter 10).

Client: No. I assumed she wouldn't want to hear from me.

Client's head is bowed.

Conduct a solution analysis after completing the chain (remember not to overwhelm the client with too many solutions from one chain; you can build over time).

Therapist: Yeah, feeling ashamed is not a good way to start the day.

Therapist offers a warm closed-mouth smile.

Therapist: What I would like us to do now is go back and look at each link on the chain and see if we can come up with skills that you might use the next time. For example, we probably need to talk about your tone of voice when asking what kept you from practicing Match + 1, and maybe what walking away from the scene communicates to others. Would you be willing to do this?

Client nods yes.

Therapist: To start, just how committed were you to genuinely practicing Match + 1 in the first place?

Therapist signals an easy manner, displays open curiosity.

The therapist is orienting the client to the next step of the chain analysis—finding solutions for each maladaptive link in the chain. She reviews several previously highlighted maladaptive links in the chain as potential areas for work and starts the solution analysis by first assessing the degree of the client's commitment to completing his homework assignment (that is, using Match + 1 skills to ask someone out on a date).

RO DBT Adherence: A Self-Assessment Checklist

Instructions: This rating scale is intended as a global self-assessment of RO DBT therapy adherence. Ideally, an independent RO DBT therapist conducts the ratings after viewing a videotaped recording of a session. The scale is designed to rate the behavior of the therapist (T), not the behavior of the client (C); therefore, in rating the scale items, it is important to distinguish, as much as possible, the behavior of the therapist from the behavior of the client in response to the therapist. Your ratings should reflect the entire session, with a higher number of checkmarks in relevant sections suggesting greater treatment adherence.

I. RO DBT Individual Treatment Physical/ Environmental Strategies

Place a checkmark in the box next to each statement that accurately describes the treatment environment.

☐ Ideally, chairs in individual therapy settings should be positioned at a 45-degree angle to each other, and in a manner that maximizes physical distance. Room temperature is set lower than normal.

☐ If there is no central air conditioning, T uses an electric fan or similar means to cool the room (people will tell others when they are cold but are less likely to reveal when they feel hot because of links between feeling hot and anxiety).

☐ T has a cup of water (tea, coffee) for himself/herself and offers C something to drink (water, tea, coffee) at the start of session.

II. RO DBT Individual Therapy, Orientation/ Commitment Phase (Sessions 1–4)

Place a checkmark in the box next to each statement that accurately describes what happens during the session.

A. Session 1

☐ T orients C to the two-way dialogue and collaborative stance between C and T in RO DBT at the very start of the first session (for example, by explaining that RO DBT involves therapeutic dialogue between C and T that may at times require T to interrupt C or direct the discussion toward particular topics).

☐ T briefly orients C to the aims and structure of the first session (for example, T obtains some important background information and determines the extent to which RO DBT represents a good treatment fit for C).

☐ T obtains agreement from C that C's personality style is best described as overcontrolled and that C is committed to target maladaptive OC behaviors as a core part of therapy.

☐ T uses the steps in the RO DBT script to guide the discussion (see "Four Steps for Identifying Overcontrol as the Core Problem in the First Session," chapter 5).

☐ The discussion is time-limited (approximately ten minutes) and conducted with an easy manner.

☐ T acts out the bodily gestures and facial expressions that typify each style in order to make it viscerally apparent to C which style best fits C.

☐ T uses dramatic, overstated, and exaggerated facial expressions, gestures, and tones of voice when describing the undercontrolled style of coping.

☐ T displays a calmer and more precise, constrained, and controlled manner when describing the overcontrolled or OC style of coping.

☐ T assesses current and past history of suicidal and self-harming behavior (typically, this assessment starts about thirty minutes into the session, to allow sufficient time for the risk assessment and suicide/self-injury prevention plan, if needed).

☐ T uses the RO DBT Semistructured Suicidality Interview (see appendix 4) to guide suicide assessment.

☐ T addresses any imminent life-threatening behavior in the moment, using principles from the RO DBT crisis-management protocol (see chapter 5) as needed to guide his/her interventions.

☐ T obtains C's commitment to return for at least one more session to discuss in person (not via email, text message, or telephone) any urges or thoughts about dropping out of therapy before actually making a decision to drop out; T tells C, "I have faith in your ability to follow through with your prior commitments."

B. Session 1 or 2

☐ T matter-of-factly orients C to the potential importance of addressing past trauma, sexual issues, and/or long-held grudges and resentments during the course of treatment (usually this discussion takes only a few minutes).

☐ T signals that he/she is comfortable discussing any issue with C.

☐ T models being openly curious and comfortable when discussing past traumas, sexual issues, or long-held grudges and resentments.

☐ T orients C to the rationale for not pursuing details about any past trauma or painful event in the first session (for example, tribes take time to build, and it is normal not to reveal too much too early in a new relationship).

☐ T highlights the importance of targeting the issue later in treatment, at a time that will be collaboratively decided (this delay is designed to allow time for the establishment of a therapeutic alliance before trauma or grief work begins).

☐ T reinforces C's self-disclosures (for example, of past trauma, sexual issues, or long-held grudges).

☐ T expresses gratitude or appreciation for C's candid and open disclosure (for example, by thanking C).

☐ T reinforces C's self-disclosure by taking the heat off (recall that OC clients dislike the limelight).

☐ T elicits C's commitment to attend RO skills training classes the following week (beginning with session 2).

☐ T communicates confidence in C's ability to attend RO classes, and does so in a manner that is not defensive, coercive, or apologetic.

☐ T reminds C (if a reminder is needed) that C already has a great deal of classroom experience (most OC clients have been highly successful in school and similar classroom settings, and attending an RO skills training class is like going back to school, with the focus on the material being taught and not on the individual being taught).

☐ T matter-of-factly emphasizes the importance of receiving the full "dose" of treatment and stresses that RO skills are essential.

C. *Sessions 3 and 4*

☐ T uses RO DBT teaching scripts to facilitate the introduction of the RO DBT neurobiosocial theory for overcontrol and RO DBT hypothesized mechanism of change.

☐ T continues, as necessary, to orient C to the overall structure of treatment and to the principles of the treatment.

☐ T identifies two to four of C's valued goals, with at least one (such as forming a romantic partnership, improving close relationships, raising a family, being a warm and helpful parent, or being gainfully and happily employed) linked to C's social connectedness; see the skills training manual, worksheet 10.A ("Flexible Mind Is DEEP: Identifying Valued Goals").

☐ T orients C to the RO DBT diary card.

III. RO DBT Individual Therapy, Working Phase (Sessions 5–29)

Place a checkmark in the box next to each statement that accurately describes what happens during the session.

A. *Timing and Sequencing Strategies*

☐ T identifies and monitors on diary cards at least three to five core social signaling targets linked to OC themes at any given time during the course of therapy (social signaling targets are expected to change slowly over time, be refined, and/or be replaced with new ones as the client improves).

☐ T conducts a chain and solution analysis of a social signaling target each session (it is recognized that at least occasionally some sessions will not include a formal chain analysis, but T should consider two or more sessions in a row without a chain analysis problematic).

☐ T introduces the importance of learning skills to activate the social safetey system in order to address core OC biotemperamental predispositions (such as heightened threat sensitivity; sessions 5–7).

☐ T explicitly teaches and practices, in session, RO skills designed to activate the social safety system (for example, the Big Three + 1; sessions 5–7).

☐ T explains the importance of the RO self-enquiry journal and shows C an example of a journal entry (by using the examples in chapter 7, for instance, or by showing C an example from T's personal RO journal; sessions 5–9).

☐ T encourages C to use the self-enquiry handouts and worksheets in the skills training manual to facilitate self-enquiry practices (see handout 1.3, "Learning from Self-Enquiry"; sessions 5–9).

☐ T introduces loving kindness meditation (LKM) and conducts an LKM practice in session for approximately fifteen minutes (sessions 7–9).

☐ T sticks to the LKM script provided in the skills training manual.

☐ T elicits observations from C after the first LKM practice and troubleshoots problems.

☐ T makes an audiorecording in session of the LKM practice (using C's smartphone, for example) and encourages C to use the recording each day to facilitate LKM practice.

☐ T monitors LKM on the diary card.

☐ T introduces the twelve questions in Flexible Mind ADOPTs that are used to assess whether to accept or decline critical feedback and encourages C to practice using them when feeling criticized (sessions 10–12).

☐ T informally teaches Flexible Mind REVEALs skills, with a particular emphasis on "pushback" and "don't hurt me" responses, and uses this to facilitate targeting indirect social signaling on the diary card (sessions 13–17).

☐ T discusses the importance of personal self-disclosure in developing relationships, practices Match + 1 skills in session, and assigns related homework (sessions 11–18).

☐ T introduces the concept of forgiveness and informally teaches Flexible Mind Has HEART skills (sessions 13–24).

☐ Ideally, by session 14 T and C will have had multiple opportunities to practice alliance rupture repairs—proof of a good working relationship in RO DBT.

☐ Each repair (even if minor) has been linked, ideally, to C's values and treatment goals.[a]

☐ T reminds C—ideally, at least ten weeks prior to the end of RO DBT therapy—that therapy will be ending soon (for example, during session 20 in the thirty-week RO DBT outpatient treatment model).

☐ T teaches C, as necessary, how to grieve the ending of relationships without falling apart (see the skills training manual, handout 29.3, "Strengthening Forgiveness Through Grief Work").

☐ T reviews key RO skills as part of a relapse-prevention plan (sessions 25–28).

☐ T uses last session to celebrate C's life and notice with C the changes C has made over time. Minor changes are celebrated as much as more major ones, and reminiscences of notable therapy moments are often shared. Food and tea or coffee may be shared, to symbolize the transition, and T, ideally, encourages C to keep in contact over time (assuming that C would like to).

B. Individual Therapy Session Agenda

☐ T warmly welcomes C back and briefly checks in (one to three minutes).

☐ T warmly greets C (for example, by offering a warm closed-mouth smile) and welcomes C back to the session.

☐ T briefly checks in with C to ensure that C is ready for the session: "Everything okay? Are you ready for our session?" T blocks prolonged storytelling or chitchat.

☐ T warmly yet matter-of-factly interrupts long-winded explanations, stories, or unrelated chitchat while highlighting the potential importance of the issue.

☐ T asks C if C would like to make the topic part of the session's agenda (to be discussed after review of the diary card and completion of chain and solution analysis).

☐ As necessary, T attends to imminent life-threatening behavior or potential alliance ruptures throughout the session.

☐ T reviews diary card (six minutes).

☐ T uses the RO DBT treatment target hierarchy to guide agenda setting.

☐ T prioritizes maladaptive OC social signaling deficits for in-session chain and solution analyses.[b]

☐ T checks in with C about how C is doing in RO skills training class, including completion of homework assigned in individual therapy the previous week (1–3 minutes).

☐ T identifies other in-session agenda items (two minutes):

    ☐ C's requests (for example, interesting stories, celebrations of success)

    ☐ Non-OC targets (for example, restricted eating, medication issues)

    ☐ Specific RO skill(s) planned to be taught during session, new OC theme, and/or adjustments in treatment targeting

    ☐ Informal exposure and grief work (for example, involving past trauma, grudges, forgiveness, praise)

    ☐ Discussion of therapy-ending issues

    ☐ Additional items

☐ T conducts behavioral chain and solution analysis of the social signaling difficulty identified during review of diary card (twenty minutes).

☐ T addresses additional agenda items set at start of session (fifteen to twenty minutes).

☐ T briefly summarizes what has been addressed during session, such as new skills learned, new self-enquiry questions, new targets, or new homework practices (two minutes).

☐ T reminds C of C's prior commitment to return in person to discuss any urges to drop out of therapy before actually dropping out.[c]

☐ T ends session with a gesture of friendship (for example, a reminder to keep in touch or practice skills, a statement of caring, or a kind tease about not being perfect).

IV. The Therapeutic Relationship

Place a checkmark in the box next to each statement that accurately describes what happens during the session.

A. RO DBT Therapeutic Stance

☐ T is responsive to and flexible regarding what is happening in the moment rather than operating from a predetermined plan or professional role (that is, T knows how to leave his/her professional "game face" at home).

☐ T has a relaxed professional style that models radical openness and self-enquiry.

☐ T treats C as a person of equal status by operating from a stance of open curiosity and willingness to learn from C who C is rather than telling C who C is.

☐ T is able to reveal vulnerability and laugh with kindness at his/her own mistakes or personal foibles.

☐ T celebrates unwanted difficulties and emotions as opportunities to receive feedback from one's tribe and practice self-enquiry.

☐ T uses dialectical thinking and behavior to enhance flexible responding (for example, T is kind yet tough, open yet firm, unpredictable yet structured, playful yet serious, self-assured yet humble).

☐ T interacts with C as he/she would with a friend or family member (when we are with friends, we tend to stretch out, lie back, or lounge around; our gestures and facial expressions are more expansive, we are less polite, and we are more likely to use slang or curse words to color our speech).

B. RO DBT Global Therapeutic Stance Checklist

The following questions are designed to assess general principles related to an RO DBT therapeutic stance, with a rating of 1 meaning "not at all" and a rating of 7 meaning "to a great extent." If possible, you should compare your ratings of a session with an independent colleague's ratings of the same session (this procedure often helps identify blind spots).

	Not at all	Very slightly	A little	Moderately	Quite a bit	Very much	To a great extent
1. To what extent did T display open curiosity?	1	2	3	4	5	6	7
2. How playfully irreverent was T?	1	2	3	4	5	6	7
3. To what extent did T appear in control of the session?	1	2	3	4	5	6	7
4. To what extent did T ask rather than tell?	1	2	3	4	5	6	7
5. To what extent did T use qualifiers when asking questions or making statements (for example, by saying, "Is it possible that…" or "Perhaps…") rather than stating absolutes or telling (for example, by saying, "I know…" or "You are…")?	1	2	3	4	5	6	7
6. To what extent did T adjust his or her emotional expressions, posture, and voice tone to fit the circumstances of the moment (for example, by expressing incredulity or amused bewilderment when encountering the absurd yet sadness upon hearing of loss)?	1	2	3	4	5		
7. To what extent was T alert to C's in-session social signaling behaviors (as evidenced, for example, by frequent check-ins)?	1	2	3	4	5	6	7
8. How often did T check in with C to confirm C's engagement with what was being discussed, or with therapy more broadly?	1	2	3	4	5	6	7
9. To what extent did T encourage self-enquiry about what could be learned from an in-session mood, discrepancy, or emotional state?	1	2	3	4	5	6	7

C. Protocol for Repairing Alliance Ruptures

Place a checkmark in the box next to each statement that accurately describes what happens during the session.

- ☐ T drops his/her agenda (that is, T stops talking about current topic as soon as he/she decides there may be an alliance rupture to attend to).

- ☐ T takes the heat off C by briefly disengaging eye contact.

- ☐ T signals friendly cooperation and affection by leaning back in his/her chair, engaging a therapeutic sigh, slowing the pace of conversation, and offering a warm closed-mouth smile and an eyebrow wag.

- ☐ While signaling nondominant friendliness (slightly bowed head, slight shoulder shrug, and openhanded gestures combined with a warm closed-mouth smile, an eyebrow wag, and eye contact), T enquires about the change observed in session. (For example, T says, "I noticed that something just changed," describes the change, and asks, "What's going on with you right now?")

- ☐ T allows C time to reply to questions, reflects back what C says, and then confirms C's agreement.

- ☐ T reinforces C's self-disclosure (for example, by thanking C).

- ☐ T practices radical openness during the repair.

- ☐ T keeps the repair short (less than ten minutes).

- ☐ T checks in with C and reconfirms C's engagement in therapy before moving back to original agenda.

- ☐ T does not apologize to C for the alliance rupture unless T has actually done something wrong (for example, forgotten an appointment or shown up late).

V. Treatment Targeting Principles and Strategies

Place a checkmark in the box next to each statement that accurately describes what happens during the session.

A. Global Principles

☐ T uses the RO DBT treatment target hierarchy to guide in-session behavior (for example, if imminent life-threatening behavior suddenly emerges in session, it will take top priority).

☐ T reminds C that RO DBT considers noncompletion of diary cards, showing up late, missing sessions, and noncompletion of homework to be social signals that are intended to communicate something.

☐ T prioritizes social signaling deficits over inner experience (such as dysregulated emotion, maladaptive cognition, lack of metacognitive awareness, or past traumatic memories) and other non–social signaling issues (such as medication or restricted eating), with the exception being imminent life-threatening behavior.

☐ T formulates problem as a relational issue.

☐ T is alert to C's in-session social signaling behavior as a potential source of new treatment targets.

B. Prioritizing of Social Signaling Targets

Targeting Social Signaling Deficits in Session

☐ T highlights potential maladaptive social signaling behavior in session, but only after it has occurred multiple times and over multiple sessions.[d]

☐ T assesses the extent to which C is aware of the repetitive nature of the social signaling behavior.

☐ T reconfirms C's commitment to targeting social signaling.

☐ T asks directly about the social signal, without assuming that he/she already knows the answer.

☐ T stays focused on social signaling target and avoids getting distracted by other potential targets.

☐ T shows C what the social signal looks or sounds like (for example, via voice tone, facial expression, or body posture).

☐ T exaggerates the social signal as part of a therapeutic tease.

☐ T assesses C's response to the social signaling demonstration.

☐ T reinforces C's engagement.

☐ T reminds C of the definition of a social signal.

☐ T links the new social signaling target to C's valued goals.

☐ T obtains commitment from C to monitor the new social signal on the diary card, and T and C agree on a label for the new target and on how it will be monitored (for example, on a scale of 0 to 5).

☐ T helps C identify one thought and one emotion that may co-occur with the new social signaling target, and T gains commitment from C to monitor the thought and the emotion on the diary card.[e]

Using OC Themes to Identify Social Signaling Targets

☐ During agenda setting at the beginning of the session, T orients C to the OC theme (such as aloof and distant relationships) planned for discussion during the session.[f]

☐ As necessary, T briefly reminds C about the purpose of OC themes in general (for example, T tells C that OC themes are guides that help improve treatment targeting).

☐ T reminds C of the definition of a social signal.

☐ T, naming one of the OC themes (such as aloof and distant relationships), asks C, "What words come to mind when you think about…?"

☐ T links the OC theme being discussed to C's valued goals; for example, T asks, "How does this theme apply to your life, and with whom? What valued goals does it prevent you from achieving or living by?"

☐ T, naming one of the OC themes (for example, aloof and distant relationships), asks C, "If I were a fly on the wall, how would I know you were behaving in an aloof and distant manner?"

☐ T verifies that the new social signaling target is relevant (for example, the social signal is preventing C from achieving valued goals) and pervasive (that is, the social signal is habitual, frequent, and/or present across contexts).

☐ Rather than just talking about the social signaling deficit, T demonstrates to C what it looks or sounds like.

☐ T and C collaboratively label (name) the new social signaling target.

☐ T helps C identify one thought and one emotion that may co-occur with the new social signaling target, and T gains commitment from C to monitor the thought and the emotion on the diary card.[g]

☐ T obtains commitment from C to monitor the new social signal and any other new targets on the diary card.

VI. Behavioral Principles

Place a checkmark in the box next to each statement that accurately describes what happens during the session.

A. Contingency-Management Strategies

☐ T helps C identify the function of a social signal by discussing the eliciting stimuli, the reinforcers that maintain the social signal, and the extent to which the social signal fits C's core valued goals.

☐ T reinforces C's candid self-disclosure and uninhibited expression of emotion in session; for example, T expresses appreciation or thanks whenever C initiates vulnerable self-disclosure, but without making a big deal of it (recall that OC clients dislike the limelight).

☐ T uses heat-off strategies to reinforce C's engagement, new learning, and/or practice of RO skills.

☐ T uses heat-on strategies to reduce, punish, or extinguish a maladaptive social signal.

B. Indirect Social Signals, Hidden Intentions, and Disguised Demands

Global Principles

☐ T educates C about indirect social signals, their function, how they can be easily misinterpreted, and how they can negatively impact relationships.[h]

☐ T encourages C to notice C's nonverbal social signaling habits (for example, how often C genuinely smiles with pleasure, how often C uses a polite smile, how often C uses a burglar smile, how often C purposefully doesn't smile, how often C uses eyebrow wags or openhanded gestures, and so on).

☐ T encourages C to use self-enquiry to examine the extent to which C's social signaling habits fit with valued goals; for example, T encourages C to use self-enquiry questions like *To what extent am I proud of how I socially signaled?* and *Would I teach a child to signal similarly?* and *What is it I need to learn?*

☐ T reflects back to C T's own perplexity or confusion regarding C's indirect social signal, but only after it has occurred repeatedly; for example, T says, "I've noticed that on multiple occasions, whenever I've asked about how you are feeling, especially about difficult topics, you seem to always respond by saying that you are fine. My question is, are you always really fine?"

☐ T teaches, models, or practices key RO social signaling skills in session, such as Flexible Mind ADOPTS and Flexible Mind REVEALs (see the skills training manual).

☐ T uses instances of indirect, incongruous, and ambiguous social signaling in session as opportunities to practice social signaling skills (for example, the skill of asserting with humility that one desires a close relationship with someone by combining nondominance and cooperative-friendly signals).

☐ T displays a nonchalant, straightforward, playful manner when discussing "pushback" and "don't hurt me" responses, disguised demands, and indirect signaling.

Managing "Pushback" and "Don't Hurt Me" Responses

☐ T teaches C explicitly about "pushback" and "don't hurt me" responses, using Flexible Mind REVEALs skills to augment teaching (see the skills training manual).[i]

☐ T obtains C's commitment to target "pushback" or "don't hurt me" responses, both in session and outside of session, via diary cards.

☐ T places "pushback" or "don't hurt me" responses on an extinction schedule by nonchalantly and cheerfully carrying on with the topic being discussed, as if nothing has happened.

☐ T is more playful and curious than serious and concerned when "pushback" or "don't hurt me" behaviors appear in session.[j]

☐ During a prolonged "don't hurt me" response (C bows head, covers face, averts gaze for longer than a minute), T matter-of-factly requests C's engagement by asking C to sit up straight, with shoulders back and chin out, and look T in the eye.

☐ T reinforces C's attempts to communicate needs, wants, desires, or emotions more directly (for example, T thanks C for the gift of truth by dropping the disliked topic for the remainder of the session).

☐ T engages the RO DBT protocol for repairing an alliance rupture when in-session "pushback" or "don't hurt me" behaviors are prolonged and/or appear unresponsive to T's intervention.

C. Behavioral Chain and Solution Analysis (Approximately Twenty to Twenty-Five Minutes)
Behavioral Chain Analyses

☐ T determines the context (who, what, when, where) in which the maladaptive social signal occurred as well as the intensity of the signal.[k]

☐ T asks C to demonstrate (if possible) the maladaptive social signal; T does not assume that he/she knows, without direct experience, what the signal looks or sounds like.

☐   T asks C to identify contributing factors (also known as vulnerability factors).

☐   T identifies the prompting event and confirms that the maladaptive social signal would not have been sent if the prompting event had not occurred.

☐   T identifies the chain of events (actions, thoughts, feelings, sensations) leading up to the maladaptive social signal.

☐   T identifies the consequences of the maladaptive social signal, including possible reinforcers.

Solution Analyses

☐   T prioritizes social signaling solutions over changing internal experience (for example, T teaches C skills of signaling friendly openness to a potential friend rather than teaching C how to feel less social anxiety).

☐   T conducts a solution analysis after or during the chain analysis.

☐   T collaboratively works with C to identify solutions for the most serious link in the chain.

☐   T links solutions to C's valued goals.

☐   T shows rather than tells C how to improve or change social signaling habits (for example, T demonstrates a new social signaling skill in session and asks C to practice it in session).

☐   T reminds C to activate the social safety system prior to social interactions (for example, via LKM practice or the Big Three + 1).

☐   T encourages C to practice self-enquiry when C appears uncertain rather than trying to convince C of T's own perspective.

☐   T and C practice the new skill or social signaling solution in session, via mini–role playing, and T ensures that solutions are specific and practical (for example, T doesn't tell C to practice a skill without first ensuring that it will actually work in C's circumstances).

☐   T encourages C to write down solutions in the RO self-enquiry journal to help facilitate practice; if necessary, T writes the solutions down for C and provides C a copy of the solutions at the end of the session.

☐   T conducts frequent check-ins to assess C's engagement.

☐   T does not overwhelm C with too many solutions in one session.[1]

☐   In individual therapy, T teaches relevant RO skills as part of solution analysis instead of waiting for an RO skills class to cover at some point in the future a skill that C needs now.

VII. Nonverbal Social Signaling Strategies

Place a checkmark in the box next to each statement that accurately describes what happens during the session.

- ☐ T adjusts his/her body posture, eye gaze, voice tone, and facial expressions according to what is happening in the moment.

- ☐ T nonverbally takes heat off C by...

  - ☐ Leaning back in his/her chair in order to increase distance from C

  - ☐ Crossing the leg nearest C over the other leg in order to slightly turn shoulders away

  - ☐ Taking a slow deep breath or therapeutic sigh

  - ☐ Briefly disengaging eye contact

  - ☐ Raising eyebrows

  - ☐ Engaging a closed-mouth smile when returning eye gaze back toward C

- ☐ To encourage candid disclosure, T signals nondominant cooperative friendliness by combining appeasement signals (slightly bowed head, shoulder shrug, and openhanded gestures) with cooperative-friendly signals (warm closed-mouth smile, raised eyebrows, direct eye contact).

- ☐ Instead of just talking about C's social signal, T demonstrates it by playfully acting it out (for example, by using a silly voice, or suddenly presenting a flat face, or feigning a burp, and so on).

- ☐ T models for C, and practices with C, universal nonverbal signals of affection, friendship, trust, and social safety (such as a warm closed-mouth smile, a genuine smile of pleasure, an eyebrow wag, an affirmative head nod, a musical tone of voice, and openhanded gestures).

- ☐ T uses role playing and in-session practices to help expand C's social signaling repertoire.

VIII. Dialectical Strategies

Place a checkmark in the box next to each statement that accurately describes what happens during the session.

A. *Playful Irreverence vs. Compassionate Gravity*

☐ T balances playful irreverence and compassionate gravity (for example, moving from playfulness to seriousness and then back again to playfulness throughout the session).

☐ T affectionately teases, cajoles, jests with, and pokes C in the manner reserved for close friends (for example, to give C critical feedback without making a big deal of it, or to help C learn how not to take himself/herself so seriously).

☐ When C turns away, frowns, or bows his/her head upon encountering something he/she dislikes, T momentarily increases playful irreverence by continuing as if all is well rather than automatically soothing or validating C.

☐ T uses compassionate gravity to reinforce C's adaptive behavior and C's candid, open, vulnerable expressions of emotion (for example, T slows pace and engages a softer voice tone, gentle eye contact, and a warm closed-mouth smile).

B. *Nonmoving Centeredness vs. Acquiescent Letting Go*

☐ T balances nonmoving centeredness with acquiescent letting go.

☐ T operates from a stance of acquiescent letting go in order to repair an alliance rupture or trigger C's healthy self-doubt and C's self-enquiry regarding a pet theory.

☐ T operates from a stance of nonmoving centeredness (for example, T remains firm in the conviction that humans are social animals or that suicide and self-injury are not options, regardless of strong opposition from C.

IX. RO Skills Training Principles

Place a checkmark in the box next to each statement that accurately describes the RO skills training environment, the training itself, and/or the behavior of the instructor(s).

A. Physical/Structural and Global Principles

☐ Instructor refers to RO skills training as a "class," not a "group."[m]

☐ RO skills class is set up to look and feel like a small classroom, with a long table in the middle, chairs positioned alongside it, and a whiteboard or flip-chart at the front of the room for the instructor to write on.

☐ Instructor and coinstructor are enthusiastic and appear to be enjoying themselves while teaching skills training class.

☐ Classroom temperature is kept cool.

☐ Instructors teach directly from the skills training manual.

☐ A skills class with four or fewer clients is taught by only one instructor rather than the usual two.

☐ Instructor uses heat-on and heat-off principles to shape clients' participation.

☐ Instructor leads at least one "participate without planning" exercise per class.

☐ Instructor uses RO protocol for maladaptive social signals that cannot be ignored in class to address a "don't hurt me" response, a personal attack, or noncompletion of homework (see the skills training manual, chapter 3).

B. When a Classroom Goes Quiet

☐ Instructor practices radical openness by directly seeking critical feedback from the class; for example, the instructor asks, "Has something just occurred to make it harder for everyone to participate or contribute to our work together?"

☐ Instructor, confronted with a classroom of blank stares and flat faces, goes opposite to his/her urges to quiet down or behave in a solemn manner by purposefully employing expansive expressions and gestures.

☐ Instructor randomly assign participants to read aloud the next point being covered on a handout or worksheet, in order to break the barrier of silence.

☐ Instructor uses bodily movements and meaningless vocalizations to break tension; for example, instructor says, without warning, "Okay, everyone, stand up and clap your hands together!"[n]

☐ Instructor takes heat off class by telling a story or using a metaphor.

C. Instructor Uses Therapeutic Induction of Social Responsibility

☐ During break or after class, instructor has a private chat or discussion with a participant in order to remind him/her of prior commitments, describe the impact that his/her behavior may be having on other class members, or encourage him/her to behave more appropriately in order to contribute to the well-being of the tribe.[o]

☐ Instructor reminds participant of his/her core values for fairness and doing the right thing, in order to help motivate more appropriate behavior in class, and gains participant's commitment to show up on time, complete homework, participate in class exercises, or contribute to discussions.

D. Instructor Effectively and Frequently Uses "Participate Without Planning" Practices

☐ The practice is always unannounced.

☐ Instructor does not orient or prepare the class for what is about to happen.

☐ The practice always involves mimicking the instructor's movements.

☐ Instructor uses one of the practices outlined in the skills training manual.

☐ The practice lasts no more than a minute.[p]

☐ In general, instructor avoids discussing or processing the practice afterward and simply carries on with his/her agenda as if nothing has happened.[q]

☐ Instructor does not let clients lead the practice.[r]

a   If there has not been an alliance rupture by the fourteenth session, the therapist should consider the possibility that the relationship with the client is superficial (see chapter 8).

b   The presence of imminent life-threatening behavior or an alliance rupture supersedes this.

c   This reminder should be given at the end of any session that has involved an alliance rupture, any session that has been challenging, and any session that has taken place right after the therapist received feedback from his or her supervisor. It can also be given randomly.

d   Refer to appendix 5, "Targeting Indirect Social Signals: In-Session Protocol" (also known as the "yawning protocol").

e   In general, a new social signal is not targeted for change during the first week; instead, the therapist encourages the client simply to observe during the first week.

f   The therapist should not attempt to review all five themes at one time (see "Treatment Targeting: Common Pitfalls," chapter 9).

g   See note e.

h   For example, a blank stare and an expressionless tone of voice, and the absence of reciprocal smiles and head nods, are universally perceived as sending a signal of threat or disapproval, regardless of the sender's actual intentions.

i   "Pushback" and "don't hurt me" responses indirectly signal nonengagement and disapproval; they function to block unwanted feedback or requests to join the community while allowing the sender of these signals to avoid admitting to having sent them (see chapter 10).

j   A playfully irreverent stance provides corrective feedback without being too heavy-handed and avoids reinforcing the maladaptive social signal while encouraging more direct communication.

k   To help prevent unnecessarily long chain analyses, the therapist should look for prompting events or triggers that, ideally, occurred no more than half an hour before the maladaptive social signal. In reality, prompting events or triggers most often occur from a few seconds to a few minutes before a maladaptive social signal.

l   Ideally, the therapist will find no more than three or four solutions per chain.

m   Using the word "class" reflects the training's primary purpose (that is, the teaching and learning of new skills).

n   In the unlikely event that a participant refuses to stand up, the instructor should simply reverse the directions and tell those participants who are still standing, "Okay, good job! Now go ahead and sit back down."

o   See chapter 5.

p   The idea is to reward participation in the tribe by ending the practice slightly before participants begin to feel too self-conscious, in order to lay down new learning—namely, that participating in a tribe can be fun.

q   Except during formal teaching of "participate without planning" practices (see the skills training manual), processing of these practices is discouraged because it often backfires by triggering increased social comparisons and/or inadvertently implying that there is a right way to participate.

r   Such an approach could quickly become a contest and generate unhelpful social comparisons, with participants vying to see who is the silliest or most creative of all.

Endnotes

Notes to the Introduction

1   Interestingly, clinical experience, my own and that of my colleagues, suggests that clients with disorders of overcontrol tend to prefer biological over psychological explanations, a preference reflecting the belief that the need for psychological help represents a personal failure of control; see also the study by Kocsis et al., 2009, p. 1185, which reports a preference for antidepressant medication over psychotherapy in a sample of chronically depressed patients who "required considerable convincing that psychotherapy was important."

2   RO DBT posits that our core values as a species are good because they function to assist our fellow humans. Even values for independence contribute to the welfare of others by lessening the need for assistance; thus, our tribal nature represents a core part of who we are as a species, and our values reflect this.

Notes to Chapter 1

3   The idea of self-control as a cross-cultural phenomenon is not new; for example, Gottfredson and Hirschi's (1990) "self-control theory" posits that all human groups value self-control qualities, such as delayed gratification and selflessness, and cross-cultural research has supported this notion (Vazsonyi & Klanjšek, 2008).

4   Cultural norms matter. In the Americas and Western Europe, eye contact is interpreted in the same way, as conveying interest and honesty; people who avoid eye contact when speaking are viewed in a negative light and seen as withholding information and lacking in general confidence. However, in the Middle East, Africa, and especially Asia, sustained eye contact is experienced as disrespectful and even challenging of one's authority, although brief eye contact is experienced as respectful and courteous.

5   Undercontrolled individuals are hypothesized to struggle with planning for the future and with inhibiting emotion-based action urges.

6   The biotemperament-based high reward sensitivity that characterizes undercontrolled coping may make it more likely for persistence in UC individuals to involve activities linked with immediate rewards, as when an artist paints for hours on end. In OC individuals, by contrast, the low reward sensitivity that characterizes overcontrolled coping may lead to persistence that is aimed at avoiding an imagined future negative consequence, as when a student dutifully studies in order to avoid receiving a bad grade.

7   Social signaling deficits are found in both undercontrolled and overcontrolled disorders, albeit how the social signal is expressed differs widely between the two. OC social signaling tends to be understated, controlled, predictable, and non-mood-dependent, whereas

UC social signaling tends to be dramatic, disinhibited, unpredictable, and mood-dependent. Inhibited expressions among UC individuals are usually temporary and secondary to aversive contingencies.

8   The first randomized controlled trial was supported by funding from the National Institute of Mental Health (R03 MH057799–01; Thomas R. Lynch, principal investigator).

9   Among the skills piloted were those that had to do with enumerating the pros and cons of being open to new experience; the myths of a closed mind; closed, fluid, and naive states of mind; steps for practicing radical openness; the path to Alive Mind; and dialectical dilemmas for OC depression.

10 Our second randomized controlled trial, like our first, was supported by funding from the National Institute of Mental Health (K23MH01614; Thomas R. Lynch, principal investigator).

11 The second RODBT-Early manual included adapted standard DBT skills for disorders of overcontrol as well as the new RO skills and targets that were piloted in the first randomized controlled trial; see T. R. Lynch et al., 2003.

12 These new skills included being more open to critical feedback; playing; signaling cooperation to others; engaging in novel behavior; activating the social safety system; and forgiving and grieving. Interestingly, the majority of the new concepts and skills that were developed and tested in our first two randomized controlled trials also appear in the RO skills training manual that accompanies the present volume, although in the new manual they are often presented and described in different words.

13 The urge-surfing of food-averse response tendencies is the only formal mindfulness practice that specifically focuses on food-related stimuli; see T. R. Lynch et al., 2013.

14 Treatment was provided by the Haldon Eating Disorder Service, an inpatient unit housing a program that is part of the Devon Partnership NHS Trust, in the United Kingdom. The Haldon program is unique in that the overall treatment approach on the unit is informed by RO DBT principles and by a transdiagnostic treatment philosophy that accounts for individual differences in self-control tendencies (see T. R. Lynch et al., 2013).

15 One of the nine participants was withdrawn from the study because of medical instability due to anorexia nervosa and the need for inpatient care, but none of the remaining eight participants required additional day treatment, inpatient care, or emergency services during treatment.

16 The RO skills training module lasted nine weeks and consisted of nine three-hour classes, each one offered twice per week, for a total of eighteen hours of skills training.

17 The demonstrated improvements were in feelings of social safety (medium effects at post-treatment) and effective use of coping skills (large effects at post-treatment, maintained at three-month follow-up), and these findings remained significant after the researchers controlled for the number of training sessions the subject had attended, whether or not the subject had received medication, and whether or not the subject was also participating in other therapies. Follow-up data were available for only nineteen of the subjects who completed the RO skills training; post hoc tests showed a statistically significant difference between pretreatment and post-treatment group scores ($p<.01$) but not between pretreatment and follow-up, or between post hoc tests and follow-up.

18 Interestingly, not only did OC offenders show no benefit, they were more likely at pre-treatment assessment to describe their violent offenses as morally driven rather than emotionally driven.

19 RO DBT conceptualizes hoarding as a form of maladaptive inhibitory control linked to the ability to delay gratification in order to obtain a more distal goal (as seen, for example, in the practice of saving for a rainy day).

Notes to Chapter 2

20 Albeit emerging epigenetic research suggests that some stress-related genes can be altered by extreme experience during key developmental periods.

21 From an RO DBT perspective, repressive coping may be more reflective of the overly disagreeable OC subtype, whereas the defensive high-anxiety coping style may be more in keeping with the overly agreeable OC subtype (see chapters 3 and 9).

22 Some discrepancies are worth noting regarding findings pertaining to reward sensitivity. For example, studies relying on self-report measures to examine reward sensitivity in anorexia nervosa (AN) have at times revealed contradictory findings, with some concluding AN-R (restrictive type) to be lower in reward sensitivity and higher in threat sensitivity, AN-P (purge type) as higher in reward sensitivity relative to AN-R and controls (I. Beck, Smits, Claes, Vandereycken, & Bijttebier, 2009; Claes, Vandereycken, & Vertommen, 2006), or AN adolescents as both high threat and high reward, regardless of type (Glashouwer, Bloot, Veenstra, Franken, & de Jong, 2014). However, none of these studies differentiated between anticipatory reward (that is, dopamine/excitatory approach) and consummatory reward (that is, μ-opiate relaxation/pleasure), and the measures used to assess reward were variable or assumed overt behavioral responses (for example, impulsivity) to be analogues of reward sensitivity. More research is needed.

23 In my opinion, distinguishing between nonsocial and social consummatory rewards is essential to understanding the range of reward responses found among OC individuals. For example, one of the clearest measures of consummatory reward is the sweet-taste task that asks participants to rate the degree of pleasure experienced following incremental increases in the concentration of sucrose (sugar) in a solution they are asked to taste. The advantage of this task is that it limits the extent to which anticipatory reward or reward learning may influence findings. Research shows that ratings by depressed subjects using the sweet-taste task are similar to those of nondepressed subjects (Amsterdam, Settle, Doty, Abelman, & Winokur, 1987; Dichter, Smoski, Kampov-Polevoy, Gallop, & Garbutt, 2010; Berlin, Givry-Steiner, Lecrubier, & Puech, 1998). Recall that depression is increasingly being recognized as a chronic condition sharing features with overcontrol and, similarly, OC individuals are predicted to exhibit low anticipatory reward and yet an intact hedonic reward system (albeit for nonsocial rewards only). However, the utility of the sweet-taste task in capturing OC hedonic responses may be limited. For example, OC clients with anorexia nervosa might be expected to respond abnormally to a sweet-taste task, simply as a function of starvation or sweetness triggering a classically conditioned aversion response.

24 As mentioned earlier, when the PNS-VVC is withdrawn and SNS-mediated fight-or-flight responses dominate, physiological responses linked to social affiliation and engagement are impaired; facial expressions become frozen, and the ability to interact flexibly with others is lost; see Porges (2001, 2003b).

25 Indeed, research shows that individuals who tend to smile when they're angry, or when they reveal negative feelings, are characterized by lower emotional empathy, whereas facial expression tends to match internal experience in people who are high in emotional empathy; see Sonnby-Borgström (2002) and Sonnby-Borgström, Jönsson, & Svensson (2003).

26 For more about this reaction to an unexpressive individual, see robust research by Boone & Buck (2003), English & John (2013), Kernis & Goldman (2006), Mauss et al. (2011), and Reis & Patrick (1996).

27 See Depue & Morrone-Strupinsky (2005).

28 The aversive consequences of social rejection are posited to activate areas of the brain (such as the amygdala and the hippocampus; see LeDoux, 2012) that are involved in encoding explicit and implicit long-term memories, and thus to make automatic defensive arousal and avoidance of social stimuli more likely in the future.

Notes to Chapter 4

29 In standard dialectical behavior therapy (DBT), enhancement of skills generalization is most frequently accomplished through the use of telephone-based coaching by the individual therapist (Linehan, 1993a). Although crisis-oriented coaching calls are frequently needed in work with undercontrolled individuals and clients with borderline personality disorder, OC clients are less likely to utilize this mode. Even though OC clients may be experiencing a great deal of inner anguish, they are strongly motivated not to let this be seen by others, even their therapists. (As one OC client explained, "I just don't *do* crisis.") Indeed, for most OC clients, keeping up appearances is a core way of behaving. In general, then, because OC clients may consider a crisis call unnecessary, socially unacceptable, or a sign of weakness, crisis calls and coaching calls can be anticipated to be less frequent in work with these individuals. However, we have found that text messaging and telephone contact are very helpful and more often used as a way for OC clients to keep in touch with their therapists or let their therapists know when an individualized homework assignment has been completed or a new skill has been tried out. In other words, OC clients more often use text messaging and phone contact to practice celebrating their successes with their fellow tribe members—in this case, their therapists. However, this pattern of responding may not hold for every OC client, a fact that has implications for the importance of additional research (with adolescents, for example).

30 Consultation team meetings serve several important functions. For example, they provide support for therapists, reduce the likelihood of burnout, improve phenomenological empathy for clients, and provide guidance for treatment planning. A major assumption in RO DBT is that therapists, in order to help their clients learn to be more open, flexible, and socially connected, must possess and practice those attributes themselves so they can model them for clients. Supervision and consultation, although not required in RO DBT, are considered an important means by which therapists can practice what they preach (and thus remain treatment-adherent).

31 Training support for therapists who are in the process of learning RO DBT can be found at http://www.radicallyopen.net. This resource provides a range of supplemental training materials, including videotaped vignettes demonstrating core treatment strategies and new updates. The website also provides links to clinical supervision options from RO DBT–certified, treatment-adherent therapists.

32 See appendix 4 for a semistructured interview and treatment protocol designed specifically for assessing and managing OC clients' suicidal behavior and self-injury; see also "Assessing OC Life-Threatening Behaviors" and "The RO DBT Crisis-Management Protocol," chapter 5.

33 Regarding the special status that a need for increased medical attention can seem to confer, a client with anorexia reported her fear that if she didn't look "fragile," she would lose her status as a "princess" (T. R. Lynch et al., 2013, p. 4).

34 Readers familiar with standard dialectical behavior therapy (Linehan, 1993a) will recognize this as a major deviation. In standard DBT, behaviors that interfere with therapy (for example, a client's refusal to show up for sessions or to speak during a session, or a client's repeated crossing of the therapist's personal limits in a way that leads to the therapist's demoralization) are considered the second-most important target in the treatment hierarchy.

Notes to Chapter 5

35 In standard DBT, there is a strong emphasis generally on what is known as the *four-miss rule*. According to this rule, a client who misses four sessions in a row for either skills group or individual therapy (not both) is considered to be out of treatment (that is, the client is considered to have dropped out of treatment). The four-miss rule is not a part of RO DBT. Although attendance at skills class and individual therapy is still expected, RO DBT considers lack of attendance to be indicative of a possible alliance rupture.

36 Standard DBT uses both "door in the face" and "foot in the door" strategies, which come directly from marketing. Essentially, the therapist is trying to sell the client on DBT (see Linehan, 1993a, pp. 288–289). As a means of gaining the largest commitment the client is willing to give, the therapist can fluctuate between asking for a tremendously large commitment (for example, that the client never again mask feelings), a request that is sure to be rejected, and asking for a smaller commitment (for example, that the client practice, once per session, revealing a critical thought about the therapist).

37 RO DBT does not utilize written commitment forms; they are impersonal, and their legalistic nature can imply that the therapist does not trust the client.

38 Clients desiring additional information can be directed to http://www.radicallyopen.net.

39 In standard DBT, if clients express uncertainty about whether their therapists really understand them or their unique problems, therapists might use the irreverent strategy of "omnipotence" (see Linehan, 1993a, p. 397) by saying, "Take it from me—this is something I know. We fully understand your problems and also how to get you out of them." This approach, used with a client who has borderline personality disorder, can function to capture the client's attention and reassure her that change may be possible, which in turn strengthens commitment. However, the same approach used with an OC client is likely to be experienced as off-putting or grandiose. Most OC clients are cautious (to a fault), and many OC clients take secret pride in being different from others or difficult to understand (see "The Enigma Predicament," chapter 10).

40 In a study of self-injurious adolescents, a subgroup (10 percent of the sample) was identified that almost exclusively cut themselves in private, and they appeared to nonimpulsively plan their self-injurious behavior (Klonsky & Olino, 2008). Thus, to reiterate a point made in chapter 3, intentional self-injury should not be viewed solely as a

mood-dependent, impulsive, attention- or sensation-seeking phenomenon; it is a complex behavior that serves a range of functions, most frequently self-punishment and regulation of negative affect (Klonsky, 2007; Nock, 2009).

41   Though to my knowledge there has been no research in this area, it is possible that the majority of religious-political acts of terrorism are either led or performed by OC individuals (these types of violent acts take a great deal of planning and are most often linked to core OC issues, such as moral certitude). People who commit suicide or combine suicide with acts of terrorism may have logically come to the conclusion that committing suicide or killing others is the best means of making a point, punishing transgressors, or calling attention to a cause.

42   Our research team is in the process of evaluating the utility of distinguishing between OC and UC self-harm behaviors, and we are currently in the process of developing a self-report questionnaire that is designed to address some of the unique features associated with OC suicidal and self-injurious behavior.

Notes to Chapter 7

43   Thus RO DBT replaces the core Zen principles found in standard DBT (Linehan, 1993a) with principles derived from Malâmati Sufism.

44   This also contrasts with the concept of Wise Mind in standard DBT, which emphasizes the value of intuitive knowledge, highlights the possibility of fundamentally knowing something as true or valid, and posits inner knowing as "almost always quiet" and as involving a sense of "peace" (Linehan, 1993a). From an RO DBT perspective, facts or truth can often be misleading, partly because we don't know what we don't know, because things are constantly changing, and because there is a great deal of experience occurring outside of our conscious awareness.

45   In skills training classes, the practices associated with outing oneself are conducted in pairs, not in front of the entire class. Demonstrations of how to out oneself in front of the class are performed only by instructors, to model or teach core principles.

46   If there has been a recent alliance rupture, the therapist should consider the possibility that his demoralization may be partly a result of the rupture never having been fully repaired and should readdress the rupture and repair with the client.

47   For an explanation of the concepts of Fixed Mind and Fatalistic Mind, see the skills training manual, chapter 5, lesson 11.

Notes to Chapter 8

48   With respect to encouraging clients to discover their own motivations, RO DBT makes an exception when life-threatening behavior occurs, in which case RO DBT will use external contingencies to elicit change (see chapter 5).

Notes to Chapter 9

49   For example, Professor Liviu Librescu sacrificed his life by blocking the door to his classroom so his students could escape from Seung-Hui Cho, the gunman whose rampage left thirty-two students and faculty members dead at Virginia Tech. It is hard to argue that Librescu's act of heroism was selfish, since it never benefited him personally.

50 The core dialectical dilemma in standard DBT is acceptance versus change (see Linehan, 1993a).

51 Our research to date shows that the vast majority of therapists lean toward an overcontrolled style (albeit not in the clinical range). For example, twenty-three of the twenty-six research therapists in our ongoing multicenter trial of RO DBT have self-identified as overcontrolled. This is not particularly surprising when one considers the competitive nature of most clinical psychology training programs and other, similar health care academic programs—entry into these programs requires excellent grades as well as superior test-taking ability, persistence, and planning, all fundamental OC characteristics.

52 Okay, I feel obligated to out myself: I made this quote up in order to make a point. However, I think it also illustrates another very important principle in RO DBT—that is, silliness is no laughing matter in RO DBT! We are *really serious* about our silliness. Laughing and frivolity are solemn occasions that represent opportunities for change. Blah, blah, blah.

53 Chapter 6 includes detailed descriptions of the most common maladaptive OC social signals as well as recommended social signaling interventions for therapists.

54 Similarly, the therapist should not provide an OC client a written document or overview of the five themes for the client to think about on his own time, mainly because this can trigger long discussions and philosophical debates about word usage or grammatical errors and prevent discussion of other topics.

55 For therapists familiar with standard DBT, it is important to remember that in RO DBT, noncompletion of a diary card is not considered a therapy-interfering behavior, as it would be in standard DBT, and would not trigger a therapy-interfering chain analysis. Instead, noncompletion of a diary card is considered to be a possible indication of an alliance rupture and is explored accordingly (see chapter 8). Diary cards should *not* be reviewed during skills training classes, because this limits the time for teaching. In RO DBT, diary cards are intended solely to be used in individual therapy.

56 The principle of avoiding handouts in individual therapy can be waived when a skill with an accompanying handout or worksheet is explicitly taught during an individual therapy session.

57 Individuals of both the overly disagreeable and the overly agreeable OC subtypes will tend to abandon relationships rather than deal with conflict directly. The primary difference is in how they communicate their intentions. Overly disagreeable individuals are more likely to be obvious about signaling their displeasure (for example, by walking out of the room or informing someone in writing that the relationship is over), whereas the social signal of an overly agreeable individual is likely to be indirect and apparently polite (for example, the overly agreeable individual will suddenly notice that she has another appointment, or she will claim to want to continue a relationship but stops returning emails and telephone calls).

Notes to Chapter 10

58 Just in case you missed it, that was a tease.

59 The point here has less to do with following the protocol for handouts than with how this aspect of the enigma predicament can show up in therapy.

60 Excellent resources for readers interested in learning more about behaviorism are available. See, for example, the textbook by Farmer and Chapman, *Behavioral Interventions in Cognitive Behavior Therapy* (2016), or Pryor's *Don't Shoot the Dog* (1999), two very different works that are (to my mind, at least) equally excellent resources for learning more about cognitive behavioral principles and strategies.

61 The research examining innate versus culturally derived social signaling is complex and rife with debate as well as with divergent findings and interpretations. Although I personally find this vast area of research fascinating, I have purposefully chosen not to review it in this book, partly because there are already decent reviews available (for example, see Russell, Bachorowski, & Fernández-Dols, 2003) but also, and more importantly, because the focus of this book about treatment is *treatment*, so as to provide clinicians with an outline of the principles and steps, informed by both clinical experience and research, that we have used to intervene with social signaling deficits among clients with disorders of overcontrol.

62 "Pushback" responses are most common among clients who can be characterized as belonging to the overly disagreeable OC subtype; see chapter 9.

Notes to Chapter 11

63 Our research team is in the process of examining the psychometric properties and identifying cutoff scores.

64 Just in case you missed it…that was a tease.

References

Abrams, R. C., & Horowitz, S. V. (1996). Personality disorders after age 50: A meta-analysis. *Journal of Personality Disorders, 10*(3), 271–281.

Achenbach, T. M. (1966). The classification of children's psychiatric symptoms: A factor-analytic study. *Psychological Monographs: General and Applied, 80*(7), 1–37.

Adams, R. B., & Kleck, R. E. (2003). Perceived gaze direction and the processing of facial displays of emotion. *Psychological Science, 14*(6), 644–647.

Adler, R. B., & Proctor, R. F. II. (2007). *Looking out/looking in* (12th ed.). Belmont, CA: Thomson/Wadsworth.

Adolphs, R. (2008). Fear, faces, and the human amygdala. *Current Opinion in Neurobiology, 18*(2), 166–172. doi:10.1016/j.conb.2008.06.006

Aloi, M., Rania, M., Caroleo, M., Bruni, A., Palmieri, A., Cauteruccio, M. A.,…Segura-García, C. (2015). Decision making, central coherence, and set-shifting: A comparison between binge eating disorder, anorexia nervosa and healthy controls. *BMC Psychiatry, 15*(6). doi:10.1186/s12888-015-0395-z

Ambady, N., & Rosenthal, R. (1992). Thin slices of expressive behavior as predictors of inter-personal consequences: A meta-analysis. *Psychological Bulletin, 111*(2), 256–274. doi:10.1037/0033-2909.111.2.256

American Psychiatric Association. (2000). *Diagnostic and statistical manual of mental disorders* (DSM-IV-TR), text revision (4th ed.). Washington, DC: Author.

American Psychiatric Association. (2006). *American Psychiatric Association practice guidelines for the treatment of psychiatric disorders: Compendium 2006.* Arlington, VA: Author.

American Psychiatric Association. (2013). *Diagnostic and statistical manual of mental disorders* (5th ed.). Washington, DC: Author.

Amsterdam, J. D., Settle, R. G., Doty, R. L., Abelman, E., & Winokur, A. (1987). Taste and smell perception in depression. *Biological Psychiatry, 22*(12), 1481–1485.

App, B., McIntosh, D. N., Reed, C. L., & Hertenstein, M. J. (2011). Nonverbal channel use in communication of emotion: How may depend on why. *Emotion, 11*(3), 603–617. doi:10.1037/a0023164

Arbib, M. A. (2012). *How the brain got language: The mirror system hypothesis.* New York, NY: Oxford University Press.

Asendorpf, J. B. (2006). Typeness of personality profiles: A continuous person-centred approach to personality data. *European Journal of Personality, 20*(2), 83–106. doi:10.1002/per.575

Ashton, M. C., Lee, K., & Goldberg, L. R. (2004). A hierarchical analysis of 1,710 English personality-descriptive adjectives. *Journal of Personality and Social Psychology, 87*(5), 707–721. doi:10.1037/0022-3514.87.5.707

Bandura, A. (1973). *Aggression: A social learning analysis.* Englewood Cliffs, NJ: Prentice-Hall.

Barlow, D. H. (1988). *Anxiety and its disorders: The nature and treatment of anxiety and panic.* New York, NY: Guilford Press.

Baron-Cohen, S., & Wheelwright, S. (2003). The Friendship Questionnaire: An investigation of adults with Asperger syndrome or high-functioning autism, and normal sex differences. *Journal of Autism and Developmental Disorders, 33*(5), 509–517. doi:10.1023/A:1025879411971

Baumeister, R. F., & Cairns, K. J. (1992). Repression and self-presentation: When audiences interfere with self-deceptive strategies. *Journal of Personality and Social Psychology, 62*(5), 851–862.

Baumeister, R. F., Heatherton, T. F., & Tice, D. M. (1994). *Losing control: How and why people fail at self-regulation.* San Diego, CA: Academic Press.

Beauchaine, T. P. (2001). Vagal tone, development, and Gray's motivational theory: Toward an integrated model of autonomic nervous system functioning in psychopathology. *Development and Psychopathology, 13*(2), 183–214.

Beck, A. T., Freeman, A., & Davis, D. D. (2004). *Cognitive therapy of personality disorders* (2nd ed.). New York, NY: Guilford Press.

Beck, A. T., Kovacs, M., & Weissman, A. (1979). Assessment of suicidal intention: The Scale for Suicide Ideation. *Journal of Consulting and Clinical Psychology, 47*(2), 343–352.

Beck, A. T., Rush, A. J., Shaw, B. J., & Emery, G. (1979). *Cognitive therapy of depression.* New York, NY: Guilford Press.

Beck, I., Smits, D. J., Claes, L., Vandereycken, W., & Bijttebier, P. (2009). Psychometric evaluation of the behavioral inhibition/behavioral activation system scales and the sensitivity to punishment and sensitivity to reward questionnaire in a sample of eating disordered patients. *Personality and Individual Differences, 47*(5), 407–412.

Beevers, C. G., Wenzlaff, R. M., Hayes, A. M., & Scott, W. D. (1999). Depression and the ironic effects of thought suppression: Therapeutic strategies for improving mental control. *Clinical Psychology: Science and Practice, 6*(2), 133–148. doi:10.1093/clipsy/6.2.133

Bendesky, A., & Bargmann, C. I. (2011). Genetic contributions to behavioural diversity at the gene–environment interface. *Nature Reviews Genetics, 12*(12), 809–820.

Berlin, I., Givry-Steiner, L., Lecrubier, Y., & Puech, A. (1998). Measures of anhedonia and hedonic responses to sucrose in depressive and schizophrenic patients in comparison with healthy subjects. *European Psychiatry, 13*(6), 303–309.

Bernstein, A., Trafton, J., Ilgen, M., & Zvolensky, M. J. (2008). An evaluation of the role of smoking context on a biobehavioral index of distress tolerance. *Addictive Behaviors, 33*(11), 1409–1415. doi:10.1016/j.addbeh.2008.06.003

Berntson, G. G., Cacioppo, J. T., & Quigley, K. S. (1991). Autonomic determinism: The modes of autonomic control, the doctrine of autonomic space, and the laws of autonomic constraint. *Psychological Review, 98*(4), 459–487.

Berridge, K. C., & Robinson, T. E. (2003). Parsing reward. *Trends in Neurosciences, 26*(9), 507–513.

Berridge, K., & Winkielman, P. (2003). What is an unconscious emotion? (The case for unconscious "liking.") *Cognition and Emotion, 17*(2), 181–211.

Bieling, P. J., & Kuyken, W. (2003). Is cognitive case formulation science or science fiction? *Clinical Psychology: Science and Practice, 10*(1), 52–69. doi:10.1093/clipsy/10.1.52

Biggs, B. K., Vernberg, E., Little, T. D., Dill, E. J., Fonagy, P., & Twemlow, S. W. (2010). Peer victimization trajectories and their association with children's affect in late elementary school. *International Journal of Behavioral Development, 34*(2), 136–146. doi:10.1177/0165025409348560

Bijttebier, P., & Vertommen, H. (1999). Coping strategies in relation to personality disorders. *Personality and Individual Differences, 26*(5), 847–856. doi:10.1016/S0191–8869(98) 00187–1

Blatt, S. J. (1974). Levels of object representation in anaclitic and introjective depression. *Psychoanalytic Study of the Child, 29*, 107–157.

Blatt, S. J., D'Afflitti, J. P., & Quinlan, D. M. (1976). Experiences of depression in normal young adults. *Journal of Abnormal Psychology, 85*(4), 383–389. doi:10.1037/0021–843X .85.4.383

Blechert, J., Michael, T., Grossman, P., Lajtman, M., & Wilhelm, F. H. (2007). Autonomic and respiratory characteristics of posttraumatic stress disorder and panic disorder. *Psychosomatic Medicine, 69*(9), 935–943. doi:10.1097/PSY.0b013e31815a8f6b

Block, J. H., & Block, J. (1980). The role of ego-control and ego-resiliency in the organization of behavior. In W. A. Collins (Ed.), *The Minnesota symposium on child psychology: Vol. 13. Development of Cognition, Affect, and Social Relations* (pp. 39–101). Hillsdale, NJ: Erlbaum.

Boehm, C. (2012). *Moral origins: The evolution of virtue, altruism, and shame.* New York, NY: Basic Books.

Bonanno, G. A., Davis, P. J., Singer, J. L., & Schwartz, G. E. (1991). The repressor personality and avoidant information processing: A dichotic listening study. *Journal of Research in Personality, 25*(4), 386–401.

Bonanno, G. A., Papa, A., Lalande, K., Westphal, M., & Coifman, K. (2004). The importance of being flexible: The ability to both enhance and suppress emotional expression predicts long-term adjustment. *Psychological Science, 15*(7), 482–487. doi:10.1111/j .0956–7976.2004.00705.x

Bond, C. F., & DePaulo, B. M. (2006). Accuracy of deception judgments. *Personality and Social Psychology Review, 10*(3), 214–234.

Bond, F. W., Hayes, S. C., Baer, R. A., Carpenter, K. M., Guenole, N., Orcutt, H. K.,…Zettle, R. D. (2011). Preliminary psychometric properties of the Acceptance and Action Questionnaire–II: A revised measure of psychological inflexibility and experiential avoidance. *Behavior Therapy, 42*(4), 676–688. doi:10.1016/j.beth.2011.03.007

Boone, R. T., & Buck, R. (2003). Emotional expressivity and trustworthiness: The role of nonverbal behavior in the evolution of cooperation. *Journal of Nonverbal Behavior, 27*(3), 163–182. doi:10.1023/a:1025341931128

Bouton, M. E. (2002). Context, ambiguity, and unlearning: Sources of relapse after behavioral extinction. *Biological Psychiatry, 52*(10), 976–986. doi:10.1016/S0006–3223(02) 01546–9

Bracha, H. S. (2004). Freeze, flight, fight, fright, faint: Adaptationist perspectives on the acute stress response spectrum. *CNS Spectrums, 9*(9), 679–685.

Bradley, M. M., & Lang, P. J. (2007). Emotion and motivation. In J. T. Cacioppo, L. G. Tassinary, & G. G. Berntson (Eds.), *Handbook of psychophysiology* (3rd ed., pp. 581–607). New York, NY: Cambridge University Press.

Brand, N., Schneider, N., & Arntz, P. (1995). Information processing efficiency and noise: Interactions with personal rigidity. *Personality and Individual Differences, 18*(5), 571–579.

Brenner, S. L., Beauchaine, T. P., & Sylvers, P. D. (2005). A comparison of psychophysiological and self-report measures of BAS and BIS activation. *Psychophysiology, 42*(1), 108–115. doi:10.1111/j.1469–8986.2005.00261.x

Brown, R. A., Lejuez, C. W., Kahler, C. W., Strong, D. R., & Zvolensky, M. J. (2005). Distress tolerance and early-lapse smokers. *Clinical Psychology Review, 25*(6), 713–733.

Brown, W. M., Palameta, B., & Moore, C. (2003). Are there nonverbal cues to commitment? An exploratory study using the zero-acquaintance video presentation paradigm. *Evolutionary Psychology, 1*(1), 147470490300100104.

Brown, W. M., & Moore, C. (2002). Smile asymmetries and reputation as reliable indicators of likelihood to cooperate: An evolutionary analysis. In S. P. Shohov (Ed.), *Advances in Psychology Research* (Vol. 11, pp. 19–36). Hauppauge, NY: Nova Science.

Buck, R. (1999). The biological affects: A typology. *Psychological Review, 106*(2), 301–336. doi:10.1037/0033–295X.106.2.301

Butler, E. A., Egloff, B., Wilhelm, F. H., Smith, N. C., Erickson, E. A., & Gross, J. J. (2003). The social consequences of expressive suppression. *Emotion, 3*(1), 48–67.

Calvo, M. G., & Eysenck, M. W. (2000). Early vigilance and late avoidance of threat processing: Repressive coping versus low/high anxiety. *Cognition and Emotion, 14*(6), 763–787. doi:10.1080/02699930050156627

Cappella, J. N. (1985). Production principles for turn-taking rules in social interaction: Socially anxious vs. socially secure persons. *Journal of Language and Social Psychology, 4*(3–4), 193–212. doi:10.1177/0261927X8543003

Carroll, K. M., & Nuro, K. F. (2002). One size cannot fit all: A stage model for psychotherapy manual development. *Clinical Psychology: Science and Practice, 9*(4), 396–406.

Carter, J. C., Mercer-Lynn, K. B., Norwood, S. J., Bewell-Weiss, C. V., Crosby, R. D., Woodside, D. B., & Olmsted, M. P. (2012). A prospective study of predictors of relapse in anorexia nervosa: Implications for relapse prevention. *Psychiatry Research, 200*(2–3), 518–523.

Cashdan, E. (1998). Smiles, speech, and body posture: How women and men display sociometric status and power. *Journal of Nonverbal Behavior, 22*(4), 209–228.

Chagnon, N. A. (1974). *Studying the Yanomamö.* New York, NY: Holt, Rinehart and Winston.

Chambers, J. C. (2010). An exploration of the mechanisms underlying the development of repeat and one-time violent offenders. *Aggression and Violent Behavior, 15*(4), 310–323.

Chambless, D. L., Fydrich, T., & Rodebaugh, T. L. (2008). Generalized social phobia and avoidant personality disorder: Meaningful distinction or useless duplication? *Depression and Anxiety, 25*(1), 8–19.

Chaplin, T. M., Cole, P. M., & Zahn-Waxler, C. (2005). Parental socialization of emotion expression: Gender differences and relations to child adjustment. *Emotion, 5*(1), 80–88. doi:10.1037/1528–3542.5.1.80

Chapman, B. P., & Goldberg, L. R. (2011). Replicability and 40-year predictive power of childhood ARC types. *Journal of Personality and Social Psychology, 101*(3), 593–606.

Cheavens, J. S., Rosenthal, M. Z., Daughters, S. B., Nowak, J., Kosson, D., Lynch, T. R., & Lejuez, C. W. (2005). An analogue investigation of the relationships among perceived parental criticism, negative affect, and borderline personality disorder features: The role of thought suppression. *Behavior Research and Therapy, 43*(2), 257–268.

Chen, E. Y., Segal, K., Weissman, J., Zeffiro, T. A., Gallop, R., Linehan, M. M.,...Lynch, T. R. (2015). Adapting dialectical behavior therapy for outpatient adult anorexia nervosa: A pilot study. *International Journal of Eating Disorders, 48*(1), 123–132. doi:10.1002/eat .22360

Chen, Y. P., Ehlers, A., Clark, D. M., & Mansell, W. (2002). Patients with generalized social phobia direct their attention away from faces. *Behavior Research and Therapy, 40*(6), 677–687.

Claes, L., Klonsky, E. D., Muehlenkamp, J., Kuppens, P., & Vandereycken, W. (2010). The affect-regulation function of nonsuicidal self-injury in eating-disordered patients: Which affect states are regulated? *Comprehensive Psychiatry, 51*(4), 386–392.

Claes, L., Vandereycken, W., & Vertommen, H. (2006). Pain experience related to self-injury in eating disorder patients. *Eating Behaviors, 7*(3), 204–213.

Clark, L. A. (2005a). Stability and change in personality pathology: Revelations of three longitudinal studies. *Journal of Personality Disorders, 19*(5), 524–532. doi:10.1521/pedi .2005.19.5.524

Clark, L. A. (2005b). Temperament as a unifying basis for personality and psychopathology. *Journal of Abnormal Psychology, 114*(4), 505–521.

Cloitre, M., Miranda, R., Stovall-McClough, K. C., & Han, H. (2005). Beyond PTSD: Emotion regulation and interpersonal problems as predictors of functional impairment in survivors of childhood abuse. *Behavior Therapy, 36*(2), 119–124. doi:10.1016/S0005 –7894(05)80060–7

Cloitre, M., Stovall-McClough, C., Zorbas, P., & Charuvastra, A. (2008). Attachment organization, emotion regulation, and expectations of support in a clinical sample of women with childhood abuse histories. *Journal of Traumatic Stress, 21*(3), 282–289.

Coid, J., Yang, M., Tyrer, P., Roberts, A., & Ullrich, S. (2006). Prevalence and correlates of personality disorder in Great Britain. *British Journal of Psychiatry, 188*(5), 423–431.

Cole, P. M., Zahn-Waxler, C., Fox, N. A., Usher, B. A., & Welsh, J. D. (1996). Individual differences in emotion regulation and behavior problems in preschool children. *Journal of Abnormal Psychology, 105*(4), 518–529. doi:10.1037/0021-843X.105.4.518

Commerford, M. C., Licinio, J., & Halmi, K. A. (1997). Guidelines for discharging eating disorder inpatients. *Eating Disorders: The Journal of Treatment and Prevention, 5*(1), 69–74. doi:10.1080/10640269708249205

Constantino, M. J., Manber, R., DeGeorge, J., McBride, C., Ravitz, P., Zuroff, D. C.,...Arnow, B. A. (2008). Interpersonal styles of chronically depressed outpatients: Profiles and therapeutic change. *Psychotherapy: Theory, Research, Practice, Training, 45*(4), 491–506.

Couch, L. L., & Sandfoss, K. R. (2009). An analysis of BIS/BAS connections to reactions after romantic betrayal. *Individual Differences Research, 7*(4), 243–254.

Couper-Kuhlen, E. (2012). Exploring affiliation in the reception of conversational complaint stories. In M.-L. Sorjonen & A. Peräkylä (Eds.), *Emotion in interaction.* (pp. 113–146) New York, NY: Oxford University Press.

Coutts, L. M., & Schneider, F. W. (1975). Visual behavior in an unfocused interaction as a function of sex and distance. *Journal of Experimental Social Psychology, 11*(1), 64–77.

Crijnen, A. A., Achenbach, T. M., & Verhulst, F. C. (1997). Comparisons of problems reported by parents of children in 12 cultures: Total problems, externalizing, and internalizing. *Journal of the American Academy of Child and Adolescent Psychiatry, 36*(9), 1269–1277. doi:10.1097/00004583–199709000–00020

Cromwell, H. C., & Panksepp, J. (2011). Rethinking the cognitive revolution from a neural perspective: How overuse/misuse of the term "cognition" and the neglect of affective controls in behavioral neuroscience could be delaying progress in understanding the BrainMind. *Neuroscience and Biobehavioral Reviews, 35*(9), 2026–2035.

Darke, S., Williamson, A., Ross, J., & Teesson, M. (2005). Non-fatal heroin overdose, treatment exposure, and client characteristics: Findings from the Australian Treatment Outcome Study (ATOS). *Drug and Alcohol Review, 24*(5), 425–432. doi: 10.1080/095952 30500286005

Darwin, C. (1872/1998). *The expression of the emotions in man and animals* (3rd ed.). New York, NY: Oxford University Press.

Daughters, S. B., Lejuez, C. W., Bornovalova, M. A., Kahler, C. W., Strong, D. R., & Brown, R. A. (2005). Distress tolerance as a predictor of early treatment dropout in a residential substance abuse treatment facility. *Journal of Abnormal Psychology, 114*(4), 729–734. doi:10.1037/0021–843X.114.4.729

Davey, L., Day, A., & Howells, K. (2005). Anger, over-control, and serious violent offending. *Aggression and Violent Behavior, 10*(5), 624–635. doi:10.1016/j.avb.2004.12.002

Davis, J. M., McKone, E., Dennett, H., O'Connor, K. B., O'Kearney, R., & Palermo, R. (2011). Individual differences in the ability to recognise facial identity are associated with social anxiety. *PloS One, 6*(12), e28800. doi:10.1371/journal.pone.0028800

De Jong, P. J. (1999). Communicative and remedial effects of social blushing. *Journal of Nonverbal Behavior, 23*(3), 197–217.

Depue, R. A., & Iacono, W. G. (1989). Neurobehavioral aspects of affective disorders. *Annual Review of Psychology, 40*, 457–492. doi:10.1146/annurev.ps.40.020189.002325

Depue, R. A., Krauss, S. P., & Spoont, M. R. (1987). A two-dimensional threshold model of seasonal bipolar affective disorder. In D. Magnusson & A. Öhman (Eds.), *Psychopathology: An interactional perspective* (pp. 95–123). Orlando, FL: Academic Press.

Depue, R. A., & Morrone-Strupinsky, J. V. (2005). A neurobehavioral model of affiliative bonding: Implications for conceptualizing a human trait of affiliation. *Behavioral and Brain Sciences, 28*(3), 313–349.

Derakshan, N., & Eysenck, M. W. (1999). Are repressors self-deceivers or other-deceivers? *Cognition and Emotion, 13*(1), 1–17.

DeScioli, P., & Kurzban, R. (2009). Mysteries of morality. *Cognition, 112*(2), 281–299. doi: 10.1016/j.cognition.2009.05.008

Dichter, G. S., Smoski, M. J., Kampov-Polevoy, A. B., Gallop, R., & Garbutt, J. C. (2010). Unipolar depression does not moderate responses to the Sweet Taste Test. *Depression and Anxiety, 27*(9), 859–863.

DiGiuseppe, R., & Tafrate, R. C. (2003). Anger treatment for adults: A meta-analytic review. *Clinical Psychology: Science and Practice, 10*(1), 70–84.

Dijk, C., Koenig, B., Ketelaar, T., & de Jong, P. J. (2011). Saved by the blush: Being trusted despite defecting. *Emotion, 11*(2), 313–319. doi:10.1037/a0022774

Dijk, C., Voncken, M. J., & de Jong, P. J. (2009). I blush, therefore I will be judged negatively: Influence of false blush feedback on anticipated others' judgments and facial coloration in high and low blushing-fearfuls. *Behavior Research and Therapy, 47*(7), 541–547.

Dill, E. J., Vernberg, E. M., Fonagy, P., Twemlow, S. W., & Gamm, B. K. (2004). Negative affect in victimized children: The roles of social withdrawal, peer rejection, and attitudes toward bullying. *Journal of Abnormal Child Psychology, 32*(2), 159–173. doi:10.1023/B:JACP.0000019768.31348.81

Dillon, D. G., Rosso, I. M., Pechtel, P., Killgore, W. D., Rauch, S. L., & Pizzagalli, D. A. (2014). Peril and pleasure: An RDoC-inspired examination of threat responses and reward processing in anxiety and depression. *Depression and Anxiety, 31*(3), 233–249.

Dixon-Gordon, K. L., Whalen, D. J., Layden, B. K., & Chapman, A. L. (2015). A systematic review of personality disorders and health outcomes. *Canadian Psychology/Psychologie Canadienne, 56*(2), 168.

Downey, G., Lebolt, A., Rincón, C., & Freitas, A. L. (1998). Rejection sensitivity and children's interpersonal difficulties. *Child Development, 69*(4), 1074–1091.

Dunkley, D. M., Zuroff, D. C., & Blankstein, K. R. (2003). Self-critical perfectionism and daily affect: Dispositional and situational influences on stress and coping. *Journal of Personality and Social Psychology, 84*(1), 234–252. doi:10.1037/0022–3514.84.1.234

Du Toit, L., & Duckitt, J. (1990). Psychological characteristics of over- and undercontrolled violent offenders. *Journal of Psychology, 124*(2), 125–141.

Ehrlich, H. J., & Bauer, M. L. (1966). The correlates of dogmatism and flexibility in psychiatric hospitalization. *Journal of Consulting Psychology, 30*(3), 253–259. doi:10.1037/h0023378

Eisenberg, N., Fabes, R. A., Guthrie, I. K., & Reiser, M. (2000). Dispositional emotionality and regulation: Their role in predicting quality of social functioning. *Journal of Personality and Social Psychology, 78*(1), 136–157. doi:10.1037/0022–3514.78.1.136

Eisenberg, N., Guthrie, I. K., Fabes, R. A., Shepard, S., Losoya, S., Murphy, B. C.,…Reiser, M. (2000). Prediction of elementary school children's externalizing problem behaviors from attention and behavioral regulation and negative emotionality. *Child Development, 71*(5), 1367–1382. doi:10.1111/1467–8624.00233

Eisenberg, N., Zhou, Q., Losoya, S. H., Fabes, R. A., Shepard, S. A., Murphy, B. C.,…Cumberland, A. (2003). The relations of parenting, effortful control, and ego control to children's emotional expressivity. *Child Development, 74*(3), 875–895.

Eisenberger, N. I., & Lieberman, M. D. (2004). Why rejection hurts: A common neural alarm system for physical and social pain. *Trends in Cognitive Sciences, 8*(7), 294–300. doi:10.1016/j.tics.2004.05.010

Ekman, P. (1972). Universal and cultural differences in facial expressions of emotion. In J. Cole (Ed.), *Nebraska symposium on motivation, 1971* (pp. 207–283). Lincoln: University of Nebraska Press.

Ekman, P. (1992). An argument for basic emotions. *Cognition and Emotion, 6*(3–4), 169–200. doi:10.1080/02699939208411068

Ekman, P., & O'Sullivan, M. (1991). Who can catch a liar? *American Psychologist, 46*(9), 913–920. doi:10.1037/0003–066X.46.9.913

Ekman, P., O'Sullivan, M., & Frank, M. G. (1999). A few can catch a liar. *Psychological Science, 10*(3), 263–266. doi:10.1111/1467–9280.00147

Ellsworth, P. C., Carlsmith, J. M., & Henson, A. (1972). The stare as a stimulus to flight in human subjects: A series of field experiments. *Journal of Personality and Social Psychology, 21*(3), 302–311. doi:10.1037/h0032323

English, T., & John, O. P. (2013). Understanding the social effects of emotion regulation: The mediating role of authenticity for individual differences in suppression. *Emotion, 13*(2), 314–329. doi:10.1037/a0029847

Fairburn, C. G. (2005). Evidence-based treatment of anorexia nervosa. *International Journal of Eating Disorders, 37*(Suppl.), S26–S30. doi:10.1002/eat.20112

Farmer, R. F., & Chapman, A. L. (2016). *Behavioral interventions in cognitive behavior therapy: Practical guidance for putting theory into action* (2nd ed.). Washington, DC: American Psychological Association.

Feinberg, M., Willer, R., & Keltner, D. (2012). Flustered and faithful: Embarrassment as a signal of prosociality. *Journal of Personality and Social Psychology, 102*(1), 81–97. doi: 10.1037/a0025403

Feldman, C., & Kuyken, W. (2011). Compassion in the landscape of suffering. *Contemporary Buddhism, 12*(1), 143–155. doi:10.1080/14639947.2011.564831

Ferenczi, S., & Rank, O. (1925). *The development of psychoanalysis* (Caroline Newton, Trans.). Washington, DC: Nervous and Mental Disease Publishing Co.

Ferguson, T. J., Brugman, D., White, J., & Eyre, H. L. (2007). Shame and guilt as morally warranted experiences. In J. L. Tracy, R. W. Robins, & J. P. Tangney (Eds.), *The self-conscious emotions: Theory and research* (pp. 330–348). New York, NY: Guilford Press.

First, M., Gibbon, M., Spitzer, R. L., Williams, J. B. W., & Benjamin, L. S. (1997). *Structured Clinical Interview for DSM-IV Axis II personality disorders* (SCID-II). Washington, DC: American Psychiatric Press.

First, M., Williams, J., Karg, R., & Spitzer, R. (2015). *Structured clinical interview for DSM-5, research version.* Arlington, VA: American Psychiatric Association.

Foa, E. B., & Kozak, M. J. (1986). Emotional processing of fear: Exposure to corrective information. *Psychological Bulletin, 99*(1), 20–35.

Forsyth, J. P., Parker, J. D., & Finlay, C. G. (2003). Anxiety sensitivity, controllability, and experiential avoidance and their relation to drug of choice and addiction severity in a residential sample of substance-abusing veterans. *Addictive Behaviors, 28*(5), 851–870. doi:10.1016/S0306–4603(02)00216–2

Fournier, J. C., DeRubeis, R. J., Shelton, R. C., Hollon, S. D., Amsterdam, J. D., & Gallop, R. (2009). Prediction of response to medication and cognitive therapy in the treatment of moderate to severe depression. *Journal of Consulting and Clinical Psychology, 77*(4), 775–787.

Fox, E. (1993). Allocation of visual attention and anxiety. *Cognition and Emotion, 7*(2), 207–215.

Franco-Paredes, K., Mancilla-Díaz, J. M., Vázquez-Arévalo, R., López-Aguilar, X., & Álvarez-Rayón, G. (2005). Perfectionism and eating disorders: A review of the literature. *European Eating Disorders Review, 13*(1), 61–70. doi:10.1002/erv.605

Frank, E., Prien, R. F., Jarrett, R. B., Keller, M. B., Kupfer, D. J., Lavori, P. W.,…Weissman, M. M. (1991). Conceptualization and rationale for consensus definitions of terms in major depressive disorder: Remission, recovery, relapse, and recurrence. *Archives of General Psychiatry, 48*(9), 851–855.

Frank, R. H. (1988). *Passions within reason: The strategic role of the emotions.* New York, NY: Norton.

Freedman, J. L., & Fraser, S. C. (1966). Compliance without pressure: The foot-in-the-door technique. *Journal of Personality and Social Psychology, 4*(2), 195.

Fridlund, A. J. (1991). Sociality of solitary smiling: Potentiation by an implicit audience. *Journal of Personality and Social Psychology, 60*(2), 229.

Fridlund, A. J. (2002). The behavioral ecology view of smiling and other facial expressions. In M. Abel (Ed.), *An empirical reflection on the smile* (pp. 45–82). New York, NY: Edwin Mellen Press.

Friesen, W. V. (1972). *Cultural differences in facial expressions in a social situation: An experimental test of the concept of display rules* (Unpublished doctoral dissertation). University of California, San Francisco.

Furnham, A., Petrides, K. V., Sisterson, G., & Baluch, B. (2003). Repressive coping style and positive self-presentation. *British Journal of Health Psychology, 8*(2), 223–249.

Furr, R. M., & Funder, D. C. (1998). A multimodal analysis of personal negativity. *Journal of Personality and Social Psychology, 74*(6), 1580–1591. doi:10.1037/0022–3514.74.6.1580

Gailliot, M. T., Baumeister, R. F., DeWall, C. N., Maner, J. K., Plant, E. A., Tice, D. M.,…Schmeichel, B. J. (2007). Self-control relies on glucose as a limited energy source: Willpower is more than a metaphor. *Journal of Personality and Social Psychology, 92*(2), 325–336. doi:10.1037/0022–3514.92.2.325

Gallagher, N. G., South, S. C., & Oltmanns, T. F. (2003). Attentional coping style in obsessive-compulsive personality disorder: A test of the intolerance of uncertainty hypothesis. *Personality and Individual Differences, 34*(1), 41–57. doi:10.1016/S0191–8869(02)00025–9

Gansle, K. A. (2005). The effectiveness of school-based anger interventions and programs: A meta-analysis. *Journal of School Psychology, 43*(4), 321–341.

Gard, D. E., Gard, M. G., Kring, A. M., & John, O. P. (2006). Anticipatory and consummatory components of the experience of pleasure: A scale development study. *Journal of Research in Personality, 40*(6), 1086–1102.

Gardner, D. L., & Cowdry, R. W. (1985). Suicidal and parasuicidal behavior in borderline personality disorder. *Psychiatric Clinics of North America, 8*(2), 389–403.

Gazelle, H., & Druhen, M. J. (2009). Anxious solitude and peer exclusion predict social helplessness, upset affect, and vagal regulation in response to behavioral rejection by a friend. *Developmental Psychology, 45*(4), 1077.

Geller, J., Cockell, S. J., Hewitt, P. L., Goldner, E. M., & Flett, G. L. (2000). Inhibited expression of negative emotions and interpersonal orientation in anorexia nervosa. *International Journal of Eating Disorders, 28*(1), 8–19.

George, L. K., Blazer, D. G., Hughes, D. C., & Fowler, N. (1989). Social support and the outcome of major depression. *British Journal of Psychiatry, 154*(4), 478–485.

Ghaziuddin, M., Tsai, L. Y., & Ghaziuddin, N. (1991). Brief report: Haloperidol treatment of trichotillomania in a boy with autism and mental retardation. *Journal of Autism and Developmental Disorders, 21*(3), 365–371.

Giesler, R. B., Josephs, R. A., & Swann, W. B. Jr. (1996). Self-verification in clinical depression: The desire for negative evaluation. *Journal of Abnormal Psychology, 105*(3), 358–368. doi:10.1037/0021–843X.105.3.358

Gladstone, G. L., Parker, G. B., & Malhi, G. S. (2006). Do bullied children become anxious and depressed adults? A cross-sectional investigation of the correlates of bullying and anxious depression. *Journal of Nervous and Mental Disease, 194*(3), 201–208. doi:10.1097/01.nmd.0000202491.99719.c3

Glashouwer, K. A., Bloot, L., Veenstra, E. M., Franken, I. H., & de Jong, P. J. (2014). Heightened sensitivity to punishment and reward in anorexia nervosa. *Appetite, 75*, 97–102.

Glisky, M. L., Tataryn, D. J., Tobias, B. A., Kihlstrom, J. F., & McConkey, K. M. (1991). Absorption, openness to experience, and hypnotizability. *Journal of Personality and Social Psychology, 60*(2), 263–272. doi:10.1037/0022–3514.60.2.263

Goldberg, L. R. (1993). The structure of personality traits: Vertical and horizontal aspects. In D. C. Funder, R. D. Parke, C. Tomlinson-Keasey, & K. Widaman (Eds.), *Studying lives through time: Personality and development* (pp. 169–188). Washington, DC: American Psychological Association.

Goldberg, L. R., & Kilkowski, J. M. (1985). The prediction of semantic consistency in self-descriptions: Characteristics of persons and of terms that affect the consistency of responses to synonym and antonym pairs. *Journal of Personality and Social Psychology, 48*(1), 82–98. doi:10.1037/0022–3514.48.1.82

Gottfredson, M. R., & Hirschi, T. (1990). *A general theory of crime.* Stanford, CA: Stanford University Press.

Gottheil, N. F., & Dubow, E. F. (2001). Tripartite beliefs models of bully and victim behavior. *Journal of Emotional Abuse, 2*(2–3), 25–47. doi:10.1300/J135v02n02_03

Grammer, K., Schiefenhovel, W., Schleidt, M., Lorenz, B., & Eibl-Eibesfeldt, I. (1988). Patterns on the face: The eyebrow flash in crosscultural comparison. *Ethology, 77*(4), 279–299.

Gray, J. A. (1987). The neuropsychology of emotion and personality structure. *Zhurnal Vysshei Nervnoi Deyatel'nosti, 37*(6), 1011–1024.

Gray, J. A., & McNaughton, N. (2000). *The neuropsychology of anxiety: An enquiry into the functions of the septo-hippocampal system.* Oxford: Oxford University Press.

Greenberg, J. R., & Mitchell, S. A. (1983). *Object relations in psychoanalytic theory.* Cambridge, MA: Harvard University Press.

Greville-Harris, M., Hempel, R., Karl, A., Dieppe, P., & Lynch, T. R. (2016). The power of invalidating communication: Receiving invalidating feedback predicts threat-related emotional, physiological, and social responses. *Journal of Social and Clinical Psychology, 35*(6), 471–493. doi:10.1521/jscp.2016.35.6.471

Gross, J. J., & John, O. P. (2003). Individual differences in two emotion regulation processes: Implications for affect, relationships, and well-being. *Journal of Personality and Social Psychology, 85*(2), 348–362. doi:10.1037/0022–3514.85.2.348

Gross, J. J., & Levenson, R. W. (1997). Hiding feelings: The acute effects of inhibiting negative and positive emotion. *Journal of Abnormal Psychology, 106*(1), 95–103. doi:10.1037/0021–843X.106.1.95

Gross, L. (2006). How the human brain detects unexpected events. *PLoS Biology, 4*(12), e443. doi:10.1371/journal.pbio.0040443

Hamilton, M. (1960). A rating scale for depression. *Journal of Neurology, Neurosurgery and Psychiatry, 23*(1), 56–62.

Hanson, R. K., Bourgon, G., Helmus, L., & Hodgson, S. (2009). The principles of effective correctional treatment also apply to sexual offenders: A meta-analysis. *Criminal Justice and Behavior, 36*(9), 865–891.

Happé, F., & Frith, U. (2006). The weak coherence account: Detail-focused cognitive style in autism spectrum disorders. *Journal of Autism and Developmental Disorders, 36*(1), 5–25. doi:10.1007/s10803–005–0039–0

Harrison, A., O'Brien, N., Lopez, C., & Treasure, J. (2010). Sensitivity to reward and punishment in eating disorders. *Psychiatry Research, 177*(1–2), 1–11.

Harrison, A., Tchanturia, K., & Treasure, J. (2010). Attentional bias, emotion recognition, and emotion regulation in anorexia: State or trait? *Biological Psychiatry, 68*(8), 755–761.

Hartmann, A., Weber, S., Herpertz, S., & Zeeck, A. (2011). Psychological treatment for anorexia nervosa: A meta-analysis of standardized mean change. *Psychotherapy and Psychosomatics, 80*(4), 216–226.

Haslam, N. (2011). The return of the anal character. *Review of General Psychology, 15*(4), 351–360. doi:10.1037/a0025251

Hawley, L. L., Ho, M. R., Zuroff, D. C., & Blatt, S. J. (2006). The relationship of perfectionism, depression, and therapeutic alliance during treatment for depression: Latent difference score analysis. *Journal of Consulting and Clinical Psychology, 74*(5), 930–942. doi:10.1037/0022–006X.74.5.930

Hayes, S. C. (2004). Acceptance and commitment therapy, relational frame theory, and the third wave of behavioral and cognitive therapies. *Behavior Therapy, 35*(4), 639–665.

Hayes, S. C., Brownstein, A. J., Haas, J. R., & Greenway, D. E. (1986). Instructions, multiple schedules, and extinction: Distinguishing rule-governed from schedule-controlled behavior. *Journal of the Experimental Analysis of Behavior, 46*(2), 137–147.

Hayes, S. C., Follette, W. C., & Follette, V. (1995). Behavior therapy: A contextual approach. In A. S. German & S. B. Messer (Eds.), *Essential psychotherapies: Theory and practice* (pp. 128–181). New York, NY: Guilford Press.

Hayes, S. C., Wilson, K. G., Gifford, E. V., Follette, V. M., & Strosahl, K. (1996). Experiential avoidance and behavioral disorders: A functional dimensional approach to diagnosis and treatment. *Journal of Consulting and Clinical Psychology, 64*(6), 1152.

Heerey, E. A., & Kring, A. M. (2007). Interpersonal consequences of social anxiety. *Journal of Abnormal Psychology, 116*(1), 125–134. doi:10.1037/0021–843X.116.1.125

Heisel, M. J., Duberstein, P. R., Conner, K. R., Franus, N., Beckman, A., & Conwell, Y. (2006). Personality and reports of suicide ideation among depressed adults 50 years of age or older. *Journal of Affective Disorders, 90*(2), 175–180.

Henderson, J. M., Williams, C. C., & Falk, R. J. (2005). Eye movements are functional during face learning. *Memory and Cognition, 33*(1), 98–106.

Henderson, M. (1983a). An empirical classification of non-violent offenders using the MMPI. *Personality and Individual Differences, 4*(6), 671–677.

Henderson, M. (1983b). Self-reported assertion and aggression among violent offenders with high or low levels of overcontrolled hostility. *Personality and Individual Differences, 4*(1), 113–115.

Henriques, J. B., & Davidson, R. J. (2000). Decreased responsiveness to reward in depression. *Cognition and Emotion, 14*(5), 711–724.

Hershorn, M., & Rosenbaum, A. (1991). Over- vs. undercontrolled hostility: Application of the construct to the classification of maritally violent men. *Violence and Victims, 6*(2), 151–158.

Hertenstein, M. J., Verkamp, J. M., Kerestes, A. M., & Holmes, R. M. (2006). The communicative functions of touch in humans, nonhuman primates, and rats: A review and synthesis of the empirical research. *Genetic, Social, and General Psychology Monographs, 132*(1), 5–94. doi:10.3200/MONO.132.1.5-94

Hess, U., & Blairy, S. (2001). Facial mimicry and emotional contagion to dynamic emotional facial expressions and their influence on decoding accuracy. *International Journal of Psychophysiology, 40*(2), 129–141. doi:10.1016/S0167-8760(00)00161-6

Hintikka, J., Tolmunen, T., Rissanen, M.-L., Honkalampi, K., Kylmä, J., & Laukkanen, E. (2009). Mental disorders in self-cutting adolescents. *Journal of Adolescent Health, 44*(5), 464–467.

Hock, M., & Krohne, H. W. (2004). Coping with threat and memory for ambiguous information: Testing the repressive discontinuity hypothesis. *Emotion, 4*(1), 65–86.

Hock, M., Krohne, H. W., & Kaiser, J. (1996). Coping dispositions and the processing of ambiguous stimuli. *Journal of Personality and Social Psychology, 70*(5), 1052.

Hofmann, W., Rauch, W., & Gawronski, B. (2007). And deplete us not into temptation: Automatic attitudes, dietary restraint, and self-regulatory resources as determinants of eating behavior. *Journal of Experimental Social Psychology, 43*(3), 497–504.

Hofstede, G. (1983). National cultures in four dimensions: A research-based theory of cultural differences among nations. *International Studies of Management and Organization, 13*(1–2), 46–74.

Hollerman, J. R., & Schultz, W. (1998). Dopamine neurons report an error in the temporal prediction of reward during learning. *Nature Neuroscience, 1*(4), 304–309.

Hollin, C. R., Palmer, E. J., & Hatcher, R. M. (2013). Efficacy of correctional cognitive skills programmes. In L. A. Craig, L. Dixon, & T. A. Gannon (Eds.), *What works in offender rehabilitation: An evidence-based approach to assessment and treatment* (pp. 115–128). Chichester, England: Wiley-Blackwell.

Horstmann, G., & Bauland, A. (2006). Search asymmetries with real faces: Testing the anger-superiority effect. *Emotion, 6*(2), 193.

Hutcherson, C. A., Seppala, E. M., & Gross, J. J. (2008). Loving-kindness meditation increases social connectedness. *Emotion*, 8(5), 720–724. doi:10.1037/a0013237

Iizuka, Y. (1992). Eye contact in dating couples and unacquainted couples. *Perceptual and Motor Skills*, 75(2), 457–461.

Ikemoto, S., & Panksepp, J. (1999). The role of nucleus accumbens dopamine in motivated behavior: A unifying interpretation with special reference to reward-seeking. *Brain Research Reviews*, 31(1), 6–41.

Jessell, T. M. (1995). The nervous system. In E. R. Kandel, J. H. Schwartz, & T. M. Jessell (Eds.), *Essentials of neural science and behavior* (3rd ed). Stamford, CT: Appleton & Lange.

John, O. P., & Robins, R. W. (1994). Accuracy and bias in self-perception: Individual differences in self-enhancement and the role of narcissism. *Journal of Personality and Social Psychology*, 66(1), 206–219. doi:10.1037/0022–3514.66.1.206

Johnson, J. G., Smailes, E. M., Cohen, P., Brown, J., & Bernstein, D. P. (2000). Associations between four types of childhood neglect and personality disorder symptoms during adolescence and early adulthood: Findings of a community-based longitudinal study. *Journal of Personality Disorders*, 14(2), 171–187.

Joiner, T. E., & Metalsky, G. I. (1995). A prospective test of an integrative interpersonal theory of depression: A naturalistic study of college roommates. *Journal of Personality and Social Psychology*, 69(4), 778–788. doi:10.1037/0022–3514.69.4.778

Kagan, J. (1994). On the nature of emotion. In N. A. Fox (Ed.), *The development of emotion regulation and dysregulation: Biological and behavioral considerations* (pp. 7–24). Ann Arbor, MI: Society for Research in Child Development.

Kagan, J., Reznick, J. S., & Snidman, N. (1987a). The physiology and psychology of behavioral inhibition in children. *Child Development*, 58(6), 1459–1473.

Kagan, J., Reznick, J. S., & Snidman, N. (1987b). Temperamental variation in response to the unfamiliar. In N. A. Krasnegor, E. M. Blass, & M. A. Hofer (Eds.), *Perinatal development: A psychobiological perspective* (pp. 421–440). Orlando, FL: Academic Press.

Kanngiesser, P., & Warneken, F. (2012). Young children consider merit when sharing resources with others. *PloS One*, 7(8), e43979.

Kasch, K. L., Rottenberg, J., Arnow, B. A., & Gotlib, I. H. (2002). Behavioral activation and inhibition systems and the severity and course of depression. *Journal of Abnormal Psychology*, 111(4), 589–597.

Kaye, W. H., Wierenga, C. E., Bailer, U. F., Simmons, A. N., & Bischoff-Grethe, A. (2013). Nothing tastes as good as skinny feels: The neurobiology of anorexia nervosa. *Trends in Neurosciences*, 36(2), 110–120.

Keel, P. K., Dorer, D. J., Eddy, K. T., Franko, D., Charatan, D. L., & Herzog, D. B. (2003). Predictors of mortality in eating disorders. *Archives of General Psychiatry*, 60(2), 179–183.

Keiley, M. K., Howe, T. R., Dodge, K. A., Bates, J. E., & Pettit, G. S. (2001). The timing of child physical maltreatment: A cross-domain growth analysis of impact on adolescent externalizing and internalizing problems. *Development and Psychopathology*, 13(4), 891–912.

Keltner, D., Capps, L., Kring, A. M., Young, R. C., & Heerey, E. A. (2001). Just teasing: A conceptual analysis and empirical review. *Psychological Bulletin, 127*(2), 229.

Keltner, D., & Harker, L. (1998). The forms and functions of the nonverbal signal of shame. In P. Gilbert & B. Andrews (Eds.), *Shame: Interpersonal behavior, psychopathology, and culture* (pp. 78–98). New York, NY: Oxford University Press.

Keltner, D., Young, R. C., & Buswell, B. N. (1997). Appeasement in human emotion, social practice, and personality. *Aggressive Behavior, 23*(5), 359–374. doi:10.1002/(SICI)1098 –2337(1997)23:5<359::AID-AB5>3.0.CO;2-D

Kendler, K. S., Hettema, J. M., Butera, F., Gardner, C. O., & Prescott, C. A. (2003). Life event dimensions of loss, humiliation, entrapment, and danger in the prediction of onsets of major depression and generalized anxiety. *Archives of General Psychiatry, 60*(8), 789–796. doi:10.1001/archpsyc.60.8.789

Kendler, K. S., Prescott, C. A., Myers, J., & Neale, M. C. (2003). The structure of genetic and environmental risk factors for common psychiatric and substance use disorders in men and women. *Archives of General Psychiatry, 60*(9), 929–937.

Keogh, K., Booth, R., Baird, K., & Davenport, J. (2016). The Radical Openness Group: A controlled trial with 3-month follow-up. *Practice Innovations, 1*(2), 129–143.

Kernis, M. H., & Goldman, B. M. (2006). A multicomponent conceptualization of authenticity: Theory and research. In M. P. Zanna (Ed.), *Advances in experimental social psychology* (Vol. 38, pp. 283–357). San Diego, CA: Academic Press.

Kiecolt-Glaser, J., & Murray, J. A. (1980). Social desirability bias in self-monitoring data. *Journal of Behavioral Assessment, 2*(4), 239–247. doi:10.1007/BF01666783

Kim, J., Cicchetti, D., Rogosch, F. A., & Manly, J. T. (2009). Child maltreatment and trajectories of personality and behavioral functioning: Implications for the development of personality disorder. *Development and Psychopathology, 21*(3), 889–912.

Kimbrel, N. A., Nelson-Gray, R. O., & Mitchell, J. T. (2007). Reinforcement sensitivity and maternal style as predictors of psychopathology. *Personality and Individual Differences, 42*(6), 1139–1149. doi:10.1016/j.paid.2006.06.028

Klonsky, E. D. (2007). The functions of deliberate self-injury: A review of the evidence. *Clinical Psychology Review, 27*(2), 226–239.

Klonsky, E. D., & Olino, T. M. (2008). Identifying clinically distinct subgroups of self-injurers among young adults: A latent class analysis. *Journal of Consulting and Clinical Psychology, 76*(1), 22–27. doi:10.1037/0022–006X.76.1.22

Klonsky, E. D., Oltmanns, T. F., & Turkheimer, E. (2003). Deliberate self-harm in a nonclinical population: Prevalence and psychological correlates. *American Journal of Psychiatry, 160*(8), 1501–1508.

Kocsis, J. H., Gelenberg, A. J., Rothbaum, B. O., Klein, D. N., Trivedi, M. H., Manber, R.,… Arnow, B. A. (2009). Cognitive behavioral analysis system of psychotherapy and brief supportive psychotherapy for augmentation of antidepressant nonresponse in chronic depression: The REVAMP Trial. *Archives of General Psychiatry, 66*(11), 1178–1188.

Kohlenberg, R. J., & Tsai, M. (1991). *Functional analytic psychotherapy: Creating intense and curative therapeutic relationships.* New York, NY: Plenum Press.

Kraus, M. W., & Keltner, D. (2009). Signs of socioeconomic status: A thin-slicing approach. *Psychological Science, 20*(1), 99–106. doi:10.1111/j.1467–9280.2008.02251.x

Krueger, R. F. (1999). The structure of common mental disorders. *Archives of General Psychiatry, 56*(10), 921–926. doi:10.1001/archpsyc.56.10.921

Krueger, R. F., Caspi, A., Moffitt, T. E., & Silva, P. A. (1998). The structure and stability of common mental disorders (DSM-III-R): A longitudinal-epidemiological study. *Journal of Abnormal Psychology, 107*(2), 216–227. doi:10.1037/0021–843X.107.2.216

Krueger, R. F., & Markon, K. E. (2014). The role of the DSM-5 personality trait model in moving toward a quantitative and empirically based approach to classifying personality and psychopathology. *Annual Review of Clinical Psychology, 10,* 477–501.

Kumar, P., Berghorst, L. H., Nickerson, L. D., Dutra, S. J., Goer, F., Greve, D., & Pizzagalli, D. A. (2014). Differential effects of acute stress on anticipatory and consummatory phases of reward processing. *Neuroscience, 266,* 1–12.

Kuyken, W., Fothergill, C. D., Musa, M., & Chadwick, P. (2005). The reliability and quality of cognitive case formulation. *Behavior Research and Therapy, 13*(9), 1187–1201. doi:10.1016/j.brat.2004.08.007

Kyriacou, O., Treasure, J., & Schmidt, U. (2008). Expressed emotion in eating disorders assessed via self-report: An examination of factors associated with expressed emotion in carers of people with anorexia nervosa in comparison to control families. *International Journal of Eating Disorders, 41*(1), 37–46. doi:10.1002/eat.20469

Lakin, J. L., & Chartrand, T. L. (2003). Using nonconscious behavioral mimicry to create affiliation and rapport. *Psychological Science, 14*(4), 334–339. doi:10.1111/1467–9280.14481

Lakin, J. L., Jefferis, V. E., Cheng, C. M., & Chartrand, T. L. (2003). The chameleon effect as social glue: Evidence for the evolutionary significance of nonconscious mimicry. *Journal of Nonverbal Behavior, 27*(3), 145–162. doi:10.1023/A:1025389814290

Lane, P. J., & Kling, J. S. (1979). Construct validation of the Overcontrolled Hostility scale of the MMPI. *Journal of Consulting and Clinical Psychology, 47*(4), 781–782. doi:10.1037/0022–006X.47.4.781

Lane, P. J., & Spruill, J. (1980). Validity of the overcontrolled/undercontrolled typology usage on criminal psychiatric patients. *Criminal Justice and Behavior, 7*(2), 215–228.

Lane, R. D., Quinlan, D. M., Schwartz, G. E., Walker, P. A., & Zeitlin, S. (1990). The Levels of Emotional Awareness Scale: A cognitive-developmental measure of emotion. *Journal of Personality Assessment, 55*(1–2), 124–134. doi:10.1207/s15327752jpa5501&2_12

Lane, R. D., Sechrest, L., Riedel, R., Shapiro, D. E., & Kaszniak, A. W. (2000). Pervasive emotion recognition deficit common to alexithymia and the repressive coping style. *Psychosomatic Medicine, 62*(4), 492–501.

Lang, K., Lopez, C., Stahl, D., Tchanturia, K., & Treasure, J. (2014). Central coherence in eating disorders: An updated systematic review and meta-analysis. *World Journal of Biological Psychiatry, 15*(8), 586–598. doi:10.3109/15622975.2014.909606

Lang, K., & Tchanturia, K. (2014). A systematic review of central coherence in young people with anorexia nervosa. *Journal of Child and Adolescent Behavior, 2*(140). doi:10.4172/2375–4494.1000140

Lawson, J., Baron-Cohen, S., & Wheelwright, S. (2004). Empathising and systemising in adults with and without Asperger syndrome. *Journal of Autism and Developmental Disorders, 34*(3), 301–310. doi:10.1023/B:JADD.0000029552.42724.1b

LeDoux, J. (2012). Rethinking the emotional brain. *Neuron, 73*(4), 653–676.

Lee, J. J., & Pinker, S. (2010). Rationales for indirect speech: The theory of the strategic speaker. *Psychological Review, 117*(3), 785–807. Retrieved from https://dash.harvard.edu /bitstream/handle/1/10226781/lee_pinker_rationales.pdf?sequence=2.

Lenzenweger, M. F. (2008). Epidemiology of personality disorders. *Psychiatric Clinics of North America, 31*(3), 395–403.

Lewis, M., & Weinraub, M. (1979). Origins of early sex-role development. *Sex Roles, 5*(2), 135–153. doi:10.1007/BF00287927

Linehan, M. M. (1993a). *Cognitive-behavioral treatment of borderline personality disorder.* New York, NY: Guilford Press.

Linehan, M. M. (1993b). *Skills training manual for treating borderline personality disorder.* New York, NY: Guilford Press.

Livingstone, M. S. (2000). Is it warm? Is it real? Or just low spatial frequency? *Science, 290*(5495), 1229–1229. doi:10.1126/science.290.5495.1299b

London, B., Downey, G., Bonica, C., & Paltin, I. (2007). Social causes and consequences of rejection sensitivity. *Journal of Research on Adolescence, 17*(3), 481–506.

Lopez, C., Tchanturia, K., Stahl, D., & Treasure, J. (2008). Central coherence in eating disorders: A systematic review. *Psychological Medicine, 38*(10), 1393–1404. doi:10.1017 /S0033291708003486

Lopez, C., Tchanturia, K., Stahl, D., & Treasure, J. (2009). Weak central coherence in eating disorders: A step towards looking for an endophenotype of eating disorders. *Journal of Clinical and Experimental Neuropsychology, 31*(1), 117–125. doi:10.1080/13803390802036092

Loranger, A. W., Janca, A., & Sartorius, N. (1997). *Assessment and diagnosis of personality disorders: The ICD-10 International Personality Disorder Examination (IPDE).* Cambridge, England: Cambridge University Press.

Losh, M., Adolphs, R., Poe, M. D., Couture, S., Penn, D., Baranek, G. T., & Piven, J. (2009). Neuropsychological profile of autism and the broad autism phenotype. *Archives of General Psychiatry, 66*(5), 518–526. doi:10.1001/archgenpsychiatry.2009.34

Low, K., & Day, A. (2015). Toward a clinically meaningful taxonomy of violent offenders: The role of anger and thinking styles. *Journal of Interpersonal Violence, 32*(4), 489–514. doi:10.1177/0886260515586365

Lundqvist, D., & Öhman, A. (2005). Emotion regulates attention: The relation between facial configurations, facial emotion, and visual attention. *Visual Cognition, 12*(1), 51–84.

Lynch, M. P. (2004). *True to life: Why truth matters.* Cambridge, MA: MIT Press.

Lynch, T. R. (2000). Treatment of elderly depression with personality disorder comorbidity using dialectical behavior therapy. *Cognitive and Behavioral Practice, 7*(4), 468–477.

Lynch, T. R. (2018). *The skills training manual for radically open dialectical behavior therapy: A clinician's guide for treating disorders of overcontrol.* Oakland, CA: New Harbinger.

Lynch, T. R., & Aspnes, A. (2001). Personality disorders in older adults: Diagnostic and theoretical issues. *Clinical Geriatrics, 9,* 64–70.

Lynch, T. R., Chapman, A. L., Rosenthal, M. Z., Kuo, J. R., & Linehan, M. M. (2006). Mechanisms of change in dialectical behavior therapy: Theoretical and empirical observations. *Journal of Clinical Psychology, 62*(4), 459–480. doi:10.1002/jclp.20243

Lynch, T. R., & Cheavens, J. S. (2007). Dialectical behavior therapy for depression with comorbid personality disorder: An extension of standard dialectical behavior therapy with a special emphasis on the treatment of older adults. In L. A. Dimeff & K. Koerner (Eds.), *Dialectical behavior therapy in clinical practice: Applications across disorders and settings* (pp. 264–297). New York, NY: Guilford Press.

Lynch, T. R., & Cheavens, J. S. (2008). Dialectical behavior therapy for comorbid personality disorders. *Journal of Clinical Psychology, 64*(2), 154–167. doi:10.1002/jclp.20449

Lynch, T. R., Cheavens, J. S., Morse, J. Q., & Rosenthal, M. Z. (2004). A model predicting suicidal ideation and hopelessness in depressed older adults: The impact of emotion inhibition and affect intensity. *Aging & Mental Health, 8*(6), 486–497.

Lynch, T. R., & Cozza, C. (2009). Behavior therapy for nonsuicidal self-injury. In M. K. Nock (Ed.), *Understanding nonsuicidal self-injury: Origins, assessment, and treatment* (pp. 211–250). Washington DC: American Psychological Association.

Lynch, T. R., Gray, K. L., Hempel, R. J., Titley, M., Chen, E. Y., & O'Mahen, H. A. (2013). Radically open–dialectical behavior therapy for adult anorexia nervosa: Feasibility and outcomes from an inpatient program. *BMC Psychiatry, 13*(293), 1–17. doi:10.1186/1471 –244x-13–293

Lynch, T. R., Hempel, R. J., & Clark, L. A. (2015). Promoting radical openness and flexible control. In J. Livesley, G. Dimaggio, & J. Clarkin (Eds.), *Integrated treatment for personality disorder: A modular approach* (pp. 325–344). New York, NY: Guilford Press.

Lynch, T. R., Hempel, R. J., & Dunkley, C. (2015). Radically open–dialectical behavior therapy for disorders of over-control: Signaling matters. *American Journal of Psychotherapy, 69*(2), 141–162.

Lynch, T. R., Hempel, R. J., Titley, M., Burford, S., & Gray, K. L. H. (2012). *Anorexia nervosa: The problem of overcontrol.* Paper presented at the annual meeting of the Association for Behavioral and Cognitive Therapies, National Harbor, MD.

Lynch, T. R., Johnson, C. S., Mendelson, T., Robins, C. J., Krishnan, K . R . R., & Blazer, D. G. (1999). Correlates of suicidal ideation among an elderly depressed sample. *Journal of Affective Disorders, 56*(1), 9–15.

Lynch, T. R., & Mizon, G. A. (2011). Distress over-tolerance and distress intolerance: A behavioral perspective. In M. J. Zvolensky, A. Bernstein, & A. A. Vujanovic (Eds.), *Distress tolerance* (pp. 52–79). New York, NY: Guilford Press.

Lynch, T. R., Morse, J. Q., Mendelson, T., & Robins, C. J. (2003). Dialectical behavior therapy for depressed older adults: A randomized pilot study. *American Journal of Geriatric Psychiatry, 11*(1), 33–45.

Lynch, T. R., Robins, C. J., Morse, J. Q., & Krause, E. D. (2001). A mediational model relating affect intensity, emotion inhibition, and psychological distress. *Behavior Therapy, 32*(3), 519–536.

Lynch, T. R., Schneider, K. G., Rosenthal, M. Z., & Cheavens, J. S. (2007). A mediational model of trait negative affectivity, dispositional thought suppression, and intrusive thoughts following laboratory stressors. *Behavior Research and Therapy, 45*(4), 749–761.

Maclean, J. C., Xu, H., French, M. T., & Ettner, S. L. (2014). Mental health and high-cost health care utilization: New evidence from Axis II disorders. *Health Services Research, 49*(2), 683–704.

Malhi, G. S., Parker, G. B., Crawford, J., Wilhelm, K., & Mitchell, P. B. (2005). Treatment-resistant depression: Resistant to definition? *Acta Psychiatrica Scandinavica, 112*(4), 302–309. doi:10.1111/j.1600–0447.2005.00602.x

Manly, J. T., Kim, J. E., Rogosch, F. A., & Cicchetti, D. (2001). Dimensions of child maltreatment and children's adjustment: Contributions of developmental timing and subtype. *Development and Psychopathology, 13*(4), 759–782.

Marean, C. W. (2015). How Homo sapiens became the ultimate invasive species. *Scientific American, 313*(2). Retrieved from http://www.phrenicea.com/ScientificAmericanMarean082015.pdf

Marlatt, G., & Gordon, J. (Eds.). (1985). *Relapse prevention: Maintenance strategies in the treatment of addictive disorders.* New York, NY: Guilford Press.

Marvel, F. A., Chen, C.-C., Badr, N., Gaykema, R. P. A., & Goehler, L. E. (2004). Reversible inactivation of the dorsal vagal complex blocks lipopolysaccharide-induced social withdrawal and c-Fos expression in central autonomic nuclei. *Brain, Behavior, and Immunity, 18*(2), 123–134.

Matsumoto, D. (1991). Cultural influences on facial expressions of emotion. *Southern Journal of Communication, 56*(2), 128–137.

Matsumoto, D., & Willingham, B. (2009). Spontaneous facial expressions of emotion of congenitally and noncongenitally blind individuals. *Journal of Personality and Social Psychology, 96*(1), 1.

Mauss, I. B., Shallcross, A. J., Troy, A. S., John, O. P., Ferrer, E., Wilhelm, F. H., & Gross, J. J. (2011). Don't hide your happiness! Positive emotion dissociation, social connectedness, and psychological functioning. *Journal of Personality and Social Psychology, 100*(4), 738–748. doi:10.1037/a0022410

McAdams, D. P. (1982). Experiences of intimacy and power: Relationships between social motives and autobiographical memory. *Journal of Personality and Social Psychology, 42*(2), 292.

McClernon, F. J., Westman, E. C., & Rose, J. E. (2004). The effects of controlled deep breathing on smoking withdrawal symptoms in dependent smokers. *Addictive Behaviors, 29*, 765–772. doi:10.1016/j.addbeh.2004.02.005

McCrae, R. R. (1987). Creativity, divergent thinking, and openness to experience. *Journal of Personality and Social Psychology, 52*(6), 1258–1265. doi:10.1037/0022–3514.52.6.1258

McCrae, R. R., & Costa, P. T. Jr. (1996). Toward a new generation of personality theories: Theoretical contexts for the five-factor model. In J. S. Wiggins (Ed.), *The five-factor model of personality: Theoretical perspectives* (pp. 51–87). New York, NY: Guilford Press.

McCrae, R. R., & Costa, P. T. Jr. (1997). Personality trait structure as a human universal. *American Psychologist, 52*(5), 509–516. doi:10.1037/0003–066X.52.5.509

McCullough, J. P. Jr. (2000). *Treatment for chronic depression: Cognitive behavioral analysis system of psychotherapy.* New York, NY: Guilford Press.

McCullough, M. E., Root, L. M., & Cohen, A. D. (2006). Writing about the benefits of an interpersonal transgression facilitates forgiveness. *Journal of Consulting and Clinical Psychology, 74*(5), 887–897. doi:10.1037/0022–006X.74.5.887

McEwen, B. S., Eiland, L., Hunter, R. G., & Miller, M. M. (2012). Stress and anxiety: Structural plasticity and epigenetic regulation as a consequence of stress. *Neuropharmacology, 62*(1), 3–12.

Megargee, E. I. (1966). Undercontrolled and overcontrolled personality types in extreme antisocial aggression. *Psychological Monographs: General and Applied, 80*(3), 1–29. doi: 10.1037/h0093894

Megargee, E. I., & Bohn, M. J. (1979). *Classifying criminal offenders: A new system based on the MMPI*. Beverly Hills, CA: Sage.

Meyer, B., Johnson, S. L., & Carver, C. S. (1999). Exploring behavioral activation and inhibition sensitivities among college students at risk for bipolar spectrum symptomatology. *Journal of Psychopathology and Behavioral Assessment, 21*(4), 275–292. doi:10.1023/A :1022119414440

Miller, W. R. (1983). Motivational interviewing with problem drinkers. *Behavioural and Cognitive Psychotherapy, 11*(2), 147–172.

Miller, W. R., & Rose, G. S. (2009). Toward a theory of motivational interviewing. *American Psychologist, 64*(6), 527.

Miller, W. R., Taylor, C. A., & West, J. C. (1980). Focused versus broad-spectrum behavior therapy for problem drinkers. *Journal of Consulting and Clinical Psychology, 48*(5), 590.

Mineka, S., and Öhman, A. (2002). Learning and unlearning fears: Preparedness, neural pathways, and patients. *Society of Biological Psychiatry, 52*, 927–937.

Mizushima, L., & Stapleton, P. (2006). Analyzing the function of meta-oriented critical comments in Japanese comic conversations. *Journal of Pragmatics, 38*(12), 2105–2123.

Moffitt, T. E., Arseneault, L., Belsky, D., Dickson, N., Hancox, R. J., Harrington, H.,…Caspi, A. (2011). A gradient of childhood self-control predicts health, wealth, and public safety. *PNAS (Proceedings of the National Academy of Sciences of the United States of America), 108*(7), 2693–2698. doi:10.1073/pnas.1010076108

Montague, E., Chen, P.-Y., Xu, J., Chewning, B., & Barrett, B. (2013). Nonverbal interpersonal interactions in clinical encounters and patient perceptions of empathy. *Journal of Participatory Medicine, 5*, e33.

Montgomery, K. J., & Haxby, J. V. (2008). Mirror neuron system differentially activated by facial expressions and social hand gestures: A functional magnetic resonance imaging study. *Journal of Cognitive Neuroscience, 20*(10), 1866–1877. doi:10.1162/jocn.2008.20127

Moody, E. J., McIntosh, D. N., Mann, L. J., & Weisser, K. R. (2007). More than mere mimicry? The influence of emotion on rapid facial reactions to faces. *Emotion, 7*(2), 447–457. doi:10.1037/1528–3542.7.2.447

Morris, D. (2002). *Peoplewatching*. London, England: Vintage.

Morse, J. Q., & Lynch, T. R. (2000). Personality disorders in late life. *Current Psychiatry Reports, 2*(1), 24–31.

Morse, J. Q., & Lynch, T. R. (2004). A preliminary investigation of self-reported personality disorders in late life: Prevalence, predictors of depressive severity, and clinical correlates. *Aging & Mental Health, 8*(4), 307–315.

Mountford, V., Corstorphine, E., Tomlinson, S., & Waller, G. (2007). Development of a measure to assess invalidating childhood environments in the eating disorders. *Eating Behaviors, 8*(1), 48–58. doi:10.1016/j.eatbeh.2006.01.003

Muraven, M., & Baumeister, R. F. (2000). Self-regulation and depletion of limited resources: Does self-control resemble a muscle? *Psychological Bulletin, 126*(2), 247–259. doi:10.1037 /0033–2909.126.2.247

Myers, L. B. (2010). The importance of the repressive coping style: Findings from 30 years of research. *Anxiety, Stress and Coping, 23*(1), 3–17.

Najavits, L. M., & Weiss, R. D. (1994). Variations in therapist effectiveness in the treatment of patients with substance use disorders: An empirical review. *Addiction, 89*(6), 679–688.

National Collaborating Centre for Mental Health. (2004). *Eating disorders: Core interventions in the treatment and management of anorexia nervosa, bulimia nervosa and related eating disorders.* Leicester, England: British Psychological Society/Gaskell.

National Institute of Mental Health. (n.d.). Research domain criteria (RDoC). Retrieved from https://www.nimh.nih.gov/research-priorities/rdoc/index.shtml.

Neal, D. T., Wood, W., & Drolet, A. (2013). How do people adhere to goals when willpower is low? The profits (and pitfalls) of strong habits. *Journal of Personality and Social Psychology, 104*(6), 959.

Neuberg, S. L., & Newsom, J. T. (1993). Personal need for structure: Individual differences in the desire for simpler structure. *Journal of Personality and Social Psychology, 65*(1), 113–131.

Nichols, K., & Champness, B. (1971). Eye gaze and the GSR. *Journal of Experimental Social Psychology, 7*(6), 623–626.

Nicolaou, M., Paes, T., & Wakelin, S. (2006). Blushing: An embarrassing condition, but treatable. *Lancet, 367*(9519), 1297–1299.

Niedenthal, P. M., Mermillod, M., Maringer, M., & Hess, U. (2010). The Simulation of Smiles (SIMS) model: Embodied simulation and the meaning of facial expression. *Behavioral and Brain Sciences, 33*(06), 417–433.

Nock, M. K. (2009). Why do people hurt themselves? New insights into the nature and func-tions of self-injury. *Current Directions in Psychological Science, 18*(2), 78–83.

Nock, M. K., Joiner, T. E., Gordon, K. H., Lloyd-Richardson, E., & Prinstein, M. J. (2006). Non-suicidal self-injury among adolescents: Diagnostic correlates and relation to suicide attempts. *Psychiatry Research, 144*(1), 65–72.

Nock, M. K., & Mendes, W. B. (2008). Physiological arousal, distress tolerance, and social problem-solving deficits among adolescent self-injurers. *Journal of Consulting and Clinical Psychology, 76*(1), 28–38. doi:10.1037/0022–006X.76.1.28

Novaco, R. W. (1997). Remediating anger and aggression with violent offenders. *Legal and Criminological Psychology, 2*(1), 77–88.

Ogrodniczuk, J. S., Piper, W. E., Joyce, A. S., McCallum, M., & Rosie, J. S. (2003). NEO-Five Factor personality traits as predictors of response to two forms of group psychotherapy. *International Journal of Group Psychotherapy, 53*(4), 417–442.

Ogrodniczuk, J. S., Piper W. E., McCallum, M., Joyce, A. S., & Rosie, J. S. (2002). Interpersonal predictors of group therapy outcome for complicated grief. *International Journal of Group Psychotherapy, 52*(4), 511–535.

Oltmanns, T. F., Friedman, J. N. W., Fiedler, E. R., & Turkheimer, E. (2004). Perceptions of people with personality disorders based on thin slices of behavior. *Journal of Research in Personality, 38*(3), 216–229. doi:10.1016/S0092–6566(03)00066–7

Oltmanns, T. F., Gleason, M. E. J., Klonsky, E. D., & Turkheimer, E. (2005). Meta-perception for pathological personality traits: Do we know when others think that we are difficult? *Consciousness and Cognition: An International Journal, 14*(4), 739–751. doi:10.1016/j.concog.2005.07.001

Olweus, D. (1992). Victimization among schoolchildren: Intervention and prevention. In G. W. Albee, L. A. Bond, & T. V. C. Monsey (Eds.), *Improving children's lives: Global perspectives on prevention* (pp. 279–295). Thousand Oaks, CA: Sage.

Osman, A., Kopper, B. A., Linehan, M. M., Barrios, F. X., Gutierrez, P. M., & Bagge, C. L. (1999). Validation of the Adult Suicidal Ideation Questionnaire and the Reasons for Living Inventory in an adult psychiatric inpatient sample. *Psychological Assessment, 11*(2), 115.

O'Sullivan, M., & Ekman, P. (2004). The wizards of deception detection. In P.-A. Granhag & L. Strömwall (Eds.), *The detection of deception in forensic contexts* (pp. 269–286). New York, NY: Cambridge University Press.

Padesky, C. A. (1993). *Socratic questioning: Changing minds or guiding discovery?* Keynote address delivered at the European Congress of Behavioural and Cognitive Therapies, London, England.

Panksepp, J. (1981). Brain opioids: A neurochemical substrate for narcotic and social dependence. *Progress in Theory in Psychopharmacology, 149*, 175.

Panksepp, J. (1982). Toward a general psychobiological theory of emotions. *Behavioral and Brain Sciences, 5*(03), 407–422.

Panksepp, J. (1986). The neurochemistry of behavior. *Annual Review of Psychology, 37*(1), 77–107.

Panksepp, J. (1998). *Affective neuroscience: The foundations of human and animal emotions.* New York, NY: Oxford University Press.

Panksepp, J. (2005). On the embodied neural nature of core emotional affects. *Journal of Consciousness Studies, 12*(8–10), 158–184.

Park, S. Y., Belsky, J., Putnam, S., & Crnic, K. (1997). Infant emotionality, parenting, and 3-year inhibition: Exploring stability and lawful discontinuity in a male sample. *Developmental Psychology, 33*(2), 218–227.

Parker, J. D. A., Taylor, G., & Bagby, M. (1993). Alexithymia and the processing of emotional stimuli: An experimental study. *New Trends in Experimental and Clinical Psychiatry, 9*(1–2), 9–14.

Parkinson, B. (2005). Do facial movements express emotions or communicate motives? *Personality and Social Psychology Review, 9*(4), 278–311.

Parr, L. A., & Waller, B. M. (2006). Understanding chimpanzee facial expression: Insights into the evolution of communication. *Social Cognitive and Affective Neuroscience, 1*(3), 221–228.

Pauls, C. A., & Stemmler, G. (2003). Repressive and defensive coping during fear and anger. *Emotion, 3*(3), 284–302.

481

Pelham, B. W., & Swann, W. B. (1994). The juncture of intrapersonal and interpersonal knowledge: Self-certainty and interpersonal congruence. *Personality and Social Psychology Bulletin, 20*(4), 349–357. doi:10.1177/0146167294204002

Perls, F. S. (1969). *Ego, hunger and aggression: The beginning of Gestalt therapy.* New York, NY: Random House.

Perren, S., & Alsaker, F. D. (2006). Social behavior and peer relationships of victims, bully-victims, and bullies in kindergarten. *Journal of Child Psychology and Psychiatry, 47*(1), 45–57. doi:10.1111/j.1469–7610.2005.01445.x

Petrie, K. J., Booth, R. J., & Pennebaker, J. W. (1998). The immunological effects of thought suppression. *Journal of Personality and Social Psychology, 75*(5), 1264–1272. doi:10.1037/0022–3514.75.5.1264

Pinto, R. Z., Ferreira, M. L., Oliveira, V. C., Franco, M. R., Adams, R., Maher, C. G., & Ferreira, P. H. (2012). Patient-centred communication is associated with positive therapeutic alliance: A systematic review. *Journal of Physiotherapy, 58*(2), 77–87.

Pittam, J., & Scherer, K. R. (1993). Vocal expression and communication of emotion. In M. Lewis & J. M. Haviland (Eds.), *Handbook of emotions* (pp. 185–197). New York, NY: Guilford Press.

Polaschek, D. L., & Collie, R. M. (2004). Rehabilitating serious violent adult offenders: An empirical and theoretical stocktake. *Psychology, Crime and Law, 10*(3), 321–334.

Porges, S. W. (1995). Orienting in a defensive world: Mammalian modifications of our evolutionary heritage: A polyvagal theory. *Psychophysiology, 32*(4), 301–318.

Porges, S. W. (1998). Love: An emergent property of the mammalian autonomic nervous system. *Psychoneuroendocrinology, 23*(8), 837–861. doi:10.1016/s0306–4530(98)00057–2

Porges, S. W. (2001). The polyvagal theory: Phylogenetic substrates of a social nervous system. *International Journal of Psychophysiology, 42*(2), 123–146.

Porges, S. W. (2003a). The Polyvagal Theory: Phylogenetic contributions to social behavior. *Physiology and Behavior, 79*(3), 503–513.

Porges, S. W. (2003b). Social engagement and attachment: A phylogenetic perspective. In J. A. King, C. F. Ferris, & I. I. Lederhendler (Eds.), *Roots of mental illness in children* (pp. 31–47). New York: New York Academy of Sciences.

Porges, S. W. (2007). The polyvagal perspective. *Biological Psychology, 74*(2), 116–143.

Porges, S. W. (2009). Reciprocal influences between body and brain in the perception and expression of affect: A polyvagal perspective. In D. Fosha, D. J. Siegel, & M. F. Solomon (Eds.), *The healing power of emotion: Affective neuroscience, development and clinical practice* (pp. 27–54). New York, NY: Norton.

Porges, S. W., & Lewis, G. F. (2009). The polyvagal hypothesis: Common mechanisms mediating autonomic regulation, vocalizations, and listening. In S. M. Brudzynski (Ed.), *Handbook of mammalian vocalizations: An integrative neuroscience approach* (pp. 255–264). San Diego, CA: Academic Press.

Powers, T. A., Zuroff, D. C., & Topciu, R. A. (2004). Covert and overt expressions of self-criticism and perfectionism and their relation to depression. *European Journal of Personality, 18*(1), 61–72. doi:10.1002/per.499

Pryor, K. (1999). *Don't shoot the dog: The new art of teaching and training* (Rev. ed.). New York, NY: Bantam.

Quinsey, V. L., Maguire, A., & Varney, G. W. (1983). Assertion and overcontrolled hostility among mentally disordered murderers. *Journal of Consulting and Clinical Psychology, 51*(4), 550.

Rachman, S. (1997). A cognitive theory of obsessions. *Behavior Research and Therapy, 35*(9), 793–802. doi:10.1016/S0005-7967(97)00040-5

Reed, B. S. (2011). Beyond the particular: Prosody and the coordination of actions. *Language and Speech, 55*(1), 13–34.

Reis, H. T., & Patrick, B. C. (1996). Attachment and intimacy: Component processes. In E. T. Higgins & A. W. Kruglanski (Eds.), *Social psychology: Handbook of basic principles* (pp. 523–563). New York, NY: Guilford Press.

Reynolds, C., Arean, P., Lynch, T. R., & Frank, E. (2004). Psychotherapy in Old-Age depression: Progress and challenges. In S. Roose & H. Sackheim (Eds.), *Late-life depression* (287–298). New York, NY: Oxford University Press.

Reynolds, W. M. (1991). Psychometric characteristics of the Adult Suicidal Ideation Questionnaire in college students. *Journal of Personality Assessment, 56*(2), 289–307.

Riso, L. P., du Toit, P. L., Blandino, J. A., Penna, S., Dacey, S., Duin, J. S.,…Ulmer, C. S. (2003). Cognitive aspects of chronic depression. *Journal of Abnormal Psychology, 112*(1), 72–80.

Ritts, V., & Stein, J. R. (1995). Verification and commitment in marital relationships: An exploration of self-verification theory in community college students. *Psychological Reports, 76*(2), 383–386. doi:10.2466/pr0.1995.76.2.383

Robbins, S. J. (1990). Mechanisms underlying spontaneous recovery in autoshaping. *Journal of Experimental Psychology: Animal Behavior Processes, 16*(3), 235–249.

Robins, R. W., John, O. P., Caspi, A., Moffitt, T. E., & Stouthamer-Loeber, M. (1996). Resilient, overcontrolled, and undercontrolled boys: Three replicable personality types. *Journal of Personality and Social Psychology, 70*(1), 157–171. doi:10.1037/0022–3514 .70.1.157

Rogers, C. R. (1959). A theory of therapy, personality, and interpersonal relationships, as developed in the client-centered framework. In S. Koch (Ed.), *Psychology: A Study of a Science* (Vol. 3, pp. 184–256). New York, NY: McGraw-Hill.

Rosenthal, M. Z., Cheavens, J. S., Lejuez, C. W., & Lynch, T. R. (2005). Thought suppression mediates the relationship between negative affect and borderline personality disorder symptoms. *Behavior Research and Therapy, 43*(9), 1173–1185.

Rosenthal, M. Z., Kim, K., Herr, N. R., Smoski, M. J., Cheavens, J. S., Lynch, T. R., & Kosson, D. S. (2011). Speed and accuracy of facial expression classification in avoidant personality disorder: A preliminary study. *Personality Disorders: Theory, Research, and Treatment, 2*(4), 327–334. doi:10.1037/a0023672

Rossier, V., Bolognini, M., Plancherel, B., & Halfon, O. (2000). Sensation seeking: A personality trait characteristic of adolescent girls and young women with eating disorders? *European Eating Disorders Review, 8*(3), 245–252. doi:10.1002/(sici)1099–0968(200005) 8:3<245::aid-erv308>3.0.co;2-d

Rothbart, M. K., Ahadi, S. A., Hersey, K. L., & Fisher, P. (2001). Investigations of temperament at three to seven years: The Children's Behavior Questionnaire. *Child Development, 72*(5), 1394–1408. doi:10.1111/1467–8624.00355

Rounsaville, B. J., Carroll, K. M., & Onken, L. S. (2001). A stage model of behavioral therapies research: Getting started and moving on from stage I. *Clinical Psychology: Science and Practice, 8*(2), 133–142.

Rubin, K. H., Bukowski, W., & Parker, J. G. (1998). Peer interactions, relationships, and groups. In N. Eisenberg (Ed.), *Handbook of child psychology* (5th ed.): Vol. 3. *Social, emotional, and personality development* (pp. 619–700). Hoboken, NJ: Wiley.

Rubin, K. H., Burgess, K. B., & Hastings, P. D. (2002). Stability and social-behavioral consequences of toddlers' inhibited temperament and parenting behaviors. *Child Development, 73*(2), 483–495.

Rubin, K. H., Hastings, P. D., Stewart, S. L., Henderson, H. A., & Chen, X. (1997). The consistency and concomitants of inhibition: Some of the children, all of the time. *Child Development, 68*(3), 467–483.

Rumi, Mewlana Jalaluddin. (1230/2004). The guest house. In C. Barks (Ed. and Trans.), *The essential Rumi: New expanded edition.* San Francisco: HarperSanFrancisco.

Russell, J. A., Bachorowski, J.-A., & Fernández-Dols, J.-M. (2003). Facial and vocal expressions of emotion. *Annual Review of Psychology, 54*(1), 329–349.

Safer, D. L., & Chen, E. Y. (2011). Anorexia nervosa as a disorder of emotion dysregulation: Theory, evidence, and treatment implications. *Clinical Psychology: Science and Practice, 18*(3), 203–207. doi:10.1111/j.1468–2850.2011.01251.x

Safran, J. D., & Muran, J. C. (2000). *Negotiating the therapeutic alliance: A relational treatment guide.* New York, NY: Guilford Press.

Salavert, J., Caseras, X., Torrubia, R., Furest, S., Arranz, B., Dueñas, R., & San, L. (2007). The functioning of the behavioral activation and inhibition systems in bipolar I euthymic patients and its influence in subsequent episodes over an eighteen-month period. *Personality and Individual Differences, 42*(7), 1323–1331. doi:10.1016/j.paid.2006.10.010

Sander, D., Grandjean, D., Kaiser, S., Wehrle, T., & Scherer, K. R. (2007). Interaction effects of perceived gaze direction and dynamic facial expression: Evidence for appraisal theories of emotion. *European Journal of Cognitive Psychology, 19*(3), 470–480.

Sarra, S., & Otta, E. (2001). Different types of smiles and laughter in preschool children. *Psychological Reports, 89*(3), 547–558. doi:10.2466/PR0.89.7.547–558

Satir, D. A., Goodman, D. M., Shingleton, R. M., Porcerelli, J. H., Gorman, B. S., Pratt, E. M.,...Thompson-Brenner, H. (2011). Alliance-focused therapy for anorexia nervosa: Integrative relational and behavioral change treatments in a single-case experimental design. *Psychotherapy, 48*(4), 401–420. doi:10.1037/a0026216

Schaie, K. W., Willis, S. L., & Caskie, G. I. (2004). The Seattle longitudinal study: Relationship between personality and cognition. *Aging Neuropsychology and Cognition, 11*(2–3), 304–324. doi:10.1080/13825580490511134

Schauer, M., & Elbert, T. (2010). Dissociation following traumatic stress: Etiology and treatment. *Zeitschrift für Psychologie/Journal of Psychology, 218*(2), 109–127. doi:10.1027/0044–3409/a000018

Schneider, K. G., Hempel, R. J., & Lynch, T. R. (2013). That "poker face" just might lose you the game! The impact of expressive suppression and mimicry on sensitivity to facial expressions of emotion. *Emotion, 13*(5), 852–866. doi:10.1037/a0032847

Schug, J., Matsumoto, D., Horita, Y., Yamagishi, T., & Bonnet, K. (2010). Emotional expressivity as a signal of cooperation. *Evolution and Human Behavior, 31*(2), 87–94. doi:10.1016/j .evolhumbehav.2009.09.006

Segal, Z. V., Williams, J. M. G., & Teasdale, J. D. (2002). *Mindfulness-based cognitive therapy for depression: A new approach to preventing relapse.* New York, NY: Guilford Press.

Selby, E. A., Bender, T. W., Gordon, K. H., Nock, M. K., & Joiner, T. E. Jr. (2012). Non-suicidal self-injury (NSSI) disorder: A preliminary study. *Personality Disorders: Theory, Research, and Treatment, 3*(2), 167–175. doi:10.1037/a0024405

Sequeira, H., Hot, P., Silvert, L., & Delplanque, S. (2009). Electrical autonomic correlates of emotion. *International Journal of Psychophysiology, 71*(1), 50–56. doi:10.1016/j.ijpsycho .2008.07.009

Shankman, S. A., Klein, D. N., Tenke, C. E., & Bruder, G. E. (2007). Reward sensitivity in depression: A biobehavioral study. *Journal of Abnormal Psychology, 116*(1), 95–104. doi:10 .1037/0021–843X.116.1.95

Shapiro, J. P., Baumeister, R. F., & Kessler, J. W. (1991). A three-component model of children's teasing: Aggression, humor, and ambiguity. *Journal of Social and Clinical Psychology, 10*(4), 459–472.

Shaw, A., & Olson, K. R. (2012). Children discard a resource to avoid inequity. *Journal of Experimental Psychology: General, 141*(2), 382–395. doi:10.1037/a0025907

Smillie, L. D., & Jackson, C. J. (2005). The appetitive motivation scale and other BAS measures in the prediction of approach and active avoidance. *Personality and Individual Differences, 38*(4), 981–994.

Smith, G. T., Fischer, S., Cyders, M. A., Annus, A. M., Spillane, N. S., & McCarthy, D. M. (2007). On the validity and utility of discriminating among impulsivity-like traits. *Assessment, 14*(2), 155–170.

Smoski, M. J., Lynch, T. R., Rosenthal, M. Z., Cheavens, J. S., Chapman, A. L., & Krishnan, R. R. (2008). Decision-making and risk aversion among depressive adults. *Journal of Behavior Therapy and Experimental Psychiatry, 39*(4), 567–576.

Soltysik, S., & Jelen, P. (2005). In rats, sighs correlate with relief. *Physiology and Behavior, 85*(5), 598–602.

Sonnby-Borgström, M. (2002). Automatic mimicry reactions as related to differences in emotional empathy. *Scandinavian Journal of Psychology, 43*(5), 433–443. doi:10.1111/1467 –9450.00312

Sonnby-Borgström, M., Jönsson, P., & Svensson, O. (2003). Emotional empathy as related to mimicry reactions at different levels of information processing. *Journal of Nonverbal Behavior, 27*(1), 3–23. doi:10.1023/A:1023608506243

Spitzer, R. L. (1983). Psychiatric diagnosis: Are clinicians still necessary? *Comprehensive Psychiatry, 24*(5), 399–411.

Steketee, G., & Frost, R. (2003). Compulsive hoarding: Current status of the research. *Clinical Psychology Review, 23*(7), 905–927. doi:10.1016/j.cpr.2003.08.002

Steklis, H., & Kling, A. (1985). Neurobiology of affiliative behavior in nonhuman primates. In M. Reite & T. Field (Eds.), *The psychobiology of attachment and separation* (pp. 93–134). Orlando, FL: Academic Press.

Stewart, S. H., Zvolensky, M. J., & Eifert, G. H. (2002). The relations of anxiety sensitivity, experiential avoidance, and alexithymic coping to young adults' motivations for drinking. *Behavior Modification, 26*(2), 274–296.

Sukhodolsky, D. G., Kassinove, H., & Gorman, B. S. (2004). Cognitive-behavioral therapy for anger in children and adolescents: A meta-analysis. *Aggression and Violent Behavior, 9*(3), 247–269.

Swann, W. B. Jr. (1983). Self-verification: Bringing social reality into harmony with the self. *Social Psychological Perspectives on the Self, 2,* 33–66.

Swann, W. B. Jr. (1997). The trouble with change: Self-verification and allegiance to the self. *Psychological Science, 8*(3), 177–180. doi:10.1111/j.1467–9280.1997.tb00407.x

Swann, W. B. Jr., de la Ronde, C., & Hixon, J. G. (1994). Authenticity and positivity strivings in marriage and courtship. *Journal of Personality and Social Psychology, 66*(5), 857–869. doi:10.1037/0022–3514.66.5.857

Swann, W. B. Jr., Rentfrow, P. J., & Gosling, S. D. (2003). The precarious couple effect: Verbally inhibited men + critical, disinhibited women = bad chemistry. *Journal of Personality and Social Psychology, 85*(6), 1095–1106. doi:10.1037/0022–3514.85.6.1095

Swann, W. B. Jr., Stein-Seroussi, A., & McNulty, S. E. (1992). Outcasts in a white-lie society: The enigmatic worlds of people with negative self-conceptions. *Journal of Personality and Social Psychology, 62*(4), 618–624. doi:10.1037/0022–3514.62.4.618

Tew, J., Harkins, L., & Dixon, L. (2013). What works in reducing violent re-offending in psychopathic offenders. In L. A. Craig, L. Dixon, & T. A. Gannon (Eds.), *What works in offender rehabilitation: An evidence-based approach to assessment and treatment* (pp. 129–141). Chichester, England: Wiley-Blackwell.

Thayer, J. F., & Lane, R. D. (2000). A model of neurovisceral integration in emotion regulation and dysregulation. *Journal of Affective Disorders, 61*(3), 201–216.

Thayer, J. F., & Lane, R. D. (2009). Claude Bernard and the heart–brain connection: Further elaboration of a model of neurovisceral integration. *Neuroscience and Biobehavioral Reviews, 33*(2), 81–88. doi:10.1016/j.neubiorev.2008.08.004

Thompson, M. M., Naccarato, M. E., Parker, K. C. H., & Moskowitz, G. B. (2001). The personal need for structure and personal fear of invalidity measures: Historical perspectives, current applications, and future directions. In G. B. Moskowitz (Ed.), *Cognitive social psychology: The Princeton Symposium on the Legacy and Future of Social Cognition* (pp. 19–39). Mahwah, NJ: Erlbaum.

Tobin, M. J., Jenouri, G. A., Watson, H., & Sackner, M. A. (1983). Noninvasive measurement of pleural pressure by surface inductive plethysmography. *Journal of Applied Physiology, 55*(1), 267–275.

Toussulis, Y. (2011). *Sufism and the way of blame: Hidden sources of a sacred psychology.* Wheaton, IL: Quest Books.

Tsoudis, O., & Smith-Lovin, L. (1998). How bad was it? The effects of victim and perpetrator emotion on responses to criminal court vignettes. *Social Forces, 77*(2), 695–722. doi:10.2307/3005544

Tsytsarev, S. V., & Grodnitzky, G. R. (1995). Anger and criminality. In H. Kassinove (Ed.), *Anger disorders: Definition, diagnosis, and treatment* (pp. 91–108). New York, NY: Taylor & Francis.

Tucker, D. M., Derryberry, D., & Luu, P. (2005). Anatomy and physiology of human emotion: Vertical integration of brainstem, limbic, and cortical systems. In J. C. Borod (Ed.), *The neuropsychology of emotion* (pp. 56–79). New York, NY: Oxford University Press.

Turkat, I. D. (1985). Formulation of paranoid personality disorder. In I. D. Turkat (Ed.), *Behavioral case formulation* (pp. 161–198). New York, NY: Plenum Press.

Turnbull, C. M. (1962). *The peoples of Africa.* Cleveland, OH: World.

Van der Gaag, C., Minderaa, R. B., & Keysers, C. (2007). Facial expressions: What the mirror neuron system can and cannot tell us. *Social Neuroscience, 2*(3–4), 179–222. doi:10.1080/17470910701376878

Vazsonyi, A. T., & Klanjšek, R. (2008). A test of self-control theory across different socio-economic strata. *Justice Quarterly, 25*(1), 101–131.

Vernberg, E. M. (1990). Psychological adjustment and experiences with peers during early adolescence: Reciprocal, incidental, or unidirectional relationships? *Journal of Abnormal Child Psychology, 18*(2), 187–198. doi:10.1007/BF00910730

Vollebergh, W. A. M., Iedema, J., Bijl, R. V., de Graaf, R., Smit, F., & Ormel, J. (2001). The structure and stability of common mental disorders: The NEMESIS Study. *Archives of General Psychiatry, 58*(6), 597–603. doi:10.1001/archpsyc.58.6.597

Vrana, S. R., & Gross, D. (2004). Reactions to facial expressions: Effects of social context and speech anxiety on responses to neutral, anger, and joy expressions. *Biological Psychology, 66*(1), 63–78. doi:10.1016/j.biopsycho.2003.07.004

Waltz, J., Addis, M. E., Koerner, K., & Jacobson, N. S. (1993). Testing the integrity of a psychotherapy protocol: Assessment of adherence and competence. *Journal of Consulting and Clinical Psychology, 61*(4), 620.

Warneken, F., & Tomasello, M. (2006). Altruistic helping in human infants and young chimpanzees. *Science, 311*(5765), 1301–1303.

Watson, D., & Naragon, K. (2009). Positive affectivity: The disposition to experience positive emotional states. In S. J. Lopez & C. R. Snyder (Eds.), *Oxford handbook of positive psychology* (2nd ed., pp. 207–215). New York, NY: Oxford University Press.

Watson, H. J., & Bulik, C. M. (2013). Update on the treatment of anorexia nervosa: Review of clinical trials, practice guidelines and emerging interventions. *Psychological Medicine, 43*(12), 2477–2500.

Wegner, D. M., & Gold, D. B. (1995). Fanning old flames: Emotional and cognitive effects of suppressing thoughts of a past relationship. *Journal of Personality and Social Psychology, 68*(5), 782–792. doi:10.1037/0022–3514.68.5.782

Weinberger, D. A. (1995). The construct validity of the repressive coping style. In J. L. Singer (Ed.), *Repression and dissociation: Implications for personality theory, psychopathology, and health* (pp. 337–386). Chicago, IL: University of Chicago Press.

Weinberger, D. A., Schwartz, G. E., & Davidson, R. J. (1979). Low-anxious, high-anxious, and repressive coping styles: Psychometric patterns and behavioral and physiological responses to stress. *Journal of Abnormal Psychology, 88*(4), 369–380. doi:10.1037/0021–843X.88.4.369

Weinberger, D. A., Tublin, S. K., Ford, M. E., & Feldman, S. S. (1990). Preadolescents' social-emotional adjustment and selective attrition in family research. *Child Development, 61*(5), 1374–1386. doi:10.2307/1130749

Wenzlaff, R. M., & Bates, D. E. (1998). Unmasking a cognitive vulnerability to depression: How lapses in mental control reveal depressive thinking. *Journal of Personality and Social Psychology, 75*(6), 1559–1571. doi:10.1037/0022–3514.75.6.1559

Wenzlaff, R. M., Rude, S. S., & West, L. M. (2002). Cognitive vulnerability to depression: The role of thought suppression and attitude certainty. *Cognition and Emotion, 16*(4), 533–548. doi:10.1080/02699930143000338

Westen, D., DeFife, J. A., Bradley, B., & Hilsenroth, M. J. (2010). Prototype personality diagnosis in clinical practice: A viable alternative for DSM–5 and ICD–11. *Professional Psychology: Research and Practice, 41*(6), 482–487. doi:10.1037/a0021555

Westphal, M., Seivert, N. H., & Bonanno, G. A. (2010). Expressibv ghfve flexibility. *Emotion, 10*(1), 92–100. doi:10.1037/a0018420

White, C. N., Gunderson, J. G., Zanarini, M. C., & Hudson, J. I. (2003). Family studies of borderline personality disorder: A review. *Harvard Review of Psychiatry, 11*(1), 8–19.

Wieser, M. J., Pauli, P., Alpers, G. W., & Mühlberger, A. (2009). Is eye to eye contact really threatening and avoided in social anxiety? An eye-tracking and psychophysiology study. *Journal of Anxiety Disorders, 23*(1), 93–103.

Williams, J. M. G. (2010). Mindfulness and psychological process. *Emotion, 10*(1), 1–7. doi:10.1037/a0018360

Williams, K. D., Shore, W. J., & Grahe, J. E. (1998). The silent treatment: Perceptions of its behaviors and associated feelings. *Group Processes and Intergroup Relations, 1*(2), 117–141.

Williams, L. M., Liddell, B. J., Kemp, A. H., Bryant, R. A., Meares, R. A., Peduto, A. S., & Gordon, E. (2006). Amygdala–prefrontal dissociation of subliminal and supraliminal fear. *Human Brain Mapping, 27*(8), 652–661. doi:10.1002/hbm.20208

Williams, L. M., Liddell, B. J., Rathjen, J., Brown, K. J., Gray, J., Phillips, M.,…Gordon, E. (2004). Mapping the time course of nonconscious and conscious perception of fear: An integration of central and peripheral measures. *Human Brain Mapping, 21*(2), 64–74. doi:10.1002/hbm.10154

Wirth, J. H., Sacco, D. F., Hugenberg, K., & Williams, K. D. (2010). Eye gaze as relational evaluation: Averted eye gaze leads to feelings of ostracism and relational devaluation. *Personality and Social Psychology Bulletin, 36*(7), 869–882. doi:10.1177/0146167210370032

Wong, S. C. P., & Gordon, A. (2013). The Violence Reduction Programme: A treatment programme for violence-prone forensic clients. *Psychology, Crime and Law, 19*(5–6), 461–475. doi:10.1080/1068316X.2013.758981.

Wright, A. G., Thomas, K. M., Hopwood, C. J., Markon, K. E., Pincus, A. L., & Krueger, R. F. (2012). The hierarchical structure of DSM-5 pathological personality traits. *Journal of Abnormal Psychology, 121*(4), 951.

Yardley, L., McDermott, L., Pisarski, S., Duchaine, B., & Nakayama, K. (2008). Psychosocial consequences of developmental prosopagnosia: A problem of recognition. *Journal of Psychosomatic Research, 65*(5), 445–451.

Zanarini, M. C., Frankenburg, F. R., Reich, D. B., & Fitzmaurice, G. (2010). The 10-year course of psychosocial functioning among patients with borderline personality disorder and Axis II comparison subjects. *Acta Psychiatrica Scandinavica, 122*(2), 103–109.

Zimmerman, M., Rothschild, L., & Chelminski, I. (2005). The prevalence of DSM-IV personality disorders in psychiatric outpatients. *American Journal of Psychiatry, 162*(10), 1911–1918.

Zucker, N. L., Losh, M., Bulik, C. M., LaBar, K. S., Piven, J., & Pelphrey, K. A. (2007). Anorexia nervosa and autism spectrum disorders: Guided investigation of social cognitive endophenotypes. *Psychological Bulletin, 133*(6), 976–1006.

Zuroff, D. C., & Fitzpatrick, D. K. (1995). Depressive personality styles: Implications for future attachment. *Personality and Individual Differences, 18*(2), 253–265. doi:10.1016/0191–8869(94)00136-g

Thomas R. Lynch, PhD, FBPsS, is professor emeritus of clinical psychology at the University of Southampton school of psychology. Previously, he was director of the Duke Cognitive-Behavioral Research and Treatment Program at Duke University from 1998–2007. He relocated to Exeter University in the UK in 2007. Lynch's primary research interests include understanding and developing novel treatments for mood and personality disorders using a translational line of inquiry that combines basic neurobiobehavioral science with the most recent technological advances in intervention research. He is founder of radically open dialectical behavior therapy (RO DBT).

Lynch has received numerous awards and special recognitions from organizations such as the National Institutes of Health-US (NIMH, NIDA), Medical Research Council-UK (MRC-EME), and the National Alliance for Research on Schizophrenia and Depression (NARSAD). His research has been recognized in the Science and Advances Section of the National Institutes of Health Congressional Justification Report; and he is a recipient of the John M. Rhoades Psychotherapy Research Endowment, and a Beck Institute Scholar.

Index

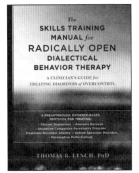
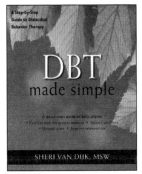
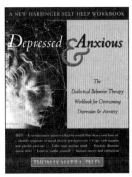
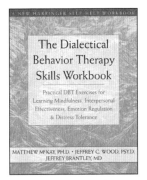
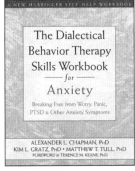
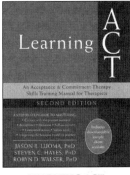

Register your **new harbinger** titles for additional benefits!

When you register your **new harbinger** title—purchased in any format, from any source—you get access to benefits like the following:

- Downloadable accessories like printable worksheets and extra content

- Instructional videos and audio files

- Information about updates, corrections, and new editions

Not every title has accessories, but we're adding new material all the time.

Access free accessories in 3 easy steps:

1. Sign in at NewHarbinger.com (or **register** to create an account).

2. Click on **register a book**. Search for your title and click the **register** button when it appears.

3. Click on the **book cover or title** to go to its details page. Click on **accessories** to view and access files.

That's all there is to it!

If you need help, visit:

NewHarbinger.com/accessories

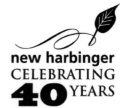

new harbinger
CELEBRATING
40 YEARS